Palliative Care Nursing
A Guide to Practice

Second Edition

Edited by Margaret O'Connor and Sanchia Aranda

Foreword by Susie Wilkinson

Radcliffe Medical Press

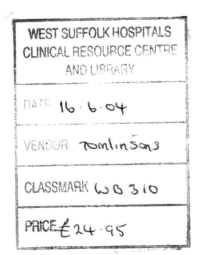
Radcliffe Medical Press Ltd
18 Marcham Road
Abingdon
Oxon OX14 1AA
United Kingdom

www.radcliffe-oxford.com
The Radcliffe Medical Press electronic catalogue and online ordering facility.
Direct sales to anywhere in the world

This book was originally published in Melbourne, Australia by Ausmed Publications Pty Ltd

©Ausmed Publications Pty Ltd 2003

Although the Publisher has taken every care to ensure the accuracy of the professional, clinical, and technical components of this publication, it accepts no responsibility for any loss or damage suffered by any person as a result of following the procedures described or acting on information set out in this publication. The Publisher reminds readers that the information in this publication is no substitute for individual medical and/or nursing assessment and treatment by professional staff.

Palliative Care Nursing: A Guide to Practice
First edition published by Ausmed Publications Pty Ltd, 1999; reprinted 1999, 2001.
This second edition (completely revised and rewritten) first published by
Ausmed Publications Pty Ltd 2003.

British Library Cataloguing in Publication Data

A catalogue record for this book is available from the British Library

ISBN 1 85775 839 0

Typeset by Egan-Reid Ltd, Auckland, New Zealand
Printed and bound by T J International Ltd, Padstow, Cornwall, UK

Contents

Foreword

Palliative Care Nursing: A Guide to Practice addresses palliative care from a nursing perspective, and will assist nurses in a variety of settings to care for people and their families with confidence and competence. Written in the main by nurses, the book presents the expertise that the contributing authors have gathered over many years of practical experience in clinical practice, backed by extensive research and an awareness of the relevant nursing and medical literature. The book is a tribute to all the contributing authors.

This book offers all nurses an evidence-based approach to handling the many difficult scenarios faced by nurses who care for dying people and their families. The World Health Organization definition of palliative care (WHO 2002) emphasises, for the first time, the importance of 'impeccable assessment' in the provision of high-quality palliative care. Each chapter of *Palliative Care Nursing* gives nurses detailed guidelines for making in-depth assessments to elicit the patients' problems, followed by relevant advice to enable them to plan effective care.

Palliative care is now accepted as an important aspect of health care by an increasing number of government health departments and by health professionals all over the world. For nurses worldwide who are contributing to new palliative-care services, as well as for those working in established service settings, this book is a must. It is an authoritative text on palliative-care nursing, and will provide up-to-date knowledge and ideas for enhancing the care that nurses provide in assisting people achieve a peaceful dignified death, and in caring for their families and loved ones.

I have great pleasure in commending this excellent book.

Dr Susie Wilkinson
Head of Palliative Care Research and Senior Lecturer in Palliative Care
Marie Curie Palliative Care Research & Development Unit, London, UK

Preface

Palliative care has been traditionally defined as '... specialised health care of dying people, aiming to maximise quality of life and assist families and carers during and after death' (PCA 1999). The long tradition of the hospice movement attests to a commitment to care for people who are dying. More recently, palliative care has developed into an active practice-based discipline aimed at improving the care of those who are facing the end of their lives. Palliative care now begins before the traditionally understood dying phase of care, and has become a multidisciplinary practice involving interactions with other relevant parts of the health-care system.

Wherever palliative care is practised, it is founded on the following values and principles (PCA 1999):

- the dignity of the patient and family;
- compassionate care of the patient and family;
- equity in access to palliative-care services;
- respect for the patient, family, and carers;
- advocacy on behalf of the expressed wishes of patients, families, and communities;
- pursuit of excellence in the provision of care and support; and
- accountability to patients, families, and the wider community.

The success of the first edition of *Palliative Care Nursing* suggests that the original goal of developing a book that would make palliative care accessible to nurses in all health settings has been realised. This second edition has been totally revised, rewritten, and redesigned to ensure that the book remains a reliable and useful practice guide for nurses, especially for those who are new to palliative care and those who work in other areas of health in which palliative-care skills are required.

This complete revision and rewriting required a comprehensive re-evaluation of the first edition. Feedback from nurses revealed that the clinically focused chapters of the earlier edition were especially useful in guiding practice, and this has resulted in an increased focus on clinical issues in this second edition. The content of the new book has therefore been refocused to incorporate a wider range of clinical problems faced by nurses in their care of dying people. Each of these new chapters has been written by a nurse with recognised expertise in the topic area and a commitment to providing recommendations that are firmly evidence-based. Many of these authors are from countries other than Australia, and this reflects a widening of content and readership from a predominantly Australian focus to a wider international scope.

This book will empower nurses through the development of their clinical knowledge, and will contribute to enhanced care for people who are dying.

Acknowledgements

Radcliffe Medical Press has received much help and advice from the UK contributors to this book, and from Susie Wilkinson, who wrote the foreword. It was on Susie's advice that we asked the following experts to review certain chapters to ensure they reflected current practice in the NHS.

Margaret Goodman, Marie Curie Palliative Care Research and Development Unit, Royal Free Hospital, London

Kath Jenkins, Marie Curie Centre, Caterham, Surrey

Carole Mula MA, Macmillan Nurse Consultant in Adult Palliative Care, Christie Hospital NHS Trust, Manchester and North Manchester Primary Care Trust

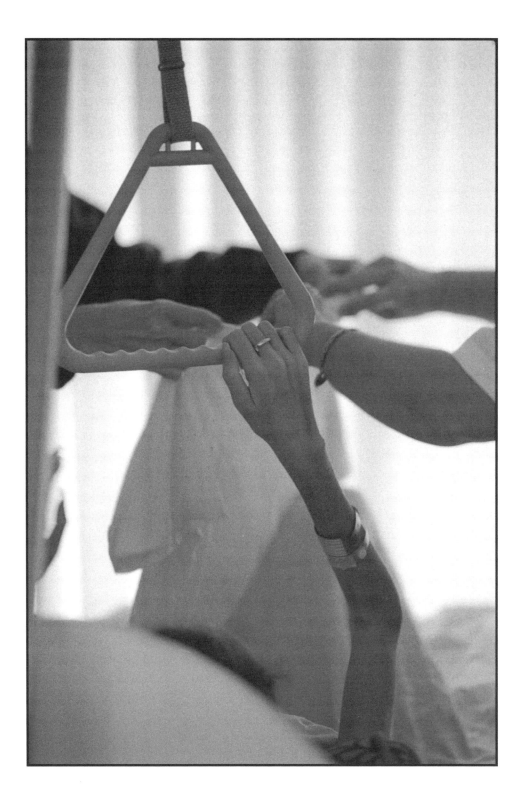

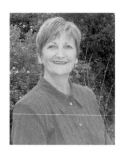

Sanchia Aranda

Sanchia Aranda is professor and director of cancer nursing research at Peter MacCallum Cancer Institute, Melbourne (Victoria, Australia). She has worked in cancer care since 1979, predominantly in the tertiary sector since 1990. Her research interests include cancer and palliative nursing in both inpatient and community settings, especially in the area of supportive care. Her research, both quantitative and qualitative, concentrates on implementing evidence into clinical practice, especially in improving the delivery of health services and the outcomes for people with cancer and their families. Current studies include workforce planning in breast care, the support needs of women with advanced cancer, symptom interventions in pain and fatigue, prevention of oral mucositis, and care of people suffering bodily decay.

Chapter 1

Framing Palliative Care

Sanchia Aranda

The purpose of this book is to disseminate knowledge of palliative-care nursing to improve the care of people at the end of their lives, and to provide care and assistance to their families, friends, and carers. It is important that knowledge of palliative care is available to nurses who care for dying people, regardless of the health-care setting or the diagnosis. Because dying people can be found in almost any setting, palliative care is increasingly a core component of all health-care roles.

Palliative care occurs at three levels (Finlay & Jones 1995):
- the palliative approach;
- specialist interventions; and
- specialist palliative care.

The *palliative approach* consists of a core set of knowledge and skills, and can be used by all health professionals who are involved in caring for people with life-threatening or terminal illnesses. At this level, all nurses can undertake basic symptom assessment and management, understand the experiences of dying people and their families, engage in communication regarding individual needs and experiences, and consult with specialist palliative-care practitioners if the needs of these people are outside the nurses' expertise.

Specialist interventions by practitioners from disciplines outside palliative care are sometimes required to assist in the management of difficult nursing problems. Examples include the involvement of a wound nurse in the care of a malignant wound or the involvement of a radiotherapy nurse in palliative radiotherapy.

Specialist palliative care is provided by practitioners who have specialist qualifications and experience in the care of dying people and their families. These practitioners might work in specialist community palliative-care services, in palliative consulting services in an acute hospital, or in a hospice. The involvement of such specialist services and practitioners is most relevant for patients with complex and difficult symptoms or care needs. Such specialist services might be involved in an advisory capacity, or can assume primary care of the patient.

This book provides a core set of knowledge that can be applied at each of these three levels of practice, but the focus of the book is to assist *all* nurses to incorporate palliative care into their work, on the premise that all nurses require access to information that will support their care of dying people and their families. The book presents palliative care as the expert, holistic, and interdisciplinary care that is offered to dying people, regardless of diagnosis or care setting. It is a continuum of practice from a generalised approach to a specialist discipline.

Even though one of the tenets of palliative care is the promotion of equitable access, there are still considerable difficulties with access to palliative care in many communities and in many settings of care, especially for people with non-cancer diagnoses. In part, this is caused by the reluctance of some health professionals to involve specialist palliative-care services in the care of people who have palliative needs. In addition, there is still some ignorance in the community about the care of people facing the end of life. Public testimonials in the media about unnecessary suffering in dying are evidence that many people still do not have ready access to expert palliative care. Despite efforts to the contrary, palliative care continues to be represented in the media in the context of discussions about the active ending of life.

The artificial separation of curative care and palliative care means that people are sometimes reluctant to recommend or receive palliative care because it infers an acceptance of inevitable death. However, there is now an increasing recognition that many people actively seek life-prolonging therapy while simultaneously requiring palliative care. In the future, especially with an ageing population, palliative care will be more closely integrated into the acute care of people with chronic life-limiting illness. Nurses who work with chronic illness will therefore require an increasing level of palliative-care knowledge. The goal of this book is to transcend settings of care and diagnosis in setting out a knowledge base that is applicable to all.

In facing the challenges of promoting the best care for people at the end of life, and support for those who are significant to them, nurses will find this approach to palliative care useful in understanding need and in promoting palliative-care practices in all environments.

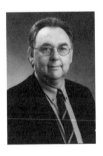

Alan Pearson

Professor Alan Pearson is head of nursing in the School of Nursing and Midwifery, La Trobe University, Melbourne (Victoria, Australia). Alan has extensive experience in nursing practice, nursing research, and academic nursing. Having qualified as a registered nurse in 1969, he has practised in a range of nursing fields in the United Kingdom, Papua New Guinea, and Australia. He has been an active researcher since 1981 and has conducted a large number of research projects in the fields of aged care, nursing history, and organ donation. Alan was instrumental in establishing the Joanna Briggs Institute for Evidence Based Nursing (of which he is currently the director) and is the foundation director of the newly established Australian Centre for Evidence Based Residential Aged Care. He has played a leading role in promoting research of evidence-based practice in Australia, New Zealand, and Hong Kong. Alan is editor of the *International Journal of Nursing Practice* and has published 20 books and numerous journal articles. He is active in developing and promoting nursing at the state, national, and international levels.

Chapter 2

Evidence-Based Practice in Palliative Care

Alan Pearson

Introduction

In the industrialised world, all areas of the health-care system are facing increasing demands and an escalation in costs. Governments and health-care professionals have responded to this in a variety of ways. Some responses focus on cost-cutting—by rationing services, by introducing measures to increase productivity, and by imposing cost-shifting exercises. This has involved serious ethical discussions of what can be afforded and what cannot, and the development of processes to provide essential health services to those who most need it. Some responses promote a 'user-pays' approach, and others simply blame others!

Another response is that of evidence-based practice (EBP). The emergence of EBP has led, in most Western countries, to a focus on best practice, based on the best available evidence.

This chapter provides an overview of the development of EBP, considers the processes of EBP, and discusses its limitations in palliative care. The view presented here is that clinical performance and professional judgment in the 'information age' must increasingly be based on exposure to summarised evidence and that, in the not-too-distant future, practice that is not based on a consideration of the evidence will be difficult to justify.

EBP: What is it?

Simply defined, EBP is a combination of individual clinical professional expertise with the best available external evidence to produce practice that is most likely to lead to a positive outcome for the person receiving care.

Although medicine and nursing are the health-care occupations that are most advanced in the EBP movement, the ideas and arguments are common to all professionals who work in health care. Sackett et al. (1996) have contended that evidence-based medicine (EBM) had its philosophical origins in the mid nineteenth century in Paris. They defined it as being 'the conscientious, explicit and judicious use of current best evidence in making decisions about the care of individual patients' (p. 71).

> 'Professional judgment in the 'information age' must increasingly be based on exposure to summarised evidence . . . practice that is not based on a consideration of the evidence will be difficult to justify.'

The establishment of the Cochrane Collaboration stemmed from the work of A.L. Cochrane. He drew attention to the lack of information about the effects of health care, with particular reference to medicine, and suggested (Cochrane 1979) that it is:

> . . . surely a great criticism of our profession that we have not organised a critical summary by specialty or sub-specialty adapted periodically of all relevant randomised controlled trials.

Cochrane argued that, because resources for health care are limited, they should be used effectively to provide care that has been shown, in valid evaluations, to result in desirable outcomes. He emphasised the importance of randomised controlled trials in providing reliable information on the effectiveness of medical interventions.

The development of EBM has been rapid—led by Professor David Sackett, formerly of McMaster University in Canada, and now of the University of Oxford, England. EBM has been defined by Sackett and colleagues (1996, p. 71) as:

The conscientious, explicit, and judicious use of current best evidence in making decisions about the care of individual patients. The practice of evidence based medicine means integrating individual clinical expertise with the best available external clinical evidence from systematic research.

Sackett and Rosenberg (1995) have suggested that EBM is concerned with five linked ideas:

▶ that clinical and other health-care decisions should be based on the best patient-based, population-based, and laboratory-based evidence;
▶ that the nature and source of the evidence to be sought depends on the particular clinical question;
▶ that the identification of the best available evidence requires the application of epidemiological, economic, and biostatistical principles, together with a consideration of the relevant pathophysiology in the context of personal experience;
▶ that this identification and appraisal of the evidence must be acted upon; and
▶ that there should be continuous evaluation of performance.

'EBM is the conscientious, explicit, and judicious use of current best evidence in making decisions about the care of individual patients.'

The Cochrane Collaboration provides systematic reviews of randomised controlled trials with respect to specific medical conditions, specific client groups, and specific interventions by health professionals. Such a systematic review of any given topic involves:

▶ determining the objectives and eligibility criteria for including trials;
▶ identifying studies that are likely to meet the eligibility criteria;
▶ tabulating the characteristics of, and assessing the methodological quality of, each study identified;
▶ excluding studies that do not meet the eligibility criteria;
▶ compiling the most complete set of data feasible, involving the investigators if possible;
▶ analysing the results of eligible studies, using a meta-analysis or statistical synthesis of data if appropriate and possible;
▶ performing sensitivity analyses if appropriate and possible; and
▶ preparing a structured report of the review that states the aims of the review, describes the materials and methods used, and reports the results.

The Cochrane Collaboration caters for other interests, including non-medical groups. In the health-care field, it assists certain categories of health-service users, different groups of health professionals, various health-care settings, and certain classes of intervention. The involvement of nurses is, however, just beginning to occur in most Western countries.

There is a small but growing body of literature on EBP in nursing. Much of the work has originated in the United Kingdom (UK), but there is a growing awareness of the importance of the subject in the United States of America (USA). In Australia, there has been considerable development of infrastructure underpinning evidence-based nursing, and there is an increasing amount of work on EBP in nursing, emanating largely from the Joanna Briggs Institute for Evidence Based Nursing & Midwifery (JBI) and its collaborating centres in Adelaide, Perth, Darwin, Toowoomba, Brisbane, Sydney, and Melbourne (where there are two centres). The institute also has collaborating centres in Auckland (New Zealand) and Hong Kong (China).

EBP in palliative care

Because the EBP movement has, in the past, focused on *effectiveness*, and because it has elevated the randomised controlled trial as the 'best' generator of evidence, many practitioners are critical of the wide application of evidence-based approaches to palliative care. As Higginson (1999, p. 462) has asserted, palliative care is essentially focused on 'a person centered approach . . . It focuses on both the quality of life remaining to patients and supporting their families and those close to them'. Keeley (1999, p. 1448) has criticised the current overemphasis on the use of evidence, and has asked:

> . . . if our loved one is dying and wishes to die at home, how much evidence do we need that skilled home nursing available around the clock would be a good idea?

Although it is true that the randomised trial is frequently an inappropriate method for the study of palliative-care interventions, it remains useful for many. Grande et al. (1999) reported on a randomised controlled trial designed to establish the relationship between the utilisation of a 'hospital-at-home' service and the place of death. Their findings suggested that there is no difference in the place of death between patients admitted to hospital and those who participate in a hospital-at-home program. They noted, however, that the randomised controlled trial is problematic in palliative care in terms of: (i) sample recruitment; (ii) the ethical difficulties associated with randomisation;

(iii) the complexities of collecting data from palliative-care patients and their significant others; and (iv) the difficulties of standardising intervention and control conditions.

Fitch et al. (1995) have argued for the adoption of evidence-based approaches to those areas of palliative-care nursing that require an evidence base, and have argued that these approaches be drawn from international research to work towards 'best practice'. They have suggested that there is a wide range of interventions for which such good evidence exists to inform the decision-making of palliative-care practitioners. For example, Gerson and Triadafilopoulos (2000) reviewed the care of people requiring palliative care for pain control, for the management of oral and skin ulcerations, for the control of nausea and vomiting, and for the treatment of psychological problems associated with inflammatory bowel disease. The review took an evidence-based approach and ranked the evidence to support various care interventions. The study included evidence-based algorithms for the management of pain and nausea in patients with inflammatory bowel disease.

Although there are large areas of palliative-care practice that will always rely on the professional judgment of the practitioner, this professional judgment will increasingly need to be seen to be informed by the best available evidence. Although the best available evidence might be a distillation of the practical experience of expert practitioners, some interventions will increasingly have a strong evidence base upon which to draw.

'Care decisions ultimately balance the needs and desires of individual patients and their families with the judgment of the caring practitioners in the light of the best available evidence.'

EBP does not imply that practitioners should slavishly follow the recommendations of a systematic review or those of an evidence-based set of guidelines. Care decisions ultimately balance the needs and desires of individual patients and their families with the judgment of the caring practitioners in the light of the best available evidence.

Health care practices and evidence-based guidelines

In response to high-profile initiatives of governments and provider agencies, health professions are increasingly embracing the use of evidence-based guidelines to inform (rather than direct) practice.

In the USA, considerable resources have been invested in high-quality, high-cost research and development programs with a view to developing appropriate clinical guidelines. The US National Institutes of Health now have a well-established strategy for reviewing international literature, and conduct meta-analyses to generate clinical guidelines based on best available evidence.

In the UK, recent policy initiatives have directed health-care provider agencies to develop research and development (R&D) strategies, to establish R&D units, and to promote practices based on the best available knowledge. The British government has also established a number of centres for EBP, supported by health research centres such as the Kings Fund.

At an international level, the Cochrane Collaboration has linked R&D sites across the world to review and analyse randomised clinical trials from an international perspective. The Cochrane Collaboration also generates reports to inform practitioners and influence practice, and acts as a resource in the development of consensus guidelines.

As a result of these and other developments, the practical application of rigorously reviewed evidence is now promoted through the development and dissemination of practice guidelines in most developed health-care systems. Clinical practice guidelines, systematically developed on the basis of consensus within expert groups, consist of statements to assist the decisions of practitioners and patients regarding appropriate health care in specific clinical circumstances. An increasing number of well-constructed, practical, evidence-based guidelines is being developed, with most of this activity emanating from the USA.

EBP is now almost institutionalised in most industrialised countries, especially in Europe, the UK, North America, and Australasia. Many of these regions have established centres for evidence-based health care, medicine, and nursing. There are, for example, Cochrane centres in all of these regions. In addition, specific centres exist for evidence-based nursing in the UK, North America, and Australia. The JBI, based in Australia, has collaborating centres in China and New Zealand.

Evidence-based practice in Australia and New Zealand

Policy-makers and health services in Australia began to focus on EBP some years ago and several developments have occurred in this area.

The Health Advisory Committee of the National Health and Medical Research Council (NH&MRC) funds the Australasian Cochrane Centre. The centre draws on the methodology and findings of the international Cochrane Collaboration to promote EBM in Australia and New Zealand. Drawing on this work, the translation of reviews into clinical practice guidelines has developed rapidly in Australia. The establishment of a national guidelines development program was first proposed by the National Health Strategy, as one of five major activities of a national focus on quality and effectiveness. This followed an earlier survey of health professional organisations in Australia by the National Health Strategy to determine whether guidelines were being developed and, if so, for which purposes. In its interim report, the Professional Indemnity Review noted that clinical practice guidelines have potential to improve the quality of services and set standards (DHHCS 1992).

In 1992, the Australian Health Ministers' Advisory Council agreed to work with the NH&MRC to develop a process for promoting best practice linked to outcomes and effective cost-management, including the development of clinical practice guidelines. In the 1995/96 Commonwealth budget, funding for clinical practice guideline development was built into the National Hospitals Outcomes Program.

The Quality of Care and Health Outcomes Committee (QCHOC) of the NH&MRC encourages and facilitates clinical colleges and other groups to develop guidelines and outcome measures. The QCHOC has stated that the development of clinical practice guidelines should be carried out within a context of worldwide concerns about:

▶ documented and unjustifiable variations in practice for similar conditions;

▶ increasing availability of new treatments and technology;

▶ lack of knowledge about effectiveness of interventions in terms of patient health outcomes; and

▶ the rising cost of health care.

'Development of clinical practice guidelines should be carried out within a context of worldwide concerns.'

Several guidelines have been developed on the basis that the health system should focus on the outcomes of patient care. The NH&MRC has recommended that clinical practice guidelines be developed through a multidisciplinary approach that includes contributions from all relevant clinicians, representatives of consumers, and other key groups and disciplines. Guidelines should provide information on the best investment for the best health outcomes, and should include an economic appraisal. They should identify known exceptions or risks, and identify the specific patient populations to which they apply. They must be comprehensive and flexible enough to apply to diverse settings and circumstances.

The multidisciplinary development process should define and recommend processes to encourage adoption of the guidelines. Implementation strategies could use the education and communication links of appropriate colleges, professional organisations, and consumer groups, and should seek to be incorporated into quality-assurance processes. They should include consideration of confidentiality and privacy (which might otherwise inhibit implementation), identify other barriers to implementation, and ensure that incentives and support for dissemination and implementation are linked to accountability.

The systematic review

The core of EBP is a systematic review of the literature on a particular condition, intervention, or issue. Such a systematic review is essentially an analysis of all of the available evidence in the literature, together with a judgment of the effectiveness of a practice. The process developed by the Cochrane Collaboration involves three steps:

▶ planning the review;
▶ the review protocol; and
▶ assessing the quality of a research report.

Planning the review

Planning of the review begins with an initial search of the Cochrane Library, especially the Database of Abstracts of Reviews of Effectiveness (DARE), to establish whether or not a recent review report exists. If this is the case, permission is sought from the originators of the existing review to use it to develop a practice information sheet. If the topic has not been the subject of a systematic review, a review protocol is developed.

The review protocol

As in any research endeavour, the development of a rigorous research proposal or protocol is vital for a high-quality systematic review, and a similar approach is required for a focused reading program. The review protocol provides a predetermined plan to ensure scientific rigour and minimise potential bias. It also allows for periodic updating of the review if necessary. Figure 2.1 (page 17) shows the format of the JBI review protocol described here.

Protocol development involves:

- a background review;
- objectives;
- inclusion criteria;
- search strategy;
- assessment criteria;
- data extraction; and
- data synthesis.
    Each of these is considered below.

Background review

The initial step is to undertake a quick, general evaluation of the literature to determine the scope and quantity of the primary research, to search for any existing reviews, and to identify issues of importance.

Objectives

As with any research, it is important to have a clear question. The protocol should state in detail the questions or hypotheses that will be pursued in the review. Questions should be specific regarding the patients, setting, interventions, and outcomes to be investigated.

> 'As with any research, it is important to have a clear question . . . regarding the patients, setting, interventions, and outcomes to be investigated.'

Inclusion criteria

The protocol must describe the criteria that will be used to select the literature. The inclusion criteria should address the participants of the primary studies, the intervention, and the outcomes. In addition to this, it should also specify the research methodologies that will be considered for inclusion in the review (for example, randomised controlled trials, clinical trials, case studies, and so on).

Search strategy

The protocol should provide a detailed strategy that will be used to identify all relevant literature within an agreed timeframe. This should include databases and bibliographies that will be searched, and the search terms that will be used.

Assessment criteria

It is important to assess the quality of the research to minimise the risk of an inconclusive review resulting from excessive variation in the quality of the studies. The protocol must therefore describe how the validity of primary studies will be assessed and any exclusion criteria based on quality considerations.

Data extraction

It is necessary to extract data from the primary research regarding the participants, the intervention, the outcome measures, and the results. Examples of sheets developed for this purpose are shown in Figure 2.2 (page 18) and Figure 2.3 (page 19) and should be included as part of the protocol.

Data synthesis

It is important to combine the literature in an appropriate manner when producing a report. Statistical analysis (meta-analysis) might or might not be used, depending on the nature and quality of studies included in the review. Although it might not be possible to state exactly what analysis will be undertaken, the general approach should be included in the protocol. The approach might be a statistical analysis. However, for some reviews, a narrative summary will suffice.

The format of the JBI review protocol is reproduced in Figure 2.1 (page 17).

Assessing the quality of a research report

A structured assessment process is used to evaluate the quality of the literature. The structured format used by the JBI is shown in Figures 2.2 (page 18) and 2.3 (page 19). There is one format for research (which follows a randomised control design) and one for research (which is observational in nature).

Effectiveness, appropriateness, and feasibility

To date, the EBP movement has focused on evidence of *effectiveness*. Although agreeing that EBP includes such an interest in research into effectiveness, Pearson (1998, pp 25–6) has argued that it is not confined to this:

> . . . evidence-based practice is not exclusively about effectiveness; it is about basing practice on the best available evidence . . . randomised trials are the gold standard for phenomena that we are interested in studying from a cause-and-effect perspective, but clearly they are not the gold standard if we are interested in how patients and nurses relate to each other, or if we are interested in how patients live through the experience of radiotherapy when they have a life-threatening illness. We have yet to

```
┌──────────────────────────────────────────────────────────────┐
│                          ((( ● )))                             │
│                                                                │
│                 THE JOANNA BRIGGS INSTITUTE                     │
│                 FOR EVIDENCE BASED NURSING                      │
├────────────────────────────────────────────────────────────────┤
│                       Review Protocol                          │
│ TITLE:                                                         │
│ BACKGROUND:                                                    │
│                                                                │
│                                                                │
│                                                                │
│ OBJECTIVES:                                                    │
│                                                                │
│                                                                │
│                                                                │
│ CRITERIA FOR CONSIDERING STUDIES FOR THIS REVIEW:              │
│ Types of Participants:                                         │
│                                                                │
│ Types of Intervention:                                         │
│                                                                │
│ Types of Outcome Measures:                                     │
│                                                                │
│ SEARCH STRATEGY FOR IDENTIFICATION OF STUDIES:                 │
│ METHODS OF THE REVIEW:                                         │
│ Selecting Studies for Inclusion:                               │
│                                                                │
│ Assessment of Quality:                                         │
│                                                                │
│ Methods Used to Collect Data From Included Studies:            │
│                                                                │
│ Methods Used to Synthesise Data:                               │
│                                                                │
│ Date Review to Commence:                                       │
│                                                                │
│ Date Review to Complete:                                       │
└────────────────────────────────────────────────────────────────┘
```

Figure 2.1
JBI review protocol
Courtesy Joanna Briggs Institute

work out how to assess the quality of alternative approaches to research other than the RCT [randomised control trial].

The diverse nature of problems in palliative care means that a diversity of research methodologies is required. Methodological approaches need to be eclectic enough to incorporate *both* the classical medical and scientific designs *and* the emerging qualitative action-oriented approaches from the humanities

Checklist for Assessing Validity of Experimental Studies

Ref No. ....

Experimental Studies	Yes	No	(if no use other checklist)		
Was the assignment to treatment groups really random?				Yes	No
Were participants blinded to treatment allocation?				Yes	No
Was allocation to treatment groups concealed from allocator?				Yes	No
Were the outcomes of people who withdrew described and included in the analysis (i.e. was the analysis by intention to treat)?				Yes	No
Were those assessing outcomes blind to the treatment allocation?				Yes	No
Were the control and treatment groups comparable at entry?				Yes	No
Were groups treated identically other than for the named interventions?				Yes	No
Were outcomes measured in the same way for all groups?				Yes	No
Were outcomes measured in reliable way?				Yes	No
Was an appropriate statistical analysis used?				Yes	No

Summary

TOTAL

Yes _____   No _____   ? _____

COMMENTS

Figure 2.2
JBI checklist for assessing validity of experimental studies
Courtesy Joanna Briggs Institute

and the social and behavioural sciences. The development of interdisciplinary research and greater understanding of the relationships among medical, nursing, and allied health interventions are also fundamental to the emergence of research methodologies that are relevant and sensitive to the health needs of the community.

There is a small, although growing, body of literature on the role of qualitative research in EBP, and there is an emerging recognition of a need to move beyond the *effectiveness* of interventions. Their *appropriateness* and *practical feasibility* also need to be considered.

Checklist for Assessing the Validity of Observational Studies

Ref No. ....

Observational Studies	**Yes**	**No**	(if no use other checklist)		
Is the study based on a random or pseudo-random sample?			**Yes**	**No**	**n/a**
Are the criteria for inclusion in the sample clearly defined?			**Yes**	**No**	**n/a**
Were outcomes assessed using objective criteria?			**Yes**	**No**	**n/a**
If comparisons are being made, was there sufficient description of the groups?			**Yes**	**No**	**n/a**
Was an appropriate statistical analysis used?			**Yes**	**No**	**n/a**

Summary

TOTAL

Yes _____   No _____   ? _____   n/a _____

COMMENTS

Figure 2.3
JBI checklist for assessing the validity of observational studies
Courtesy Joanna Briggs Institute

Lemmer, Grellier and Steven (1999), in conducting a systematic review in the area of health visiting, focused on the assumption that the randomised controlled trial (RCT) should be taken as the 'gold standard'. They reported a paucity of such trials in the field under study, and argued that clinical complexity demands the integration of qualitative methods into systematic reviews. They argued (1999, p. 323) that the 'comprehensiveness and synthesis of a systematic review are more important to emphasise than whether the literature is outside the clinical remit of an RCT'.

The need to integrate the results of qualitative research more fully into the systematic process was well argued by Popay (1998, p. 32), who asserted that 'there are many proponents of evidence-based decision making within health care who cannot and/or will not accept that qualitative research has an important part to play'. She went on to insist that qualitative research does more than simply enhance quantitative studies, and stated that qualitative research is capable of generating evidence that:

▶ explores practices that are taken for granted;
▶ increases understanding of consumer and clinical behaviour;
▶ develops interventions;
▶ illuminates patients' perceptions of quality and appropriateness;
▶ gives guidance to understanding organisational culture and change management; and
▶ evaluates complex policy initiatives.

In the same vein, Green and Britten (1998, p. 1230) have noted that qualitative studies might appear to be:

> . . . unscientific and anecdotal to many medical scientists. However, as the critics of evidence-based medicine are quick to point out, medicine is more than the application of scientific rules.

Green and Britten (1998, p. 1231) went on to argue that qualitative research provides rigorous accounts of treatment regimens in everyday contexts and that there is an increasing need within EBP for an awareness that different research questions require different kinds of research. They were unequivocal in asserting that ' . . . "good" evidence goes further than the results of meta-analysis of randomised controlled trials'.

'Medicine is more than the application of scientific rules.'

The Cochrane Qualitative Methods Network, established in 1998, is currently exploring the scope for incorporating qualitative research into Cochrane reviews, and a number of protocols and checklists has been developed by the group (Qualitative Methods Network 1999).

However, there are still no internationally reviewed approaches to assessing the quality of specific qualitative methods, and no accepted method of rating or ranking qualitative research findings reported in the literature. Nevertheless, there have been several attempts to synthesise the results of similar qualitative studies (as a form of meta-analysis), and these have been well described by Sandelowski, Docherty and Emden (1997). These authors have also developed an indepth theoretical approach to the systematic metasynthesis of qualitative findings, while maintaining the integrity of individual studies. Drawing on this work, together with that of the Cochrane Qualitative Methods Network and that of Popay (1998) and Lemmer, Grellier and Steven (1999), an approach to qualitative research could be developed that takes account of qualitative meta-analysis, quality assessment, and the development of a quality rating scale. This would add the dimensions of *appropriateness* and *feasibility* to a systematic review process that is currently oriented towards *effectiveness*.

Conclusion

There are signs that the EBP movement is beginning to develop a more comprehensive view of 'evidence'. Research initiatives that attempt to assess and synthesise the results of interpretive and critical research are being developed, and these forms of evidence are becoming an integral part of the systematic reviews that inform practice. Such an approach to EBP will help palliative-care practitioners to perform to the highest standards, using their professional judgment in association with appropriate evidence.

'Palliative-care practitioners, to perform to the highest standards, [must use] their professional judgment in association with appropriate evidence.'

Rejection of EBP by practitioners or researchers because of its current obsession with *effectiveness* is not in the best interests of either health-care professionals or those in their care. What is required is a constructive critique of the over-emphasis on effectiveness, and the development of approaches that systematically review other forms of evidence.

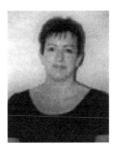 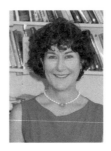

Annabel Pollard

Annabel Pollard has been a registered psychologist for five years, and completed an MA in clinical psychology in 2001. Annabel is currently employed as a psychologist at the Peter MacCallum Cancer Institute, Melbourne (Victoria, Australia), as coordinator of patient support programs in which she is responsible for the development and management of psychosocial supportive care programs for groups, patients, and families. Annabel also consults as a psychologist to individual patients and families through the psycho-oncology clinic at Peter MacCallum. Her research and clinical interests focus on staff training and patient care, as well as psychosocial issues (especially survivorship). Annabel is a member of the medical and scientific advisory board of the Leukaemia Foundation of Victoria, and of the Cancer Connect Advisory Committee at the Cancer Council of Victoria (CCV).

Kathleen Swift

Kathleen Swift has been a lecturer in nursing since 1992 and is now a member of staff of the La Trobe University and Austin & Repatriation Clinical School, Melbourne (Victoria, Australia). Kathleen's experience in cancer nursing began in 1981 and she has since held management and staff development positions within this specialty. Her work in community-based cancer care led to an interest in home-based palliative care. Kathleen is on the Committee of Management of the Banksia Palliative Care Service, a large domiciliary service in metropolitan Melbourne. She also serves on the executive of the Cancer Nurses Society of Australia, Melbourne Regional Group.

Chapter 3

Communication Skills in Palliative Care

Annabel Pollard and Kathleen Swift

Doctors and nurses need specific additional training . . . to help them acquire the knowledge and skills which will enable them to identify and respond to cancer patients needs for information, establish and resolve their concerns, and adequately assess psychological or psychiatric problems (Parle, Maguire & Heaven 1997, p. 231).

Introduction

Over the past few decades, research has shown that good communication is central to the interactions between health-care professionals and people with terminal illnesses. Research suggests that good communication can not only positively affect the psychological status and quality of life of people with such illnesses, but also assist in the resolution of physical symptoms (Faulkner & Maguire 1994; Maguire 1999; Stewart 1995).

This chapter focuses on the importance of communication skills as a central aspect of the nursing assessment and management of patients and families receiving palliative care. As the quotation at the beginning of the chapter suggests, additional specific training is required if therapeutic outcomes are to be optimised.

Such communication skills are often taken for granted. The self-evaluation questionnaire illustrated in Figure 3.1 (below) is a useful means of assessing personal skills in this area.

Therapeutic communication

A significant trend in the literature on palliative care has been a growing emphasis on communication skills as a core factor in improving patient outcomes. In the past, words such as 'counselling' and 'communication' have often been used interchangeably by nurses and other health professionals, as if they had similar meanings. However, the use of the word 'counselling' to refer

Self-evaluation—a chance to reflect on your skills	
Question	Self-evaluation score Rate as 1–10 where 1 = not at all confident; 10 = very confident
How confident are you in your knowledge about the impact of communication on patients in the palliative-care setting?	
How confident do you feel discussing psychological problems with patients who have a terminal disease?	
How confident do you feel in communicating with distressed patients?	
How confident do you feel making a referral to another health professional for a patient who is experiencing psychological distress?	
How confident do you feel in communicating with a patient who is anxious?	

Figure 3.1 Self-evaluation of communication skills
Adapted from Fallowfield, Saul & Gilligan (2001)

to general interactions between nurses and patients is a misnomer. Rather, this chapter uses the term 'therapeutic communication' to refer to the conscious, deliberate, and purposeful use of verbal and non verbal communication skills within the nurse–patient interaction to assess problems, attend to emotional cues, and elicit patient concerns. Although such therapeutic communication is a first step in identifying and clarifying patient concerns, it is emphasised that referral for skilled intervention, such as psychological counselling, might be a necessary next step.

Lack of training, lack of skills, and lack of time inhibit communication in many health-care settings. Communication in the setting of palliative care is frequently *ad hoc*, incidental to the nurse–patient interaction, and lacking in any purpose.

There is evidence that many nurses (and other health-care professionals) do not have sufficient communication skills to assist patients in discussing their concerns. Very few nurses receive more than rudimentary education about psychosocial issues, and such education as they do receive usually addresses theories of counselling and psychiatric problems in a superficial fashion. Nursing education, both general and advanced, rarely focuses on the development of knowledge and skills regarding the psychosocial distress experienced by people in times of crisis or transition (McCorkle, Frank-Stromberg & Pascreta 1998). Most nurses therefore develop their own individual approaches through trial and error, within environments that are often not conducive to effective communication.

Effects of poor communication on patient outcomes

Psychological distress in persons with terminal illness is a significant clinical problem. If the concerns of such people remain hidden, distress can be manifested as a more serious affective disorder. Such affective disorders can include a spectrum of depressive, anxiety, adjustment, and grief reactions. Among cancer patients, for example, studies have consistently indicated that about 30% of people experience an affective disorder as a result of diagnosis and/or treatment (Derogatis et al. 1983; Razavi et al. 1990). The risk of developing an affective disorder appears to be positively correlated with the

> 'About 30% of cancer patients experience an affective disorder as a result of diagnosis and/or treatment.'

complexity of treatment interventions, adverse side-effects, and various unidentified concerns (Devlen et al. 1987).

The incidence of affective disorders in the palliative-care setting can be as high as 77% during advanced disease, with psychiatric problems being exacerbated by medications and distressing symptoms such as pain (Breitbart & Passik 1997). In addition, organic disorders producing confusion and delirium account for a higher percentage of psychiatric consultations in the terminally ill and elderly than in the general population (Breitbart & Passik 1997).

Diagnosis and treatment of terminal illness is associated with a variety of concerns for the persons afflicted, and for their families. These vary, depending on the nature of the disease and the treatment received. Responses to these concerns are mediated by individual preferences for information and styles of coping. Unresolved concerns regarding psychosocial, physiological, and practical matters can have deleterious effects on patient outcomes (Maguire 1999). For example, Weisman and Worden (1997) showed that the number of patient concerns at the time of diagnosis could be correlated with later levels of emotional distress at six months. Other researchers have shown that the number and severity of concerns at diagnosis is strongly related to coping, and to levels of anxiety and depression at later stages (Parle, Jones & Maguire 1996).

Studies have indicated a relationship between disclosure of concerns by patients and levels of distress. For example, hospice patients who had more concerns were more anxious or depressed (Heaven & Maguire 1998). When hospice patients are anxious or depressed they have been shown to be less likely to talk about their concerns (Heaven & Maguire 1997). The same researchers (1998) have investigated how hospice patients disclosed their concerns and how nurses identified these concerns. They concluded that hospice patients were more likely to disclose physical concerns than psychosocial concerns, and that more than 60% of overall concerns were withheld. The researchers suggested that non-disclosure did not mean that the patient had no concerns; rather, non-disclosure was likely to be associated with an increased number of unexpressed concerns and increased distress.

In the palliative-care setting, depression and hopelessness have been shown to be associated with an increased desire for death. In one study, depressed patients were four times more likely to have a higher desire for death compared with non-depressed patients (Breitbart et al. 2000). These findings have important implications for the skills and abilities of health-care professionals in identifying patient distress and concerns in the palliative-care setting.

Communication as an effective tool

Effective communication is vital. To make meaningful decisions about their care, patients (and their families) require information about treatment options, prognosis, and side-effects (Jeffrey 1998). Patients and families require information and expert advice from nurses and other health professionals to facilitate decision-making, to reduce uncertainty regarding treatment outcomes, to engage in realistic appraisals of their situations, and to make necessary cognitive and emotional adjustments about the future.

Effective communication requires knowledge. Nurses require knowledge of the likely causes of patient distress in a given situation, as well as the ability to make educated guesses about underlying concerns. Furthermore, effective communication requires excellent communication skills if clinical interactions are to be therapeutic.

According to Maguire (1999), the use of effective communication results in:

> 'Effective communication requires excellent communication skills if clinical interactions are to be therapeutic.'

▶ eliciting patients' key problems and feelings;
▶ assisting with coping with bad news;
▶ being able to manage treatment decisions; and
▶ monitoring adverse reactions (both physical and psychological).

Barriers to effective communication

Barriers to effective communication can be due to difficulties experienced by the patient or to difficulties experienced by the nurses and other health professionals providing care.

Barriers related to patients

Patient-related communication difficulties can be considered under the following headings:
▶ reluctance to disclose concerns;
▶ individual preferences for modes of communication; and
▶ cross-cultural issues affecting communication
Each of these is considered below.

Reluctance to disclose concerns

For a variety of reasons, people are frequently reluctant to disclose their concerns to nurses and other health professionals, and are especially reluctant to talk about psychological issues. Patients often believe that nurses are too busy to address any more than the physical aspects of illness and treatment, or they might be concerned about the stigma associated with psychiatric problems (Maguire 1999).

It has been suggested that, perhaps because of the nature of terminal illness, patients often assume that psychological concerns are an inevitable part of their situation, and that nothing can be done to help them (Maguire 1999). For example, in one study of women with cervical cancer, researchers found that only 40% of patient concerns had been disclosed during the first year after diagnosis (Stewart, Walker & Maguire 1988). Heaven and Maguire (1997) also showed that hospice patients selectively disclosed information and were more likely to disclose physical problems than psychosocial concerns.

Discussing psychological concerns carries a risk of confronting difficult and painful emotions. For people with terminal illnesses these emotions sometimes seem so distressing that they cannot be disclosed to family members or carers. When emotional concerns remain unresolved, the result can be anxiety, depression, social isolation, and hopelessness. Palliative-care nurses play a key role in facilitating preparation for dying. In helping patients speak about what they most fear, the communication skills of nurses can have a significant positive effect on quality of life.

'In helping patients speak about what they most fear, the communication skills of nurses can have a significant positive effect on quality of life.'

Individual preferences for modes of communication

Confusion about what patients want to know about their diagnosis and treatment has also affected communication. Evidence suggests that patients require individualised approaches to disease-related information, and that such approaches must take into account personal preferences for high or low levels of information. Anxiety can result from a mismatch of patient needs with information received (Fallowfield et al. 1990). However some studies suggest that most cancer patients, for example, want to know about their diagnosis and prognosis (Maguire 1999). Although some evidence suggests that palliative-care patients prefer a collaborative approach to decision-making, other research has produced variable results regarding the extent to which patients wish to be involved in decision-making (Maguire 1999; Rothenbacher, Lutz & Porsolt 1997).

Patient disclosure of important information or concerns is facilitated by the use of a combination of open and 'directive' questions, and a focus on psychosocial problems using empathic statements and sensitive intuition (Maguire, Faulkner et al. 1996).

Cross-cultural issues affecting communication

Cultural diversity and related issues are to be expected in palliative care. Major life events are times when cultural heritage is relied upon and acted out. A contentious issue in palliative care is whether diagnoses should be withheld from patients of certain ethnic and cultural origins. For example, a study conducted in a large Chinese population found that the practice of withholding information from the patient was not supported by 95% of the sample (Fielding & Hung 1996). However, in some cases, family members might wish that their dying relative be not informed of the prognosis. This makes decision-making difficult and presents a challenge for nurses.

Egan (1998) has provided guidelines for dealing with diversity and multiculturalism in helping relationships. Although he acknowledged the need to learn as much as possible about different cultural groups, Egan has cautioned that the helper should:

- place the needs of the patient above all other considerations;
- ensure that the carer's own values do not adversely effect the patient's best interests; and
- avoid cultural stereotyping and generalisations by recognising that differences within groups are often more extensive than those between groups.

Barriers related to health professionals

Communication difficulties related to health professionals can be considered under the following headings:

- values, attitudes, and beliefs of health professionals; and
- skills deficits.

Each of these is considered below.

Values, attitudes, and beliefs

The extent to which a consultation is patient-centred will affect the course and outcome of communication. A patient-centred encounter is characterised by the use of skills including open questions, acknowledgment of emotional concerns, and a collaborative approach to decision-making (Jenkins & Fallowfield 2002). However, these skills are not easily employed without some self-knowledge on the part of the nurse or other health-care professional involved. Indeed, the values and beliefs held by the carer will inevitably intrude on the clinical interaction. Such values often form a tacit set of criteria in making decisions. Egan (1998) has noted that ' . . . it has become increasingly clear that helpers' values influence clients' values over the course of the helping process'. For example, if the nurse values stoicism there is a decreased likelihood that the patient will disclose emotional distress.

The attitudes and beliefs of carers will thus affect the degree to which their consultations are patient-centred. For example, a lack of self-awareness among nurses has been shown to be associated with an increased use of blocking behaviours to control communication with patients (Wilkinson 1991). In fact, patient behaviour is reinforced by the communication styles of health-care professionals (Wilkinson 1991), and patients frequently perceive that nurses and other health professionals are unwilling to explore their concerns (Maguire 1999). Some authors have suggested that values regarding death and fear of losing composure in front of patients (Maguire 1985), or fear of dying and the unknown (Razavi & Delvaux 1997), affect the attitudes and willingness of health-care professionals to discuss emotionally laden topics. However, such attitudes and beliefs can be modified by training (Jenkins & Fallowfield 2002).

Skills deficits

Nurses and other health-care professionals have been shown to engage in a variety of unhelpful behaviours that can block communication (Heaven & Maguire 1997; Faulkner & Maguire 1994; Wilkinson 1991; Wilkinson, Roberts & Aldridge 1998). A lack of skills, or fears about being unable to respond to patient questions, can adversely communication (Maguire, Booth et al. 1996).

A problem in this respect is that nurses and other health professionals often lack insight into their own limitations. They often rate their skills as high when, in fact, they are not. Behaviours that inhibit communication include the following:

▶ 'distancing' from the patient (that is, using physical barriers such as standing at the end of a bed, or avoiding particular patients on a ward round);

▶ ignoring emotional cues from patients (such as tears);

▶ providing false reassurance or colluding with denial;

▶ using avoidance tactics (such as changing the subject or focusing on physical tasks);

- focusing on physical symptoms rather than on emotional concerns;
- failing to recognise problems;
- lacking knowledge of common patient concerns; and
- possessing poor assessment skills.

Facilitating therapeutic communication
Awareness of concerns

People with terminal illness are confronted with some important questions. Who am I? Why am I here? What has my life been about? Has my life been worthwhile? Have I done everything I should have done? Meaningful communication about significant life events is vital for every person at every stage of life. The telling of stories is a way of 'reifying' events—a process of making meaning. Without this process, there is no opportunity to reflect upon, and resolve, problems with relationships or other important aspects of life.

Palliative-care nurses are often the key providers of care and support to patients and families. They are frequently required to act as care coordinators and to communicate effectively with a multitude of other professionals, including hospital staff, hospice staff, general practitioners, pharmacists, and community service providers, as well as with relatives. Nurses are well positioned to assess and explore the physical and psychosocial concerns of patients and family members.

Clinical interactions associated with advanced disease, dying, and death require effective communication. Common concerns of patients and families include worries about the future, fear of loss of control, anxiety regarding recurrence of disease, fear of dying, management of distressing symptoms, decision-making about treatment options, and advice regarding informed consent (Razavi & Delvaux 1997). Identifying and addressing the concerns of patients and their families is essential for effective palliation.

'Nurses are well positioned to assess and explore the physical and psychosocial concerns of patients and family members.'

Use of communication skills

Therapeutic communication utilises many of the skills of formal counselling. Most nurses are familiar with these skills from a theoretical perspective. However, without practical specific training in communication skills, it is

Checklist of skills

A checklist of skills for effective therapeutic communication includes:
- setting the scene—ensuring privacy and sufficient time;
- clarifying the purpose of the interaction;
- establishment of trust;
- eliciting information;
- active listening and exploring of verbal and non-verbal cues from patients;
- use of empathy;
- clarification of issues; and
- facilitating an outcome (for example, referral to another health professional).

Adapted from Lugton & Kindlen (1999)

impossible to provide important caring functions such as effective assessment, assistance with informed consent, and the provision of appropriate education and information. However, expertise in these skills requires more than clinical supervision and feedback. Discipline and critical self-reflection are also required, and these are often lacking in the training and ongoing support of palliative-care nurses and other clinicians.

Implications for nursing practice

The above discussion has certain implications for modern nursing practice in palliative care, including:
- the role of therapeutic communication in assessment skills;
- strategies and training for improving skills in communication;
- organisation and system issues;
- clinical supervision; and
- self-awareness, attitudes, and beliefs among nurses.
  Each of these is considered below.

Therapeutic communication and assessment skills

Good communication is central to effective assessment. To provide optimum care all health-care professionals must be able to assess the needs of patients and families accurately. Proper diagnosis and appropriate treatment obviously depend on accurate assessment of physical status or psychosocial concerns, and poor assessment skills can adversely affect patient outcomes. Although essential skills such as physical observation and appropriate nursing responses are routinely taught (for example, how to respond to a high temperature or how to undertake a certain technical intervention), such teaching has not traditionally extended to the art and science of communication.

In the context of palliative care, effective communication skills are essential for the comprehensive assessment of a variety of clinical parameters, including the emotional concerns of patients and families. How well do nurses perform when confronted with such issues? Wilkinson, Roberts & Aldridge (1998) studied nurses' assessment skills before and after a training course. Before training, the nurses' assessment skills scores were found to be low in all core areas of assessment and were oriented towards physical complaints. However, following an extended program in com-

'Although essential skills such as physical observation are routinely taught, such teaching has not traditionally extended to the art and science of communication.'

munication skills, their knowledge and confidence in their skills had increased.

In a study of palliative-care nurse training, Heaven and Maguire (1997) found that 60% of patient concerns remained undisclosed. Patients with more psychological distress (anxiety and depression) were even less likely to disclose concerns. In the same study, nurses registered only 40% of concerns disclosed to them and only 20% were correctly identified. This study concluded that nurses needed to improve their skills in both eliciting and identifying concerns. Evidence suggests that effective communication skills are essential for the identification of unmet needs and ongoing distress, and that those who practise such skills have the potential to improve quality of life in this high-risk patient group.

Although the number of evidence-based skills programs in communication is increasing, Fallowfield, Saul & Gilligan (2001) have suggested that nurses' communication have not improved in recent decades. Nurses fail to identify key patient concerns and tend to focus on physical issues, rather than psychosocial issues, (Heaven & Maguire 1997; Wilkinson 1991). Wilkinson (1991) investigated factors that affected nurse communication with cancer patients. She concluded that nurses routinely used strategies (such as ignoring or informing) to block communication with patients. In addition, difficult issues such as disease recurrence appeared to pose the most challenges to nurses.

In the setting of palliative care, it must be acknowledged that the distress and needs of patients might have existed for a significant length of time as the patient moves from diagnosis through various stages of treatment. In addition, patients learn a style and develop a 'framework' within which to deal with health professionals. Therefore, the palliative-care nurse might have to 'reorient' the patient and family to a health-care service that does acknowledge and address emotional experience and concerns.

Many of these findings have been replicated across other professional groups, with doctors having received the most attention in the literature. Roter and Fallowfield (1998) have presented an excellent review of the issues in which they concluded that health professionals, including oncologists, frequently lack the necessary skills to elicit and deal with emotional distress. These authors also acknowledged the personal cost to the health professional of continuing to ignore this 'hidden' or 'blocked' aspect to providing health care. Although detachment from the patient might temporarily reduce distress in medical practitioners, research has indicated that effective therapuetic relationships between doctors and patients form an important component of job satisfaction.

The implications of this discussion for practice are:

▶ that therapeutic communication skills are fundamental to comprehensive assessment;
▶ that assessment must go beyond the physical to identify emotional distress and other concerns;
▶ that nurses and other health professionals must recognise the importance of the outcomes of clinical interactions (for example, referrals);
▶ that health professionals must acknowledge the power they exert, and must take the lead in directing how the therapeutic relationship unfolds; and
▶ that an interpersonal relationship based on acknowledgment of therapeutic outcomes can promote job satisfaction.

Strategies and training for improving skills in communication

Training in patient-centred communication skills is an important aspect of improving therapeutic communication. Roter and Fallowfield (1998) have stated that successful training results from skills development. Such skills development requires practical application, role play, peer discussion, and rehearsal. After reviewing several studies aimed at changing communication skills among doctors, Roter and Fallowfield (1998) concluded that lectures on targeted communication skills had little effect on how doctors interacted with patients. Furthermore, these authors found that skills development alone was inadequate in producing long-term behavioural changes. The learner must value the need for change, be motivated to change, and be supported in that change.

Some of the skills that have been found to be valuable in working with people with cancer are: (i) the use of open direct questions with a psychological focus (for example, 'How are you feeling today?'); (ii) the clarification of psychological cues; and (iii) the summarising of issues. Parle, Maguire and Heaven (1997) found that participants who acquired skills in these areas were able to move beyond a physical focus in their clinical interactions. One caveat should be noted—once patient concerns have been elicited, referral to appropriate supports must be made. Therapeutic communication is primarily about identifying and acknowledging patient concerns; it is not always about resolving them.

It is not always possible to participate in skills training. In addition, once training has been completed, the motivation to continue patient-centred communication can wane in the routine of daily work, especially in the absence of significant ongoing feedback. One personal strategy to assist in maintaining a continuing emphasis on therapeutic communication skills in practice is to use a diary to reflect on the practice. The 'dialogue' that develops with oneself can also be shared with peers for further discussion. Difficult communication scenarios encountered can become the subject of role plays, discussion, and rehearsal—just as they would be in a formal workshop. Assistance from a skilled facilitator is preferable.

'Therapeutic communication is primarily about identifying and acknowledging patient concerns; it is not always about resolving them.'

Considerable research has focused on the question of which training methods best facilitate behavioural changes in communication skills. This research has investigated the best ways of conducting role plays in training scenarios in a safe, trusting, and confidential environment, and most formal training workshops now reflect this evidence-based approach (Maguire 1999; Razavi & Delvaux 1997).

Organisation and system issues

As previously stated, many nurses have received little specific education (and even less practice) in the application of therapeutic communication skills. Some nurses have pursued personal training in this area but find it is difficult to sustain a commitment to a practice that is relatively undervalued and unrecognised in the field. Shifting the professional focus of workplaces would be an important first step in raising nurses' awareness and in changing attitudes. This, in turn, would facilitate the re-ordering of priorities in palliative care such that the *whole* experience of the dying person is emphasised.

McCorkle, Frank-Stromberg and Pasacreta (1998) described an education program that promoted such a shift in practice. It focused on assessments and interventions for the psychosocial needs of people with cancer. One of the outcomes of this program was the development of a 'gaps and contracts' strategy that identified organisational gaps in psychosocial services for patients. Gaps that were identified included lack of assessment tools, lack of psychosocial standards of care, and poor coordination of psychosocial resources. After participants had completed the program they were empowered to participate actively in organisational changes to address these gaps, including the implementation of communication skills training. Other organisational issues known to affect communication adversely include a lack of time and the culture and environment of particular wards (Wilkinson 1991).

Improving awareness of, and access to, additional communication skills training in orientation programs and continuing education programs can facilitate successful organisational change. Development of appropriate screening tools can guide nurses to elicit information effectively, prioritise patient needs, and refer appropriately.

Clinical supervision

Clinical supervision is an efficient way to improve personal communication skills and promote therapeutic outcomes. Frequent meetings with an experienced and skilled communicator (for example, a nurse consultant, a psychologist, or a social worker) can be helpful in this respect. Supervision provides an opportunity to reflect on issues relating to clinical encounters and to develop personal skills and insights into clinical interactions. Egan (1998, p. 343) has stated that 'supervision is an extremely important part of the learning process. Indeed, effective helpers never stop learning about themselves, their clients and the helping process itself.'

Supervision is not formally recognised in nursing. However it is one way to develop an effective set of skills with which to approach and manage the serious and often confronting issues raised in the palliative-care setting.

Self-awareness, attitudes, and beliefs

Self-awareness involves becoming aware of one's own values, motivations, attitudes, and beliefs. To understand and empathise with patients and families who are confronting the reality of suffering and death, palliative-care nurses need to identify their own values about existential issues such as death and suffering. Supervision or peer support can assist with this process. However, these must be structured within a confidential and effective learning framework. Opportunities to share experiences and to encounter conflicting interpretations can be stimulating and can extend one's knowledge base.

Sample plan for improving communication skills

A useful sample plan for improving communication skills is shown in Figure 3.2 (below). This should be considered in association with Figure 3.1 (page 24) which began this chapter. A comparison of initial self-evaluation and self-evaluation after completing this chapter provides a useful basis for implementing a plan to improve the essential skills of therapeutic communication.

Sample plan for improving communication skills	
Supervision	Set up structured supervision with skilled personnel—for example, nurse consultant, psychologist, social worker
In partnership with patient and family preferences	Routinely ask the patient if you have addressed all of his or her concerns
Diary	Commence a personal diary of your experiences what you think you did well and what you think you can improve
Peer support	Seek peer supervision when conducting interviews with patients and share your diary with a supervisor
Case discussion	Introduce communication-related case discussions in team meetings
Clarification of concerns	Identify patient concerns routinely at each patient encounter
Referral	Routinely consider and discuss referral options for every patient
Education	Ensure that your knowledge and skills are maintained
Balance	Ensure that your own life is balanced; take time out

Figure 3.2 Sample plan for improving communication skills
Author's presentation

Conclusion

Palliative-care nurses are in a unique position to identify patients concerns and facilitate resolution of those concerns as the patient moves towards death. However, evidence indicates that nurses typically lack skills in eliciting such concerns and often fail to identify them accurately. Therapeutic communication is not counselling. The misuse of the term 'counselling' has led to an assumption that anyone can do it. This is a profound error that encourages a situation in which nurses and other health-care professionals assume that they have skills which, in fact, they often do not possess. Improving nursing knowledge about the strategies used by patients dealing with life-threatening illness, and improving nurses' assessment and communication skills through specific and additional training, have the potential to improve patient outcomes at this vulnerable time. Therapeutic communication is a purposeful intervention used to assess and identify patient concerns, but it requires a willingness to develop expert practice skills. Valuing the difference that palliative-care nurses can make requires a belief that therapeutic communication is a core clinical intervention requiring self-reflection and ongoing development.

Palliative-care nurses are great people! But working with people at the end of their lives, and confronting the existential dilemmas associated with death and dying are not easy tasks. Palliative-care nurses can make a substantial difference to the ability of patients to deal with these difficult experiences and to achieve some resolution of their concerns.

> 'Palliative-care nurses can make a substantial difference to the ability of patients to deal with difficult experiences and to achieve some resolution of their concerns.'

Palliative-care nurses share part of a journey with patients and families—a journey that is characterised by coping with advanced disease, reduced quality of life, uncertainty, grief, loss, and death. In these circumstances, patients and families are often confronted with a need to communicate about issues that are painful to experience and difficult to share. Speigel (1994) has suggested that terminally ill patients and their families are challenged to 'speak the unspeakable'. If they develop the necessary communication skills, palliative-care nurses are ideally positioned to assist patients and families to meet this challenge.

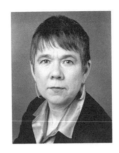

Mary Vachon

Dr Mary Vachon is a nurse, clinical sociologist, and psychotherapist in private practice. She is associate professor in the Departments of Psychiatry and Public Health Sciences at the University of Toronto (Ontario, Canada) and clinical consultant at Wellspring, a community-based support program for persons with cancer. Mary has published more than 120 professional articles and chapters, and has lectured in numerous countries. She is the recipient of many awards, and was named as the Distinguished Scientist of 2001 by the National Hospice and Palliative Care Organization (USA) for her lifetime contribution to the field of palliative care.

Chapter 4

Occupational Stress in Palliative Care

Mary Vachon

Introduction

Caring for patients and families during the palliative stages of disease can be both stressful and rewarding. Dealing with the total experience of suffering of patients and families, and assisting them to come to terms with impending death, present the caregiver with many challenges and stresses. Walking with patients and families during the most difficult time in their lives, and participating in decreasing the suffering they experience, can be extremely rewarding for the caregiver. However, constant exposure to suffering and loss does take its toll if the caregiver is unaware of the need for caring for self as one cares for others. Indeed, much of the stress in the palliative-care field comes from issues related to the personal circumstances of the caregiver—including the caregiver's work environment, team conflicts, issues of power and control, role conflict, and role strain, with much less of the stress being due to dealing with dying patients and their families (Vachon 1995, 2001, 2002a, 2002b).

The author's personal experience with a life-threatening cancer led to a new awareness of the importance of the concept of the 'wounded healer' (Nouwen

1972) and the importance of self-reflection in caring for palliative-care patients. The ability to enter into a space of personal healing can enable the nurse to be more fully available to patients and families without 'burning out'. This chapter explores the search for meaning in palliative caregivers, the 'wounded healer', sources of suffering in clinical work, and coping strategies.

The search for meaning in palliative care

Spiritual and religious belief systems have been found to be helpful in oncology and palliative care (Vachon 1995). A sense of spirituality can be helpful to caregivers as they struggle to find meaning in the work they are doing (Heim 1991; Vachon 2001). Nurses attracted to hospice work have been found to be more religious than others (Amenta 1984; Vachon 1987, 1995). Compared with oncology nurses, hospice nurses reported a greater sense of personal spirituality, more frequent spiritual caregiving, and more positive perspectives regarding spiritual caregiving (Taylor, Highfield & Amenta 1999).

In a study at Memorial Sloan Kettering Cancer Center (Kash et al. 2000), nurses were found to be more religious than others. Those 'quite a bit to extremely religious' had significantly lower scores on diminished empathy or depersonalisation and had lower emotional exhaustion on the Maslach Burnout Inventory (Maslach & Jackson 1986). For many caregivers a spiritual or religious philosophy, centred on a commitment to serve others, can be helpful and vital to deriving a sense of meaning in difficult times (Vachon 1987).

> 'A sense of spirituality can be helpful to caregivers as they struggle to find meaning in the work they are doing.'

Remen (1996), a physician who left the practice of academic paediatrics to focus her energies on working with people with cancer and their professional caregivers, has spoken of the power of a personal sense of meaning to change the experience of work, relationships, and, even, of life. As Remen (1996, p. 162) has observed:

> Competence and expertise are two of the most respected qualities in the medical subculture, as well as in our society. But important as they are, they are not sufficient to fully sustain us ... Competence may bring us satisfaction. Finding meaning in a familiar task often allows us to go beyond this and find in the most routine of tasks a deep sense of joy and even gratitude.

Suffering and healing in palliative care

Kearney (2000) has noted that although we can speak of curing another's *pain*, the *suffering* of another is beyond pain; it is the experience that results from damage to the *whole person*. In a similar vein, Cassell (1991, p. 33) has noted that: 'Suffering occurs when the impending destruction of the person is perceived'. In the same passage, Cassell defined suffering as being 'the state of severe distress associated with events which threaten the intactness of the person'.

Healing can occur within suffering. Healing has been defined by Kearney (2000, p. ixx) as 'the process of becoming psychologically and spiritually more integrated and whole: a phenomenon which enables persons to become more completely themselves and more fully alive'. Such healing can come only from the depths of the individual's psyche. Caregivers can, however, help to create an environment that fosters inner healing within a person. Kearney (2000, p. 5) has put it this way:

> In practice this happens when a combination of effective care and human companionship helps to establish a secure, inner space for that person to be in. The process is further facilitated if the carers themselves have found ways of staying with, and being in, their own experience of suffering.

The wounded caregiver and vulnerability to burnout

In *The Wounded Healer* (1972), the theologian Henri Nouwen (1932–96) hypothesised that successful caregivers are often 'wounded healers', with wounds sustained in childhood, or in adulthood, or both. In trying to heal their own wounds, these caregivers have been drawn, consciously or not, to healing others. The concept of the 'wounded healer' is derived from ancient universal shamanic stories of tribal priests: 'the original wounded healers, whose ability to heal others was seen as being directly linked to their having journeyed in depth into their own wounded selves' (Kearney 1996, p. 45).

Pines (2000) has suggested that career decisions can enable people to gratify needs that were ungratified in childhood, and to actualise dreams passed on by family heritage. Caregivers can, therefore, enter their careers with very high hopes and expectations, significant ego involvement, and much passion. If successful in their careers, such people can derive a sense of existential significance that partially heals their childhood wounds. However, if they feel that they have failed to do their work in the way that it 'should' be done, or when work does not give their lives a sense of meaning, these people 'burn out'. A lack of existential significance is the hallmark of burnout (Pines 2000).

Sulmasy (1997, p. 48), a physician, philosopher, and Franciscan friar has contended:

> All health care professionals are wounded healers. They cannot escape suffering themselves. Moments of pain, loneliness, fatigue, and sacrifice are intrinsic to the human condition. The physician or nurse's own bleeding can become the source of the compassion in the healer's art . . . The physician's or nurse's wounds can become resources for healing.

Wounded healers must not, however, become so overwhelmed with the suffering of others that they are unable to offer effective care. As Sulmasy (1997, p. 48) has observed: 'Competence remains the first act of compassion'.

If the caregiver has the impression that weakness, illness, and wounds belong only to the patient, and that the caregiver is secure against them, Guggenbühl-Craig (1971, p. 92) has observed that:

> . . . the poor creatures known as patients live in a world completely different from [the caregiver's] own. He develops into a physician without wounds and can no longer constellate the healing factor in his patients.

However, much as the patient has a physician (or nurse) within himself or herself, so too does the caregiver have a patient inside himself or herself.

The healing experience

During the twentieth century, the relativity and variability of Quantum mechanics significantly modified the certainties and rigidities of classical Newtonian physics. Kearney (2000) has used the concepts of this 'new physics' to describe an integration between the traditional 'medical model' and a new 'healing model'. Such a healing model can be applied in palliative care through its relevance to the relationship between the caregiver and the patient. As Kearney (2000, p. 24) expressed it:

> The quantum idea that ours is a participatory universe has implications for carers. Although there are still subjects and objects within the healing model, the boundaries may not be as clear as they were within the medical model. Caring now becomes a dynamic event. While the roles of 'carer' and 'patient' remain, there is also an interweaving of the two. The term 'clinical objectivity' is joined by that of 'clinical subjectivity', acknowledging a shared dimension to the healing encounter.

Sources of suffering in the work environment

Constant exposure to death and dying

Not unexpectedly, the most problematic source of stress reported by hospice nurses and nursing is 'death and dying' (Payne 2001). Coming to terms with dying is the main concern of nurses working in acute care, hospice, and community settings (Copp & Dunn 1993). There can also be difficulties when people do not want to die in the way that nurses feel they 'should' die (Hart et al. 1998). The difficulties associated with the care of dying persons are also due, in part, to the close connections that palliative-care nurses often develop with their patients.

> 'Coming to terms with dying is the main concern of nurses working in acute care, hospice, and community settings.'

Barnard et al. (2000, p. 5) have noted that:

> . . . palliative care is whole-person care, not only in the sense that the whole person of the patient (body, mind, spirit) is the object of care, but also in that the whole person of the caregiver is involved. Palliative care is, *par excellence*, care that is given through the medium of a human relationship.

They have also noted that education for palliative care involves the art of building and sustaining relationships and in using the self as a primary instrument for diagnosis and treatment. This involves a degree of psychological risk-taking that is distinctive in the health field.

Barnard (1995, p. 26) has also spoken of the need to give full weight to both the promise and the fear of intimacy in palliative care:

> We live in the tension between the promise of intimacy and the fear of our own undoing. Surprised by intimacy, we are exhilarated and lifted beyond ourselves, as if we have not only made contact with another person but also with another dimension of living. At the same time we are brought face to face with forces of chaos and destructiveness, internal as well as external, and we fear that we ourselves shall be destroyed.

Boston, Towers and Barnard (2000) have noted that dying persons experience the disruption of the essence of day-to-day living, and that their perception of who they are is challenged. Through this process they can gain new wisdom and the sense of meaning in their lives can be reshaped. A different way of knowing the world can evolve, characterised by an inner know-how and tacit knowledge that defines such persons in relationship with others. Caregivers and others around them 'are perceived to be in another place, or don't seem to be there at all' (Boston, Towers & Barnard 2001, p. 248). Patients and caregivers can feel that they just don't 'connect'. These authors speak of palliative care taking caregivers into emotional realms that are neither easy nor comfortable. The caregiver can be permanently changed through such an encounter.

Kearney and Mount (2000) have observed that dealing with the dying person, particularly those in spiritual pain, requires 'active listening'—that is, deliberately and consciously 'tuning in' to that patient's unique wavelength, and attending to both the factual content and the feeling content of what is being communicated. This closeness, however, demands that the caregiver risks being open to developing intimacy with the dying person, and this potentially involves a cost to the caregiver, as it requires going beyond the traditional biomedical caregiver–patient relationship.

Identification with a suffering individual

Identification with a particular person who reminds the caregiver of someone from his or her own life can present particular challenges involving issues of transference and countertransference. For example, a palliative-care nurse might have lost her mother as a result of breast cancer, and might wonder if she is genetically predisposed to the disease. Such a nurse can have difficulty when dealing with a woman who reminds her of her mother and her own vulnerability. In addition, caregivers who have, themselves, experienced cancer, can find it difficult to care for others with the same diagnosis, wondering if their fate will one day be the same.

Feelings of inadequacy or helplessness

Nurses can feel inadequate and helpless in situations in which they feel responsible for alleviating the pain of a palliative-care patient, but do not have a physician willing to order medication sufficient to control pain. In addition, with the current trend towards earlier discharge of sicker patients, nurses with limited experience can be expected to care for seriously ill palliative-care patients in the patients' homes, without access to physicians skilled in effective palliative care and symptom management (Coyle 1997).

'Nurses can feel inadequate and helpless in situations in which they feel responsible for alleviating the pain of a palliative-care patient.'

Nurses in intensive care units in the United Kingdom were asked about the stress of decision-making in the context of the cessation of active therapeutic treatment and a switch to a palliative approach (Schneider 1997). They were asked to identify the best and worst aspects of the situations. The worst aspects involved feelings of loss and helplessness because the nurses often had a close empathic relationship with the patient and family, and had difficulty witnessing their pain and suffering. Nurses also experienced feelings of failure after days of intensive treatment.

Feelings of lack of control and failure

Nurses can have trouble with an unexpected turn of events when those they are caring for are expected to get well, but suddenly take a turn for the worse. They can find it difficult not to be able to organise and control events related to the withdrawal of active support and the move to measures of comfort. They want to be able to give the family time to come to terms with the change of plans but, at the same time, they do not want to prolong suffering unnecessarily. They can experience difficulty when they cannot predict the timing of death—particularly if the patient dies during the temporary absence of family members (Schneider 1997).

In an Australian study by Hart et al. (1998), a sense of professional inadequacy and powerlessness marked many of the incidents identified by palliative-care nurses. The nurses had high expectations of their own performance and did not always take into account the organisational and professional constraints on their practice. Much energy was expended in maintaining harmony within family groups, and the organisation and conflict was often 'viewed negatively and avoided rather than welcomed as a creative force for personal growth and organizational change' (Hart et al. 1998, p. 253).

Palliative-care practitioners have traditionally prided themselves on having time to spend with those in their care and the families of those in their care. However, as financial constraints have become increasingly tight, hospice staff, like professionals in many other specialties, are finding themselves more and more stretched to provide the type of care they want to provide (Vachon 2001).

Multiple loss and grief

The concept of 'multiple loss' was recognised with the sudden increase in the number of AIDS sufferers in the late twentieth century. Many caregivers were caring for dying patients while, at the same time, partners, friends, and acquaintances were also dying (Vachon 2001).

Caregivers in palliative care can be caring for many people who die within a short time of each another. This grief can accumulate over the years leading to significant depression (Vachon 1987, 2001). Multiple losses can result in chronic grief because there is no time to finish grieving for one loss before another one occurs (Cho & Cassidy 1994).The sense of loss can extend beyond the deaths of patients. Papadatou (2000) has characterised the losses as:

▶ loss of a close relationship with a particular patient;
▶ loss due to the professional's identification with the pain of family members;
▶ loss of one's unmet goals and expectations;
▶ losses related to one's personal system of beliefs and assumptions about life;
▶ past unresolved losses or anticipated future losses; and
▶ the death of self.

Constant exposure to death and loss can leave caregivers with grief overload and considerable distress.

Team issues

Team issues as a source of stress have been documented in numerous studies (Vachon 1987, 1995; Graham et al. 1996; Florio, Donnelly & Zevon 1998; van Staa, Visser & van der Zouwe 2000). A lack of support from team members has been implicated in significant levels of depression (Bené & Foxall 1991), and conflict with staff has contributed to emotional exhaustion and de-personalisation on the subscales of the Maslach Burnout Inventory (Maslach & Jackson 1986).

Rivalry and anger often surface in hospice team relationships. Many palliative-care teams have difficulty dealing with anger directly, and can use a variety of obstructive behaviours. These might include careerism and rivalry in which there is a concentration on personal achievement and advancement. Some team members' competitive instincts and energies thus become channelled into rivalry among colleagues rather than into teamwork and effective patient care (Heming 1988; Vachon 1996).

Coping

Teamwork

Kearney (2000) has agreed with the chaplain and psychotherapist Peter Speck (1996) in stressing that the ability to 'contain' powerful reactions and strong emotions is an essential part of all caring relationships. As Kearney (2000, p. 88) has observed:

The most significant factor in creating containment for the person in suffering is the web of caring relationships that establish security and trust with that person. However, the containment that is created by inter-professional teamwork does not simply come about because a number of different disciplines happen to be involved in that patient's care and treatment. The container has to be built, a process which involves deliberate and conscious effort.

Each discipline involved in the person's care must have a clear sense of its own professional identity, including its profession's strengths and limitations. There must also be an acknowledgment of, and respect for, the contribution that other professions have to offer. As Kearney (2000, p. 88) has noted:

> There must also be an awareness of shared areas of care, where close communication and cooperation are essential to avoid duplication of effort, interdisciplinary territorialism, and confusion or 'flooding' of the patient . . . The process of team self-awareness comes through individual disciplines meeting together and with regular interdisciplinary team meetings . . . Such competence helps to create trust with patients, to lessen their sense of fear, and to increase their sense of security.

Kearney (2000) has suggested that the presence of an outside facilitator, experienced in team management and psychodynamics, can be valuable in the early stages of team-building, as well as when dealing with difficult issues arising from the care of a particular patient.

Personal

To participate in the healing of others, the caregiver must be aware of his or her own needs and must pay serious attention to self-care and reflection. The box on page 50 lists a number of lifestyle management techniques that are helpful for continuing to work in stressful situations.

Cumes (1999) has noted the importance of the caregiver achieving personal balance if more effective healing is to occur. Healers who have been 'wounded' through various life experiences, including negative experiences in education, clinical encounters, and the workplace, need to be able to replenish themselves if they are to bring their healing potential into clinical encounters. This requires some form of inner practice—physical or mental—such as prayer, meditation, imagery, yoga, tai chi, qi gong, or breath work.

Lifestyle management techniques

Here is a list of lifestyle management techniques that are helpful for those working in stressful situations:

- maintain good nutrition;
- practise meditation;
- maintain a spiritual life;
- grieve losses;
- decrease overtime work;
- exercise regularly (aerobics, yoga, qi gong, tai chi);
- undertake regular energy work (reiki, healing touch, therapeutic touch);
- maintain a sense of humour;
- balance work and home lives to allow sufficient time off;
- have a good social support system, personally and professionally;
- recognise and monitor personal symptoms, and seek consultation if symptoms are severe;
- discuss work-related stresses with others who share the same problems;
- visit counterparts in other institutions; look for new solutions to problems; and
- spend time with nature.

Author's presentation

Conclusion

Remen (2000, p. 205) has observed:

> Compassion begins with the acceptance of what is most human in ourselves, what is most capable of suffering. In attending to our own capacity to suffer, we can uncover a simple and profound connection between our own vulnerability and the vulnerability in all others. Experiencing this allows us to find an instinctive kindness toward life which is the foundation of all compassion and genuine service.

Remen (2000, p. 197) has also noted: 'Basically service is about taking life personally, letting the lives that touch yours touch you'.

This concept recognises the reciprocity that is inherent in the caring relationship. Watson (1989, p. 132), a nurse theoretician, has stated:

> When both care providers and care receiver are co-participants in caring, the release can allow the one who is cared for to be the one who cares, through the reflection of the human condition that in turn nourishes the

humanness of the care provider. In such connectedness they are both capable of transcending self, time and space.

The service of people in a caring relationship is a relationship between equals. When we serve, the work itself keeps us from burnout. Unless we let the patients touch us, we will never last in this work. Protecting ourselves from loss, rather than grieving and healing our losses, is one of the major causes of burnout.

As Remen (1996, p. 52) has observed:

> We burn out not because we don't care but because we don't grieve. We burn out because we have allowed our hearts to become so filled with loss that we have no room left to care.

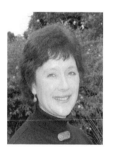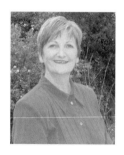

Margaret O'Connor

Dr Margaret O'Connor lectures in cancer and palliative care at La Trobe University, Melbourne (Victoria, Australia), within a unit that is dedicated to academic and clinical studies of cancer and palliative care, in association with a tertiary referral hospital. Margaret's doctoral thesis in nursing explored discourses about care of the dying in residential aged care. Her ethical interests have evolved from the work of her first degree in theology. Margaret is board member of Eastern Palliative Care, a large domiciliary service in Melbourne, and she chairs the Clinical Standards Committee and the Ethics Committee of that organisation.

Sanchia Aranda

Sanchia Aranda is professor and director of cancer nursing research at Peter MacCallum Cancer Institute, Melbourne (Victoria, Australia). She has worked in cancer care since 1979, predominantly in the tertiary sector since 1990. Her research interests include cancer and palliative nursing in both inpatient and community settings, especially in the area of supportive care. Her research, both quantitative and qualitative, concentrates on implementing evidence into clinical practice, especially in improving the delivery of health services and the outcomes for people with cancer and their families. Current studies include workforce planning in breast care, the support needs of women with advanced cancer, symptom interventions in pain and fatigue, prevention of oral mucositis, and care of people suffering bodily decay.

Chapter 5

Ethical Decision-making

Margaret O'Connor and Sanchia Aranda

Introduction

Decision-making at the end of life necessarily occurs within an ethical framework. Dying and death occur in a context of personal values and beliefs about suffering, the meaning of death, and the place of an individual within family and society. Palliative care promotes the importance of comfort and quality of life, and emphasises that the direction of care is determined by the individual concerned. However, the achievement of comfort and quality of life in association with patient-directed care often brings into focus differences in views between patients and prac-

> 'Palliative care promotes the importance of comfort and quality of life, and emphasises that the direction of care is determined by the individual concerned.'

titioners regarding various practices. Questions can arise regarding such matters as the use of morphine, physician-assisted suicide, and terminal sedation.

Although significant advances in clinical care mean that practitioners can now alleviate most physical suffering, their skills are challenged by a small proportion of patients who have intractable symptoms or significant existential distress. Caring for these people requires a sensitive appreciation of the ethical, legal, and moral perspectives of the patient, the family, and the clinical team. This requires an understanding of the context of suffering within which palliative care is often provided.

The ethical context of suffering

The underlying focus of all health care is the sick or dying person, and in palliative care the goal is principally the relief and prevention of suffering. However, understanding the unique and subjective experience of suffering for each individual is always difficult—partly because of the lack of emphasis on suffering in health-care education (Cassell 1991). As Cassell (1991, p. ix) has noted:

> Doctors do not deal with suffering in the abstract, they treat persons who are afflicted by something that leads to the suffering. The separation of the disease that underlies the suffering from both the person and the suffering itself, as though the scientific entity of the disease is more real and more important then the person and the suffering, is one of the strange intellectual paradoxes of our times.

Nurses and other palliative-care practitioners accompany a person to the conclusion of life, motivated by respect for each person's journey to death, and the inherent dignity of each individual at every stage of life. This means that nurses must always view the decisions that are made at the end of life as more than clinical decisions related to the person's disease. Rather, end-of-life decisions must not only take account of the desire to relieve suffering, but also the possibility of inflicting suffering when decisions are made that are not in keeping with each person's life context—including cultural, philosophical, and religious beliefs. All of these beliefs influence the person's understanding of suffering, and taking account of this calls for greater wisdom on the part of nurses and other practitioners than is provided by conventional health-care approaches to ethics.

Ethical studies in palliative care draw substantially on traditional concepts— such as doing good (beneficence) and doing no harm (non-malificence). Although such concepts are useful in thinking globally about ethical issues in palliative care, in practice they offer background guidance rather than pragmatic direction to the clinician.

This chapter introduces a framework for ethical clinical pragmatism in end-of-life care. This framework seeks to understand the specific context of the clinical decision, and enables the care team to consider care options with attention to patient preferences, open discussion, and legal imperatives (O'Connor, Kissane & Spruyt 1999).

Clinical pragmatism

Clinical pragmatism, as a systematic framework, arose from a perception that there was confusion arising from the differing arguments regarding euthanasia and related end-of-life issues. In particular, there was a sense of 'false agreement' on issues when considered from traditional ethical frameworks (Fins & Bacchetta 1995, p. 564). As the term implies, 'clinical pragmatism' arises from the clinical encounter and is concerned with the clinician's understanding of his or her role in relation to the person who is suffering, disabled, or dying. The framework seeks to embed ethical theory in clinical practice and has an overriding concern with *context*. Clinical pragmatism has been described by Fins & Bacchetta (1995, p. 564) as:

> . . . a deliberate process that seeks to deepen our understanding of the clinic, the care of patients, and the role of the practitioner through observation, and professional self-reflection.

In using clinical pragmatism, the nurse or other clinician sets aside particular ethical perspectives and seeks to understand the person at the centre of the decision in the context of that person's situation. This understanding is gained through interactions among all involved such that all perspectives are understood and discussed. These situation-specific interactions drive the decision-making process. Clinical pragmatism thus seeks a dynamic exchange and entails 'a collaborative search for meaning in the face of pain, suffering, and the need to maintain control at the end of life' (Fins & Bacchetta 1995, p. 567). It is very important to understand that the goals of care (and treatment options) frequently alter as the clinical picture unfolds, and that ongoing dialogue is therefore required regarding care decisions, their outcomes, and potential changes in goals and options. Ethical principles, such as 'doing no harm', are a guide to the resolution of clinical

> 'Clinical pragmatism seeks to embed ethical theory in clinical practice and has an overriding concern with *context*.'

dilemmas, but such principles require a closer focus to include an understanding of the effect of clinical decisions on all involved.

To illustrate the concepts of clinical pragmatism, the chapter discusses three important end-of-life issues that are commonly faced by palliative-care nurses, using case studies to illustrate the issues raised. These three issues are:

▶ the use of sedation;
▶ dealing with requests to hasten death; and
▶ working with differing desires for end-of-life care.

The use of sedation
The ethical problem

Discussion of the subject of 'euthanasia' is marked by polemical argument and emotive language. For example, proponents of euthanasia use terms such as 'a good death' or 'mercy killing'—implying a social good in which the end justifies the means. Conversely, terms such as 'destruction of life' or, simply, 'killing', are used by opponents of euthanasia—implying that euthanasia can be equated with other forms of killing, such as murder.

Language can be used in provocative ways to describe the use of sedation at the end of life. The term 'pharmacological oblivion' is an example of this, whereby proponents of euthanasia argue that to fill a dying person with an array of drugs is simply 'slow euthanasia'. They use this argument to advocate a simpler and faster alternative. It is imperative that terms be clearly defined to separate the use of sedation in response to clinical need from the deliberate use of sedation as 'slow euthanasia'. For example, Mount (1996, p. 25) has defined 'slow euthanasia' as the ' . . . clinical practice of treating a terminally ill patient in a fashion that will assuredly lead to a comfortable death, but not too quickly'. However, Mount has argued that unless this process hastens the patient's death, it is inaccurate to describe this as 'euthanasia'.

Sedation is certainly used at the end of life for a small number of people with intractable symptoms and for whom no other relief of suffering is available. In some situations, it is not possible to control refractory symptoms—that is, symptoms that cannot 'adequately be controlled despite aggressive efforts to identify a tolerable therapy that [does] not compromise consciousness' (Cherney & Portenoy 1998). In the face of such refractory symptoms, a negotiated and stepped approach is undertaken using moderate doses of tranquillising medication to assist in stabilisation. In such cases, sedation is used as a last resort. The term 'pharmacological oblivion' is sometimes used to describe such sedation, but the term is often used pejoratively, implying 'deep sleep therapy' or coma

(Syme 1999). Cherney and Portenoy (1998) have argued that the use of sedation for intractable symptoms is undertaken on the same basis as any other clinical practice—whereby the goal is relief of suffering, rather than the death of the person. Sedation can be offered on a trial basis to people with intractable symptoms who have exhausted all other options. After several hours the person's sedation is lightened to allow a discussion on the effectiveness of the treatment and an informed decision on whether to continue for a further trial period. Clinical pragmatism can thus be used to make difficult clinical decisions in the context of unrelieved suffering.

Case study

Janine

Janine had struggled with the diagnosis and treatment of aggressive breast cancer for six years. The 36-year-old mother of two young children was determined to avail herself of all available life-prolonging treatments. Episodes of recurrence required surgery, chemotherapy, and radiotherapy, but Janine retained a busy life and was involved with her children's school and community activities.

Eventually, a large ulcerating tumour developed over her chest and upper neck, creating a malodorous wound, dangerously close to major vessels. The palliative-care service visited twice daily for dressings and other care requirements. Janine's pain was well controlled with continuous subcutaneous analgesia.

Nursing staff had difficulty dealing with Janine's degree of disfigurement and her increasing dependence, and were also involved in supporting her children and husband. Counsellors organised regular debriefing and support sessions for the palliative-care team and the family.

Janine treasured time with her family and, although she was increasingly dependent, she valued her time in the family home. Although she not want to die, Janine understood that her increasing frailty indicated that her life was drawing to a close. She openly grieved the reality of not seeing her children reach adulthood.

Over time, the wound became deeper and extended further up her neck, and nurses expressed their concern that a major blood vessel might be eroded. Sensitive discussion with Janine confirmed that she was aware that this was how she might die, but she was determined to remain at home to die. Fortunately, Janine lived not far from some of the home-care nurses, so they were consoled that if a bleed occurred during the night, they would be within easy reach. Detailed discussions were held among members of the care team, with a view to assisting Janine and her family to prepare for such a death. Anticipating the likelihood of a massive haemorrhage and the distress that this would produce for Jane and her family, Janine agreed to receive

(Continued)

(Continued)

an injection of a tranquilliser if this occurred. A subcutaneous butterfly needle was inserted, the family was instructed on its use, and a dose of midazolam was left drawn up in the refrigerator. Janine's husband agreed that, if Janine bled, he would administer this under instruction.

Late one afternoon Janine's husband rang to say that there was an unusual amount of blood on the dressings and that Janine was not responding. He was immediately instructed to administer the midazolam. The nurse arrived to find Janine experiencing a catastrophic bleed and decided that she was dying. Green towels and drapes were used to minimise the visual impact of the haemorrhage, and Janine's husband and family gathered around her bedside as she died peacefully.

Discussion of the case study

The story of Janine (see Box, pages 57 and 58) explores the use of sedation when the terminal event is a potentially distressing, catastrophic haemorrhage. The dilemma in this situation is whether midazolam should be given to sedate Jane when this might be seen as hastening her death. By discussing the decision in the overall context, the clinical team understood that Janine's death was due to major haemorrhage resulting from the progression of her cancer. This haemorrhage was not preventable, and no attempt to stop the haemorrhage was likely to be successful. Indeed, it might have prolonged Janine's death and caused significantly more suffering. Although it is not certain that the sedation hastened Janine's death, it is clear that it eliminated the panic and distress that was likely to be associated with catastrophic haemorrhage, and that it contributed to Janine's peaceful death.

The important elements of this case are that Janine and her family were involved in all decisions about her care as her clinical condition changed. The clinical team used its knowledge of the likely nature of Janine's death to prepare in advance for decisions that would otherwise be more difficult to make at the time of a critical event. All parties agreed with the plan of action, including the use of sedation in the event of a catastrophic bleed, and this minimised the risk of distress associated with different ethical perspectives.

Principles from the case study

Janine's story suggests some basic principles for the use of sedation at the end of life. These are:

▶ a thorough assessment of the clinical situation should be undertaken;
▶ the findings of this assessment should be discussed openly and frankly;
▶ a clear goal of care should be identified;

- a time period for review of sedation usage should be established at the outset;
- novice practitioners involved in the use of sedation at the end of life require ongoing support and mentoring; and
- sedation use in emergency situations can often be predicted and some planning undertaken in advance.
  These are discussed below.

Thorough assessment of the clinical situation

A thorough assessment of the clinical situation should be undertaken by the health-care team, taking into account solutions that have been previously attempted, and the effect that they have had. Alternative treatments should be discussed, as well as the views of the person and his or her family, and the likely effects and side-effects of the sedation. It is important to clarify whether the presenting symptoms are really refractory, or merely difficult. Expertise in complex symptom management should be readily available, and nurses should be willing to seek guidance when confronted with situations that test the limits of their knowledge.

Findings of assessment discussed openly and frankly

The findings of the assessment should be discussed openly and frankly within the health-care team, and with the person and his or her family, and a decision should be reached regarding the use of sedation. If there is disagreement, the involvement of someone external to the situation, such as a person skilled in clinical ethics, might assist in resolving differences.

A clear goal identified

A clear goal of care should be identified against which the effect of the sedation can be assessed, and from which a decision to continue or withdraw the sedation can be made. The goal of care should be articulated in terms of quality of life, relief of suffering, and the promotion of comfort and personal dignity.

A time period for review established

A time period for review of sedation usage should be established at the outset and review should occur on a frequent and agreed basis. The clinical situation can change if symptoms reach a plateau after a period of relief. The findings of the review should be shared with the person (if possible) and his or her family, and their ongoing reaction to the use of sedation should be monitored.

Novice practitioners ongoing support and mentoring

Novice practitioners involved in the use of sedation at the end of life require ongoing support and mentoring through these difficult clinical situations. This might include discussion of intent and the principle of 'double effect' (see below).

Sedation use in emergency situations predicted and planned

The use of sedation in emergency situations, such as a catastrophic haemorrhage, can often be predicted, and some planning can be undertaken in advance. If this is possible, documentation of discussions and decisions is essential to ensure best management at the time of the emergency situation.

The principle of 'double effect'

A critical issue raised by Janine's clinical management is that of intention and the principle of 'double effect'. Intention refers to what was in the clinician's mind at the time of the decision (in this case, to use sedation) and whether the intention included the death of the person. The principle of 'double effect' refers to the idea that a clinician might use a treatment with one intention (in this case, relief of anxiety) but, in so doing, might legitimately cause another effect (in this case, hastening death). In honouring the right of the person to have relief from unbearable symptoms, the clinician might calculate that there is a risk of unintended death. This is described as 'double effect'.

In practice, it is almost impossible to determine intention precisely or to ascribe consequences fully to particular actions. Whether the sedation hastened Janine's death is uncertain. Ongoing discussion with those concerned is important to ensure that decisions are made openly, honestly, and in accordance with agreed goals of care. Such discussion allows the principle of 'double effect' to be openly canvassed, and offers clinicians a framework for rational decision-making, rather than being in fear that the hastening of death—albeit unprovable and without intent—will result in litigation against them. In Janine's story, a central feature was open conversation with Janine and her family, thus ensuring that the use of sedation was understood and agreed.

'In practice, it is almost impossible to determine intention precisely or to ascribe consequences fully to particular actions.'

The issue of intention and the principle of 'double effect' are commonly used in reference to debates about euthanasia. In his submission to the Australian

Senate on the Euthanasia Laws Bill, Dr Michael Ashby noted a distinction between euthanasia and the cessation of futile treatment. In making this distinction, he referred to the use of 'strong intuitive moral and clinical distinctions' (Senate 1996, p. 64). These comments are indicative of confidence in the clinical encounter, and the use of this context to decide upon actions that are right for the particular situation. Ashby went on to say (Senate 1997, p. 64):

> . . . whilst a doctor's intention may not always be easy to validate, evaluation of intention and motive are fundamental to legal analysis, and many would argue that intention is also determinative of the moral character of medical interventions.

The clinical application of intention that underlies 'double effect' can be tested thus: that if the person wakes after the administration of sedation and the symptom has been stabilised, there is no indication to continue sedation. If the intention is for the person to die, sedation would be sustained without respite. The Council on Ethical and Judicial Affairs of the American Medical Association has claimed (AMA 1992, p. 2229):

> The ethical distinction between providing palliative care that may have fatal side effects and providing euthanasia is subtle, because in both cases the action that causes death is performed for the purpose of relieving suffering. The intent of the former is to relieve suffering despite the fatal side effects, whilst the intent of the latter is to cause death as a means by which relief of suffering is achieved.

Requests to hasten death
The ethical problem

Perhaps the most common dilemma facing nurses who care for those who are dying relates to requests to hasten death. Debates about euthanasia in the media commonly portray euthanasia and palliative care as representing opposing views about the end of life. In fact, the clinical goal of a 'good death' is common to both. Although it is important that nurses be familiar with the public debate about euthanasia, nurses also require advice on how to deal with the requests that they receive from people for assistance to die. Nurses also need to ensure that their own viewpoint is represented.

Nurses are commonly involved in conversations about care and treatment options with patients and their families, and are often required to care for people whose views differ from their own. Nurses must be able to respond in ways that are respectful of patients and families, while remaining true to their own moral and legal position.

Case study

Mary

Mary, aged 80, had recently been diagnosed with lung cancer and brain metastases. Her assessment on admission to the community palliative-care program was undertaken by Karen, a nurse who worked as a member of the team.

Mary began the conversation by stating her wish to end her life as soon as possible and she asked Karen if the palliative-care service could arrange this. Mary was apparently surprised to learn that euthanasia was illegal, and could not be performed by the palliative-care team.

Karen spent considerable time with Mary discussing her outlook on life and the options she faced. Mary did not appear depressed and was resolute in wanting to know more about euthanasia as an option. Because Mary was almost blind, Karen complied with her request for assistance in finding the telephone number of the Voluntary Euthanasia Society to support her desire to gain more information. Karen then left, having negotiated a formal agreement for the involvement of the community palliative-care service to provide comfort for Mary. They also agreed to meet again in the following week. Mary's parting words were: 'If I am still here'.

In discussion with her colleagues, Karen reflected on the issues raised by her interaction with Mary, and on her response to them. She rang Mary's local doctor to talk about her situation. According to the doctor, Mary had been a positive person. However, since separating from her husband, she had struggled with depression as well as her other health problems.

On her next visit Karen learnt that Mary had indeed contacted the Voluntary Euthanasia Society. The society had been of little practical assistance, given that euthanasia was illegal. They offered no other advice or support, leading Mary to the conclusion that the society had little interest in, or understanding of, the care needs that she was experiencing. Mary had spoken to her local doctor and he had reassured her that she would experience slow deterioration, become increasingly sleepy, and eventually go into a coma and die. Karen was able to reinforce this information.

After further discussion, Mary told Karen there were worse ways to die and that at least this did not suggest that she was in danger of losing control of her mind. Mary decided not to pursue euthanasia and accepted the support of the palliative-care service.

Discussion of the case study

The case of Mary provides a clinical example of a palliative-care nurse caring for a person seeking assistance to hasten her death. Karen, despite her own beliefs against euthanasia, was able to support Mary's desire for information. By establishing a relationship with Mary, Karen became privy to Mary's desires and, without compromising her own position, was able to offer assistance, even to the point of finding the telephone number of the Voluntary Euthanasia Society.

The trusting relationship that developed provided a context in which Karen was able to provide ongoing support and symptom management without the difference in their views creating a barrier to care. The involvement of the palliative-care team did not exclude the ongoing involvement of Mary's trusted family doctor and, together, they were able to help Mary feel less desperate about her situation and able to continue living her life.

With support from her colleagues, Karen respected Mary's stance and sought an understanding of her story. Karen's goal was to alleviate Mary's symptoms and to understand her suffering, and this required a balancing of different ethical views. Because Karen recognised that their differences in beliefs did not present a barrier to the provision of ongoing support, successful negotiation of palliative care was achieved.

Principles from the case study

Open discussion about requests to die can help to ensure that such requests are taken seriously, respected, and responded to in ways that do not compromise the legal or moral position of nurses and other health practitioners. Because of the intimate relationship that nurses have with those in their care, they are often in a position to assess the vulnerabilities of people at the end of life and to identify cues that indicate a desire to die. They are well placed to note signs and symptoms that indicate depression or feelings of demoralisation, and can offer support and intervention.

Nurses often identify when a person is feeling burdened by treatment or its side-effects, and can initiate open discussions about patients' concerns and feelings, and their right to refuse treatment. Conversely, nurses also have an important advocacy role in protecting the vulnerable from pressure to request or receive euthanasia.

> 'Nurses have an important advocacy role in protecting the vulnerable from pressure to request or receive euthanasia.'

Symptom management

Although unrelieved symptoms are only one cause of the desire of some people for a hastened death, palliative-care nurses have a responsibility to maintain their expertise in symptom management at the end of life.

Symptoms such as pain can be managed effectively with current available treatment options, and the World Health Organization (WHO 1999) has suggested that cancer pain can be controlled in more than 90% of people. Apart from pain, other commonly experienced symptoms at the end of life include dyspnoea, fatigue, confusion, nausea, cachexia, restlessness, and agitation, as well as symptoms of grief and depression. Although many of these symptoms can be relieved, the degree of suffering is unique to each individual's experience at the end of life's journey. This is the unknown and unknowable aspect of caring for a person in the context of an holistic framework that values his or her psychospiritual being. Ethical management of patients with significant symptoms includes frameworks for assessment and documentation of symptoms so that progress and the effectiveness of interventions can be critically evaluated.

Differing desires for end-of-life care
The ethical problem
One of the commonest clinical dilemmas confronted by nurses is a situation in which the patient and his or her family have different desires regarding end-of-life care. These disparate views can complicate the situation and can create clinical difficulties in balancing the competing needs and wishes. The work of the nurse in such situations is often difficult and draining, but careful communication and negotiation of care can result in successful outcomes.

Case study

Frederick

Frederick, a 64-year-old retired general practitioner, had been diagnosed with cancer of the prostate, and had initially been treated with surgery. The diagnosis came as a shock to this positive, outgoing man—especially as it came so soon after a long-anticipated retirement. About two years later, Frederick was found to have bony metastases, and was treated with palliative radiotherapy.

Because he valued his independence and retained his sense of adventure, Frederick set about doing all the things he had planned for his retirement—even though it now appeared that this retirement was to be relatively shorter than anticipated. On a trip overseas with his wife, Frederick began to notice increasing pain in his back, and altered sensation in his left leg. A hasty return to home led to a diagnosis of impending cord compression due to spinal secondaries. Further radiotherapy was advised. Frederick

(Continued)

(*Continued*)

went home from hospital knowing that his prognosis was poor. He refused further treatment.

Frederick contacted an old friend, Dr N, a well-known euthanasia campaigner, and discussed plans for his death, including access to the necessary drugs.

'I don't want to die as a cripple in a bed', Frederick said. 'I want an "out" if this all gets too much.'

Frederick's wife, Amelia, a retired nurse, was a feisty advocate for her husband's care. She gained the support of their two children in disagreeing strongly with his dismal evaluation of his life and insisting that all treatment should be accepted.

The palliative-care nurses knew of Frederick's plans, and the family differences. With each passing day they noted Frederick's progression towards lower-limb paralysis. On each visit to his home, the nurses listened to the different opinions, and tried to facilitate open conversation.

Frederick did progress to complete cord compression, necessitating almost complete bed rest. But Amelia, determined to keep him at home, organised specialist equipment (such as a hospital bed) and arranged for Frederick to be in the lounge room—a well-lit, airy room with doors that opened onto an attractive back garden. In some ways, Frederick appeared to enjoy controlling his life from the confines of his bed, being in the centre of the house, and having his telephone, fax, and computer within easy reach.

Frederick eventually developed a bowel obstruction, and this required admission to the local hospice. Discussions with Frederick and his family about treatments such as nasogastric and intravenous therapy centred around Frederick's continuing wish for no further treatment. He was therefore treated palliatively, although Amelia and the children still objected strongly. A family conference was convened, and this concluded with agreement that the goal of care was comfort. Dr N continued to visit and observe all that was happening to his friend.

A week after admission to the hospice, Frederick lapsed into unconsciousness and died—with the family still wondering if something could have been done. However, their concerns were somewhat tempered by the consolation of being present at his peaceful death.

Discussion of the case study

The case of Frederick presents the difficulties involved in the care of a man whose desire to abandon treatment was inconsistent with his family's desire to have him live as long as possible.

By facilitating opportunities for all involved to discuss these different perspectives—formally and informally, individually and collectively—an agreed goal of care was reached. This case shows that it is possible to respect a patient's autonomy (in this case, Frederick's plan for euthanasia), while working with the patient and family to create care outcomes that negated the need for this plan. The nurses worked alongside Frederick and his family—effectively 'holding' his plan and not denying the depth of his need for control, while still recognising the family's desire for him to live. This was achieved in a context of mutual respect that facilitated discussion of the difficulties involved for everyone.

Clinical pragmatism emphasises a collaborative search for a resolution in which all views are respected as circumstances change.

Principles from the case study

Frederick's peaceful death does not deny the complexity of this kind of work with patients and families. However, individual and family meetings are a useful way to identify and clarify the differing perspectives of those involved, and can often reveal common ground—such as ensuring patient comfort. The following are some steps that nurses might find useful when working with patients and families in this way.

- Arrange a meeting of all parties with an agreed facilitator, with or without the patient.
- Facilitate the disclosure of all views so that each individual feels that his or her views are heard and respected. It is sometimes useful to record these views for all to see.
- Facilitate discussion to clarify views and ensure understanding.
- Provide an opportunity for each individual to clarify his or her goal of care for the patient. Perhaps record these also.
- Provide additional information if this is requested or helpful—particularly treatment options, prognostic issues, and so on. The role of food in someone who is close to death is an example of such an issue that might benefit from discussion.
- Identify points of agreement with respect to goals of care.
- Reinforce palliative-care principles in terms of being able to help with distressing symptoms, and a focus on quality of life.
- Summarise the points of agreement and points of remaining disagreement. The facilitator (if present) is the best person to do this.
- Establish a plan of care to meet agreed goals, no matter how general.
- Consider further formal meetings if points of disagreement are significant, and are likely to cause ongoing conflict.

Conclusion

End-of-life decision-making and the related questions of the active ending of life are complex and important. These difficult problems require nurses and other team members to pause and consider their response.

Clinical pragmatism offers a useful ethical framework for clinical care because it allows for a full consideration of the individual and his or her unique context when assessing the need for intervention and the type of intervention that is appropriate. The journey towards death takes place in a socio-cultural context that includes the care needs of the individual and his or her family. If the palliative-care goals of comfort, dignity, and quality of life are to be met, nurses need a workable ethical framework in which the team can work towards its goals.

'Clinical pragmatism offers a useful ethical framework for clinical care because it allows for a full consideration of the individual and his or her unique context when assessing the need for intervention.'

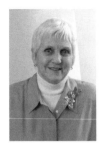 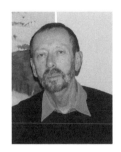

Rosalie Hudson

Dr Rosalie Hudson's varied nursing and theological career is now focused on aged care and palliative care. As an aged-care consultant her aim is to explore end-of-life issues for people in residential aged care, and to raise the profile of gerontic nursing both in Australia and internationally. Her PhD thesis covered the themes of personhood, death, and community, exploring the transforming power of relationships observed during her twelve years of experience as a director of nursing of a 50-bed nursing home. She has published articles in nursing and theological journals on subjects of spirituality, palliative care, and pastoral care. She has co-authored two books on death and dying, is lead author for *Clinical Approaches to Dementia* (Ausmed Publications, 2003), and has contributed chapters to several other Ausmed publications. Rosalie is the Victorian project manager for the Australian Palliative Aged Care Project, which is developing guidelines for palliative care in residential aged care.

Bruce Rumbold

Dr Bruce Rumbold is a senior lecturer in the Palliative Care Unit at La Trobe University, Melbourne (Victoria, Australia). He holds postgraduate qualifications in physics, pastoral care, and health social science, and has published in all three fields. His longstanding interest in palliative care began with doctoral work in England in the mid 1970s, and has continued as palliative care has developed in Australia and elsewhere. Spiritual care is a particular focus of his work. He is author of *Helplessness and Hope: pastoral care in terminal illness*, SCM Press, 1986, and editor of *Spirituality and Palliative Care: social and pastoral perspectives*, OUP, 2002.

Chapter 6
Spiritual Care

Rosalie Hudson and Bruce Rumbold

What is spiritual care?

Sacred moments occur in the midst of the ordinary, and that which might be considered deeply spiritual to one person might be no more than social to another. The notion of 'sacred' is thus profoundly personal.

According to Kaufmann (1970, p. 134), the notion of the sacred occurs in what Martin Buber has described as the 'I–thou' relationship of one person's listening presence with another. To enter a person's history is to engage at a level beyond the immediate present, or, in Polanyi's (1969) terms, to 'indwell' his or her story. To 'know' someone in these very personal terms involves our accepting a framework from outside our

> ' . . . the 'I–thou' relationship of one person's listening presence with another.'

rational, positivist world, and our entering unknown territory where facts are not immediately observable.

This chapter is jointly written by two people with complementary views—a nurse with pastoral care interests, and a pastor with an interest in nursing. Sometimes differences in perspective will show through, but the combined perspective offers useful practical guidance on the nature of spiritual care at the end of life.

Sacred moments in the midst of the ordinary

The story of Ben and Alice (see Box, below) is an illustration of how sacred moments occur in the midst of the ordinary.

Ben and Alice

In the nursing home Ben suddenly became breathless and complained of chest pain. In distress, he told his trusted charge nurse: 'Alice, I think this is it!'. Alice summoned another nurse to stay with Ben while she phoned his doctor.

As they discussed the options, the doctor was a little surprised when Alice asked him to 'please hold' while she returned to check with Ben. Ben decided that he did not want to die with ambulance sirens ringing in his ears. As long as he could have the pain relieved, and as long as Alice could '. . . spare a few minutes to sit with me and give me one of your famous back rubs', he didn't want to go to hospital. 'You know me pretty well,' he said to Alice. 'I'd rather stay here than be with strangers.'

Alice called her team together.

'Ben is aware he's dying. He's made the decision not to go to hospital. He doesn't want me to call a priest and he doesn't want the doctor to come. I have a phone order for morphine and Ben has asked me to stay with him. He doesn't want me to phone his wife. He's aware of her painful arthritis and how long it would take her to get ready to come in. They discussed this with each other yesterday in preparation for this scenario. Ben's care is my immediate priority for the next hour or so. I know I can count on you to re-order your priorities in caring for the other residents.'

Alice later confided in a colleague. 'That's the finest nursing I've ever done. And do you know what? I even heard Ben's confession! He didn't want a priest, but he wanted to tell me some things in confidence. We spoke frankly during that last hour. He apologised for being demanding and I asked his forgiveness for the times I'd been abrupt and impatient with him.'

Of course, this story is merely the bare outline of a relationship that has a much longer and richer history than that presented here. It would be easy to find fault with Alice. Some might ask whether it really is best practice to allow a person to decide against hospitalisation in these circumstances. Others might wonder whether other members of the team might resent the extra work thrust upon them: 'It's all very well for Alice to take the time to sit with Ben, but that's why we have a chaplain. What about the work she's leaving us to do short-handed?' Others might mutter: 'Does Ben really know his own mind or is Alice just taking over?'.

In the actual situation on which this scenario is based, these questions, and others like them, had already been resolved. The team members shared an understanding of the principles of palliative care. They knew that those in their care could choose their site of death, and that a staff member or other person would remain with them. It was accepted that carrying an extra nursing load in circumstances like this was part of the job. Through regular case review it had become clear that Alice was Ben's primary caregiver, and that their relationship went beyond the functional relationship of nurse and patient. The team members knew that Ben was adamant about not being 'religious'. He had met the chaplain but had not warmed to her, and he was forthright about what he believed to be the hypocrisy of calling for a minister or priest at the point of death when he had never 'never needed one before'.

Through the relationship that they had developed, Alice knew what was of ultimate importance to Ben as he confronted death. Physically, he feared the pain. Socially and emotionally, he knew what was important in his marriage and other relationships. Psychologically, he knew the back rub was as important as the morphine. And spiritually? Spiritually, he had certain things on his mind that many would call 'spiritual'. He wanted to sum up his life: 'I've not been a bad bloke but I've not been perfect either!'.

These factors correlate neatly with what Cobb (2001, p. 1) has called the 'quadrilateral' of holistic care—physical, psychological, social, and spiritual. But the reality is that such categories overlap with each other, and Alice was able to meet Ben's overlapping needs through her personal presence and her technical knowledge and skill. Ben could not have made his own decisions about his death without a living partnership with his trusted nurse.

> 'The "quadrilateral" of holistic care—physical, psychological, social, and spiritual.'

What Alice offered Ben in his last hours of life was *spiritual* care. In this caring relationship:

- there was genuine human encounter in which mutual benefit was given and received;
- Ben was enabled to reflect upon the meaning and purpose of his life, and was able to review commitments and relationships that were important to him; and

▶ Alice was enabled to undertake a corresponding review of her own personal and professional life.

Ben was given an opportunity to talk about what life had meant to him, and to express some regret about things he might have done differently. Alice did not presume to provide answers or offer false consolation. She entered into the dialogue to reveal some of her own regrets as they related to her care for Ben. As Kemp (2001, p. 408) has observed: 'Note that the goal in spiritual care is not to provide one's own answers to ultimate questions or for the patient to achieve a particular belief'.

It is also important to note that Alice was able to offer care with a spiritual dimension because she practised in a professional setting in which staff members were encouraged to build trusting relationships with those in their care and with each other. The spiritual care that became explicit in Ben's last hours was implicit within the relationship that Alice had formed with Ben over the preceding months. Because of this relationship, she was able to deliver technical nursing care, able to provide emotional and social support, and able to offer spiritual companionship. She led a team in which nurses are encouraged to use all their faculties, including intuition. Such a philosophy recognises that the care offered by one nurse will never be exactly the same as that of another. Members of the team appreciate each other's abilities and are aware of each other's limitations. They practise reflectively—that is, they review what is happening in their caring relationships, and discuss each other's initiatives (as appropriate) in a spirit of exploration, challenge, and support. This residential care facility was able to provide holistic palliative care because its services were both comprehensive and flexible—thus allowing individual members of the team to lead as appropriate.

> 'The goal in spiritual care is not to provide one's own answers to ultimate questions or for the patient to achieve a particular belief.'

The story of Ben and Alice raises further issues for consideration. What training, resources, and self-understanding do nurses need to work with spiritual issues? The team's care provided 'space' in which spiritual issues could emerge, but could the team have been more intentional in offering spiritual care? If so, what would such intentional spiritual care mean in practice, including such matters as documentation and care plans? What aspects (if any) of Ben's 'confession' should be documented? What differences might we have seen if Ben had been a 'religious' person? The rest of this chapter deals with these and related issues.

Religion and spirituality

The complex question of the relationship between the concepts of 'religion' and 'spirituality', and how this can produce difficulties in palliative care, is well illustrated in the story of Janet (see Box, below).

Janet

Janet, a patient in a palliative-care unit, was 35 years of age and was dying from disseminated bone cancer. Janet was unmarried, but was surrounded by numerous friends. She nurtured these relationships and appreciated the presence of her many friends until a few days before her death.

'I've said my goodbyes now,' she told the nurse. 'I don't want any more visitors. The only person I want is John. He knows what's important to me and I know he'll be with me right to the end.'

John was Janet's close friend and parish priest but, unfortunately, when Janet's death was imminent, he was on two days' leave. He had advised the nursing staff that the priest from the next parish would be on call during his absence. 'I've told him about Janet and he will come if needed.'

Janet was barely conscious and the nurses were hoping she would 'wait' until her own priest returned. However, Janet indicated she would like the other priest to be called. Most of the staff knew how important the priest's daily visits were to Janet, including the familiar rituals of daily Holy Communion and reading of the scriptures. John had also developed warm and friendly relationships with many staff members.

When the 'on-call' priest arrived he appeared hesitant and uncertain. The charge nurse directed him to Janet's room, before discreetly leaving. Barely two minutes later, the charge nurse passed the room again and saw the priest standing at the foot of the bed. As she watched, he quickly made for the door.

'I think she's asleep', he said, rather apologetically. 'Anyway, I have a dreadful cold and I didn't want to get too close to her.'

By the time the priest had reached the front door, Janet had died.

The members of the nursing team in the palliative-care unit where this event took place met frequently to reflect on their practice. Not surprisingly, this incident provoked considerable discussion. Responses ranged from: 'It's not our business to tell the clergy what to do' to 'It's our responsibility to ensure that our patients receive proper care from every member of the team'. The team quickly recognised that this episode raised important questions about referral, liaison, and accountability. The following conclusions were reached.

◗ In an ideal situation John would have been with Janet at the time of her death to offer her the pastoral consolation that had been so important to her throughout her life. As it turned out, her dying was far short of this ideal, largely because John's on-call arrangements had proven to be inappropriate.

▸ It is seldom possible to predict the time of death accurately, and it is therefore unrealistic for any carer to 'promise to be there'.

▸ The on-call priest's response was understandable. Many people, including some chaplains, clergy, and pastoral carers, are not comfortable when they see a relatively young person like Janet at the point of death.

▸ It is important to refer specific religious needs to an appropriate religious practitioner. But it is also important to remember that the team's responsibility for spiritual care does not end with such a referral. Nurses should continue to review spiritual-care issues, and should professionally support the contribution of religious-care providers by recognising, complementing, informing, and challenging their role.

▸ The team needs to have strategies in place to deal with similar events should they recur in future, as well as strategies to prevent such events taking place.

After further discussion, the team decided that, in similar circumstances, the following strategy should be implemented.

▸ Before an on-call priest was directed to the patient's room, a nurse would offer a few words of explanation and preparation, including relevant portions of the care plan (which, in Janet's case, had included her clearly articulated request for daily Holy Communion in the last week of her life).

▸ If a visiting priest appeared unsure of the patient's conscious state, or was concerned about other matters (as in Janet's story, about the effect of his presence and his 'dreadful cold'), a perceptive nurse might recognise this as a 'cover' for nervousness, and offer reassurance and some words of practical advice about communicating with the patient.

▸ Each locum priest would receive a follow-up telephone call and an offer of further conversation with a palliative-care nurse.

▸ John, and other regular visiting clergy, would be asked to review their on-call arrangements to ensure that any locum was appropriately skilled and adequately briefed.

▸ Whenever possible, all regular 'non-team' carers, such as John, were to be invited to participate in the preparation of care plans and the review of cases of people with whom they were involved.

The team agreed that this strategy should assist with liaison and referral, and should clarify the accountability of visiting professionals. In essence, they were accountable to the patients through the team.

However, team members recognised the limitations of their proposed strategy. In particular, they recognised that, although they were able to set up contexts in which spiritual care could take place, and although they could initiate and support referrals of patients such as Janet who expressed explicit religious commitments, they had still not identified means by which spiritual care could become an integral part of every patient's care plan.

Intentional spiritual care

The spiritual care of people receiving palliative care can be as 'intentional' as other aspects of the nursing task. Spiritual care for Ben (Box, page 70) was implicit within his care team as a result of the team's commitment to a particular quality of nursing relationship. Spiritual care for Janet (Box, page 73) was carried out, albeit less than adequately as it transpired, through referral to a religious practitioner. Both approaches have their place, but such spiritual care can be made more 'intentional' by adopting approaches that parallel other

> 'The spiritual care of people receiving palliative care can be as "intentional" as other aspects of the nursing task.'

aspects of the professional nursing task—that is, planned methods of assessment that identify and document spiritual needs, leading to strategies that are incorporated into an overall care plan.

Identifying spiritual needs

There is no lack of assessment tools in the academic literature on the subject, and it is easy enough to add a spiritual assessment schedule to existing admission procedures, although this would lengthen an already lengthy process. However, despite the plethora of such assessment tools, it should be noted that there are few comparative evaluations of these tools in the literature (CICD 2001), and it is by no means clear that the adoption of such assessments would achieve the desired objectives.

Problems with assessment tools

As suggested above, assessment tools in spiritual care are not without their problems. Palliative-care nurses should carefully consider the following issues before adopting such tools as part of their practice of care.

First, most tools seem to share an ideal of making an *objective* assessment of spiritual needs. But, as palliative-care nurses are well aware, it is the *quality of relationship*, not *objectivity* that is of paramount importance. Such quality of relationship brings an appreciation of people's *possibilities*, as well as their *problems*.

Secondly, assessment tools tend to assess people in terms of abstract qualities, rather than practical considerations. For example, Johnston Taylor (2001, p. 397) has defined spiritual needs as 'transcendence, interconnectedness, and meaning'. Johnston Taylor differentiated these concepts from religion, which she defined as 'the organized, codified, and often institutionalized beliefs and practices that express one's spirituality'. Furthermore, she included in her assessment criteria '. . . the need for purpose and meaning, forgiveness, love and relatedness, hope, creativity, religious faith and its expression'. In her list of patients' spiritual needs that need be identified, Johnston Taylor included 'fear of death or abandonment . . . unresolved past experiences, and the need for reconciliation, comfort, or peace'. Although Johnston Taylor did recognise the importance of personal relationship by including such positive elements as 'joy about sensing closeness to others . . . activities that allow expression of creative impulse', it must be said that many of her concepts and criteria are somewhat nebulous, and nurses might understandably wonder how such assessments can be translated into the everyday practicalities of nursing care.

Thirdly, the incorporation of spiritual assessment into a process of clinical assessment runs the risk of using clinically derived authority to expose patients' personal lives in ways that can be intrusive.

Fourthly, it must be acknowledged that staff members who are called upon to carry out such spiritual assessments might not have the skills to deal with the issues they provoke.

Finally, the association of strategies for spiritual care with other forms of problem-solving runs the risk that staff will feel obliged to *deliver*, rather than *offer*, such spiritual care.

Overcoming the problems with assessment tools

The theme behind the concerns noted above is the possible abuse of power that can occur when practitioners with expertise in one area of care expand their interest to include another, such as spiritual care. It needs to be reiterated that spiritual care takes place in mutual human encounters.

To overcome the problems inherent in tools of spiritual assessment, the following should be considered in the implementation of any program of intentional spiritual care.

▶ Spiritual assessment tools should be regarded with caution. It is important that dialogue is not replaced by the ticking of boxes and that spiritual matters are not reduced to a 'once-only' exercise.

▶ The focus should therefore be on *process*. As McSherry (2001, p. 112) has observed: 'Perhaps the term "assess*ing*" would be more appropriate in the context of spirituality, indicating a need for continual surveillance and vigilance by all health care professionals'.

▶ Spiritual assessment tools should be used as a means for opening-up conversation, raising the consciousness of patients, families, and staff, and indicating that spiritual issues are legitimate topics of conversation in this place. That is, the fact or the *intent*, more than the *content*, of spiritual assessment is what matters most.

Documenting spiritual care

There are ways of documenting spiritual needs and developing strategies to address them that preserve the primacy of mutual relationships in spiritual care. Such approaches are more process-oriented and less prescriptive than the objective assessment approaches discussed above. This might not appeal to practitioners who desire a standardised procedure to implement. However, although not rejecting procedure as such, the strict letter of a standard procedure can eliminate the spirit of care.

When the notes of Ben's case (Box, page 70) were reviewed after his death, it was apparent that the box for 'religion' was marked 'nil'. Moreover, although there were many pages of comprehensive notes on his care plan, these concentrated on his physical symptoms, and nothing was recorded of the events of the last hour of his life. This absence of any reference to Ben's spiritual needs implies that questions such as the following were not asked (or that the answers had not been documented):

▶ Has your experience of this illness changed your priorities—for example, the places, things, and causes that are important to you?

▶ Has your experience of this illness changed your family relationships and other relationships?

▶ Has this illness changed your sense of 'self'?

▶ Has this illness changed your view of life?

▶ If so, which of these changes are most significant to you?

▶ What is your greatest wish or hope at this stage of your life?

It does not matter if questions are not expressed in these exact words. As already indicated, prescriptive spiritual-care assessment forms can be a mixed blessing. What does matter is that nurses gain some sense of how the person in their care is connected to people and what matters to this person. In particular, it is important to know whether relationships and connections have been broken due to the person's illness and its consequences. Lartey (1997) has suggested that spirituality involves various relationships—with self, others, groups, causes, places, and with 'transcendence', a sense of possibility (or power or relationship) beyond ourselves.

Having gained some sense of these connections and disconnections, nurses should be alert to opportunities to follow them up in the conversations that take place during other nursing care. During these conversations, some questions could focus upon life review:

▶ Would you like to tell me your most cherished memory?
▶ Do you have any serious regrets as you look back on your life?
▶ Do you have any fears or anxieties that you would like to talk about with me, or with our pastoral care worker?
▶ Have you given any thought to what death means for you?
▶ How can we best assist you and your family now and in the future?
  Other questions might enquire more directly about belief:
▶ I noticed that you marked 'nil' for 'religion' on your admission form. Has that always been the case, or have your beliefs changed over your lifetime?
▶ Is it important to you to discuss your beliefs?

Recording the notes of these conversations—with due regard for confidentiality concerning details offered in trust—can assist in making an assessment of a person's spiritual needs, resources, and possibilities. Sometimes these spiritual concerns will become evident through a nurse's conversation with the person. At other times it might be helpful to invite a person with specific skills, such as a qualified pastoral-care worker, to read the notes or talk with the person to look for patterns of thought or behaviour. As in Ben's story (Box, page 70), the fact that the 'religion' box was marked 'nil' did not mean that he was uninterested in spiritual issues.

Strategies for spiritual care

In developing strategies for spiritual care it must be recognised that spiritual issues become apparent through particular situations, particular stories, or particular beliefs. Sometimes people find themselves in situations in which they don't know where to turn, and they need committed personal support as they struggle to find the resources to cope. Sometimes people find themselves unable to make sense of their lives because their beliefs about themselves and their place in the world have been dashed through an illness that seems to have taken over their identity. They need people who can help them contact other parts of their story—other resources within themselves—so that they can create fresh meanings. Sometimes they find that their beliefs are inadequate to explain their changed circumstances. They need support in reviewing and re-evaluating their belief systems.

In looking at possible strategies for spiritual care, nurses therefore need to ask about situations, stories, and systems.

▶ *Situations*: Are there ways in which this situation can be changed to make it more bearable for the person involved? For some people, access to beloved possessions provides a renewed sense of belonging. For others, getting out into the garden for a while might help. For others, it might be access to music (or protection from someone else's music!).

> 'Spiritual issues become apparent through particular situations, particular stories, or particular beliefs.'

▶ *Stories*: Are there resources within this person's life story that might help him or her to see the current situation in fresh ways, or find the strength to live with hope (rather than merely exist)?

▶ *Systems*: Does this person need the support of a skilled person who shares his or her religious or philosophical beliefs? Such a person might assist to interpret the changed circumstances or confirm the patient in his or her commitments.

Implications for the nursing process

The process outlined in the previous sections involves the whole team. Nurses are central in ensuring that the process is followed because, in most contexts, they provide the interface between the person receiving care and the team providing it. The information and insights they gather and record are crucial for the development of a spiritual-care plan. They also play a key role in implementing such a plan, by creating an environment of care in which spiritual themes can emerge, including conversation and other interactions in which they pursue the strategy agreed by the team.

The nursing process usually focuses on objective realities associated with a diagnosis or identified need. But there are more subtle factors at work in spiritual care, which involves a relationship between person and carer that cannot be plotted in a chart, and has no quantifiable outcome. This primary condition of relationship should be supported by attention to related issues, including the following:

- raising consciousness;
- intentional conversation and documentation;
- holistic practice;
- accountability; and
- reflective practice.

Each of these is discussed below.

Raising consciousness

Nurses have an important part to play in maintaining the consciousness of the team regarding the importance of spiritual care. The team's knowledge of the patient, the adequacy of team practice, and the broader issues of accountability are all assisted if the following questions are borne in mind, and raised in reviews:

- Does the team understand enough about this person's life history to provide appropriate care as he or she approaches death?
- Has the team ascertained the most important issues, including cultural issues, for this particular person at this particular time and in this particular place?
- Is the whole team agreed on the goal of care as documented in collaboration with the patient and family?
- Are there any team members who are acting unilaterally in decision-making, rather than carrying out the agreed plan of care?
- Have appropriate referrals been made, or is the patient being offered less than optimal resources from within the team?
- What is inhibiting the best care for this patient and what is maximising that care?
- Are there any areas in which justice and fairness are being denied this person and family?
- Are confidential matters respected, allowing for the requirements of legal documentation?
- How are outside practitioners held accountable to the referring team?
- Are there different criteria for accountability according to the site of care (home, aged-care facility, acute setting, palliative-care unit)?

If the answer to any of these questions is unclear, a 'care review' meeting might be needed to clarify goals, and strategies for achieving them.

Intentional conversation and documentation

Although issues of spirituality can arise spontaneously, comprehensive spiritual assessment requires an intentional conversation aimed at developing a relationship rather than ticking boxes. It involves an appreciation of life narrative rather than a collection of facts in an information sheet. But assessment might consist of fragments over time, rather than a cohesive uninterrupted narrative. The skilled palliative-care nurse ensures the narrative is returned to, or left aside, according to the person's wishes. As Cobb (1998, p. 108) has observed: 'Becoming acquainted with another person's spirituality requires more than a knowledge of facts to be systematically processed'. The two scenarios presented in the Box below illustrate the significance of this distinction.

There is an increasing recognition that spiritual care is too important *not* to be subject to rigorous scrutiny. Not everything that takes place under the banner of palliative care needs to be carried out by professionals. However, as Cobb (2001) has noted, the spiritual dimension of humanity is a sufficiently weighty matter, especially in the face of death, to require considerable care and the utmost caution.

'More than facts to be processed'

As noted in the text, effective spiritual care involves an appreciation of life narrative rather than a collection of facts in an information sheet. Cobb (1998, p. 108) put it this way: 'Becoming acquainted with another person's spirituality requires more than a knowledge of facts to be systematically processed'.

The following two scenarios illustrate the point.

Nurse A following a home visit:

'I've given Mary's husband the spiritual assessment form to fill in. I get all embarrassed when I have to ask those awkward questions. Anyway, I reckon they're private issues and none of our business. Filling in the form will give us the facts we need.'

Nurse B with Mrs Brown, recently admitted to the palliative care unit:

'Mrs Brown, I know you've had a lot of questions asked of you recently. I wonder if you're feeling comfortable enough right now for me to discuss your spiritual assessment form? In palliative care, we believe spiritual issues are just as important as physical, psychological, and social issues. We'll find a private place to talk, and hopefully we'll get to know each other a little better in the process. Let me know if you find any of the questions uncomfortable, or if you become tired. I can always come back later and complete it.'

Comment:

For some practitioners, such as Nurse A, spiritual matters are always subjective, private, and potentially embarrassing. For Nurse A, there is no need to commit such comments to paper.

Nurse B, in contrast, follows a set procedure, but knows that useful information and insights will emerge only through mutual exploration of the issues raised. With a blend of care and caution she sets out to explore the narrative.

It must be recognised that even the very best assessment tool is only a springboard for nurse and patient to explore together the spiritual component in palliative care. For many persons (such as in the cases of Ben and Janet, see Boxes earlier in this chapter), issues arise that are not covered in the documented assessment forms and documented care plans. In the process of reflecting on practice, staff members can identify implications for the nursing process and their own nursing formation, thus demonstrating a relational understanding of spiritual assessment.

Although there are many examples of good documentation showing holistic care (Hudson 1997), this field of spiritual assessment remains ripe for further research (McGrath 2002).

Holistic practice

The hallmark of holistic practice is cooperation. No individual can offer holistic care alone. No single practitioner has a full complement of skills and insights. Holistic care can thus be offered only by a team, and although individual team members can contribute their skills, insights, and personalities to this holistic caring enterprise, holistic care is something in which each of them participates, not something that any one person can control.

'The hallmark of holistic practice is cooperation.'

According to Rumbold (1986), it follows that:

▶ individual practitioners should offer who they are and what they have, while being aware that their individual contributions are not all that this person requires;

▶ a team needs to foster the same sort of internal openness, respect, and mutuality that it hopes to offer its patients; and

▶ having the right answers becomes less important than being present appropriately to the other.

When both the person receiving care and the person offering care are seen as whole persons in relation, there is an invitation for the sharing of life's experiences. In this relationship one person does not exert power over the other; the carer is not merely the 'provider' of a service. When such mutuality exists there are no defined signposts to perfection. Rather, 'there will be ambiguity, humility and uncertainty' (Cobb & Robshaw 1998, pp 4–5).

Although there is always ambiguity and uncertainty, even mystery, in the presence of death, skilled palliative-care nurses have the opportunity to bring to the dying person not only the necessary technical expertise and knowledge, but also their own presence and humanity. Nuland (1994, p. 255) has observed that this is a profound source of hope:

> . . . a restoration of certainty that when the end is near, there will be at least this source of hope—that our last moments will be guided not by the bioengineers but by those who know who we are.

Accountability

To ensure the highest standards of quality care, palliative-care nurses are guided in their management of most areas of symptom control by current standards, contemporary research, and bench-marking. But how is quality ensured in the provision of spiritual care?

'This source of hope—that our last moments will be guided not by the bioengineers, but by those who know who we are.'

Quality assurance requires that proper processes are in place. When a nurse makes an assessment of a dying person's spiritual needs, what processes are in place to ensure that those needs are met? In the management of physical symptoms, such processes are well established. Having assessed the level of pain being suffered by a patient, a competent nurse would provide a timely response by appropriate referral, and would ensure that the documentation is accurate and that the intervention is effective. Is spiritual care given the same attention? Having established, for example, that a patient wishes to explore 'unfinished business' before dying, a professional palliative-care nurse should not neglect to address this need. It should not be assumed that someone else will take responsibility, and nor should a referral be made to another person without following up the outcome.

The presence of appropriate partnerships in the team's provision of spiritual care is an important measure of quality. As indicated in the Standards for Palliative Care Provision (PCA 1999), spiritual care involves not only assessment and strategy within the team but also access to an involved network of referral possibilities in the community. Nurses need to work closely with the team's pastoral-care (or spiritual-care) coordinator to ensure that a full range of options is explored with the patient and the patient's family.

Palliative-care agencies should develop proven standards and processes of spiritual care. However, even if such formal standards of care have not been developed, the issue of knowledge, skills, and training remains paramount for those engaged in spiritual care as part of care of the whole person. A palliative-care nurse would not presume to offer adequate physical symptom control without the necessary expertise. Spiritual care should demand the same rigour.

Reflective practice

Reflective practice extends nurses' capacity to attend to the patient's experience, rather than being preoccupied with their own performance. Reflective practice thus facilitates the offering of expertise flexibly and effectively in the best interests of the patient (Burns & Bulman 2000; Johns & Freshwater 1998). Kellehear (2000, pp 76–7) has suggested that carers can acquire this insight into another's experience by asking themselves certain questions:

- What is it like to die?
- How do I feel about farewells that might be forever, or for a long time?
- How do I react to being seriously ill, to nausea, to pain, and to immobility?
- How do I react to unpredictable threats in life?
- How would I feel in such unfamiliar surroundings? Would I feel confident, hesitant, fearful, or isolated?
- Where do I look for meaning in the face of death, for myself as well as for the patient?
- Am I willing to share my reflections with others?

If nurses identify their own issues, reluctances, fears, and hopes, this helps to sensitise them to the issues that confront the patients with whom they work. Knowledge of how their own awareness shifts, and how their own answers change, should prevent their presuming that they now know the issues confronting their patients and no longer need to enquire of them how life is in the present moment.

In this respect, as in other areas of palliative care, studies of expert practice emphasise the importance of good process and mutual relationship (Fook, Ryan & Hawkins 1997). However, although professional competence is expected of every palliative-care nurse, perfection is not required. A person who is dying might be prepared to forgive a hesitant nurse who fumbles for answers, rather than trusting a super-confident nurse who presumes to know it all. Neuhaus (2000, p. 16) has asked how one can work with death and not be affected by it. He had timely advice for busy, task-centred nurses as they consider their own feelings and those of others in the face of death:

> A measure of reticence and silence is in order. There is time simply to be present to death—whether one's own or that of others—without any felt urgencies about doing something about it or getting over it . . . The worst

thing is not the sorrow or the loss or the heartbreak. Worse is to be encountered by death and not changed by the encounter.

Practice principles

From the above discussion, the following practice principles emerge.

▶ Individual openness and team commitment are essential for holistic palliative care. A necessary precondition for providing spiritual care is an atmosphere of partnership, companionship, and trust.

▶ Spiritual care is not a separate set of interventions to be distinguished from other caring tasks. Rather, spiritual care is implicit in all acts of genuine care for people.

▶ Expertise in spiritual care includes the capacity to see beyond the horizons of a particular discipline, and to respect the roles of others when appropriate.

▶ Spiritual care involves review and affirmation of the patient's current circumstances, beliefs, and relationships. This can occur naturally within the caring relationships offered by the team, or can be facilitated by a process of assessment and intervention by the team.

▶ Spiritual assessment includes identification of the needs to be met by professional carers, and of the resources and possibilities available to the patient.

▶ Assessment requires conversational skills and personal interest to engage with a patient's story, together with discernment to refrain from intruding and assuming the right to hear that story.

▶ Spiritual interventions include changing situations to support connections important to the person, encouraging stories that heal disruptions and nurture connections, and involving others to support the patient's belief systems.

▶ To practise reflectively means to be aware of the spiritual concerns of the carer, as well as those of the patient.

▶ To offer the best in spiritual care it is necessary to be familiar with current literature, resource materials, and training programs.

Conclusion

The quality of relationship is the key to spiritual care. In forming such relationships, nurses are often the primary providers of personal support in response to spiritual crisis. Furthermore, nurses should be intimately involved in a palliative-care team's assessment and development of spiritual-care plans. These contributions require cooperation with patients and with other members of the team, in particular with those with have expertise in spiritual care. Nurses make an indispensable contribution to spiritual care, but they do not own it and direct it. Nor does any other profession. Spiritual care can take place only in active partnership with the patient.

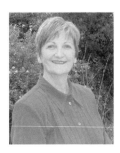

Sanchia Aranda

Sanchia Aranda is professor and director of cancer nursing research at Peter MacCallum Cancer Institute, Melbourne (Victoria, Australia). She has worked in cancer care since 1979, predominantly in the tertiary sector since 1990. Her research interests include cancer and palliative nursing in both inpatient and community settings, especially in the area of supportive care. Her research, both quantitative and qualitative, concentrates on implementing evidence into clinical practice, especially in improving the delivery of health services and the outcomes for people with cancer and their families. Current studies include workforce planning in breast care, the support needs of women with advanced cancer, symptom interventions in pain and fatigue, prevention of oral mucositis, and care of people suffering bodily decay.

Chapter 7

A Framework for Symptom Assessment

Sanchia Aranda

Introduction

Symptom control is a key component of comprehensive palliative care, and is a major emphasis of this book. This chapter aims to provide a generic framework for the assessment and understanding of symptoms in advanced disease. The chapter emphasises an integrated approach, recognising that various symptoms are often related. Unfortunately, most symptoms and their management are studied individually, and understanding of this relationship is therefore currently limited, underscoring the need for further research in this area.

Defining symptoms

The word 'symptom' is derived from the medieval Latin *synthoma* ('happening' or 'mischance'), a term that came into common usage with reference to the symptoms of disease in the 1600s (Rhodes & Watson 1987). In medieval thinking *synthoma* ' . . . was usually used as a "sign" of something evil' (Rhodes & Watson 1987, p. 242). The term 'sign' later came to be understood as that which can be noted by the senses of the observer, whereas a symptom related to changes in function experienced by the unwell person. For example, whereas cyanosis is a *sign* of disease that is visible to the health practitioner, breathlessness is a related *symptom* experience that only the patient can understand. Symptoms indicate to people that something is amiss and that medical aid should be sought. In the context of palliative care, symptoms move beyond 'usefulness' to become, commonly, an ever-present and distressing reminder of advanced disease that has a major negative impact on quality of life and the capacity to engage in daily activities. Thus the alleviation of symptoms is intimately tied to the palliative-care goal of maximising quality of living. Symptom assessment—defined here as systematic attention to the physical, emotional, social, and spiritual impact of advanced disease—creates the platform from which alleviation of symptoms can begin.

> 'Systematic attention to the physical, emotional, social, and spiritual impact of advanced disease . . . creates the platform from which alleviation of symptoms can begin.'

Symptom occurrence versus symptom distress

Rhodes and Watson (1987, p. 242) have argued that 'symptoms are composed of unique elements, components, or dimensions that produce subjective data . . . that can be perceived and verified only by the person experiencing the event', although they can be understood through comprehensive assessment. The most commonly understood example of this perspective is that pain is what the experiencing person says it is and that it occurs when and where that person says it does. However, this perspective applies equally well to other symptoms.

In understanding symptom assessment, the distinction between symptom *occurrence* and symptom *distress* is important. Symptom *occurrence* refers to perceptions about the frequency, duration, and severity of a symptom. This might also include the way in which a symptom relates to other symptoms or experiences, and it can be rated in terms of the level of discomfort that the symptom causes—for example, mild, moderate, or severe breathlessness. In contrast, symptom *distress* refers to the impact of the symptom on the person in terms of the degree to which that person has to alter his or her daily life in response to the symptom, and the extent to which the symptom or its impact causes physical or mental suffering (Rhodes & Watson 1987). For example, does the symptom interfere with the person's capacity for self-care, and to what extent is this individual bothered by this? People vary in terms of both the occurrence of a symptom and the extent to which the symptom causes distress. Thus the experience of a symptom can be defined as ' . . . the expression of the patient's reality of an experience', involving perception, evaluation, and meaning, as well as that person's *response* to the symptom (McDaniel & Rhodes 1995).

Successful management of symptoms requires attention to all aspects of the symptom experience. It is important to remember that the symptom experience in palliative care occurs in a multidimensional context that includes confrontation with dying and death, the experience of loss, changing social roles, and altered personal relationships. Three key influences should be kept in mind when assessing symptoms in such a context. It should be noted that:

▶ the person's emotional state, and the meaning given to both the illness and the symptom, profoundly influence the perception and experience of symptoms;

▶ the person might not always report symptoms honestly because of fears of being hospitalised, requiring medication, or acknowledging a worsening condition; and

▶ the meaning that the person applies to the symptoms influences his or her willingness to act in accordance with recommended interventions.

> 'Successful management of symptoms requires attention to . . . confrontation with dying and death, the experience of loss, changing social roles, and altered personal relationships.'

The problem of symptoms in advanced disease

The prevalence of symptoms in people receiving palliative care has been extensively studied, although the emphasis of such study has been on people with cancer. However, people with end-stage diseases other than cancer experience similar symptoms to those of people with cancer—in particular, nausea and anorexia (NCHSPCS 1998). Research consistently shows that fatigue, anorexia (which, together with weight loss, is often referred to as 'asthenia'), and pain are common symptoms that occur in 70–90% of people with advanced cancer. Other common symptoms include weight loss, nausea, constipation, confusion, and breathlessness (Bruera 1998). Psychological symptoms, such as anxiety and depression, are increasingly understood to be common experiences for people who are dying. The type of cancer also influences the symptom profile. For example, cancers that metastasise to bone, such as breast cancer, are commonly associated with pain, whereas gastro-intestinal cancers are commonly associated with nausea and vomiting. The treatment of cancer pain is often associated with the experience of other symptoms, such as constipation, dry mouth, and confusion, especially at the commencement of opioid therapy, and the presence of pain should therefore be a cue to enquire about these related symptoms. Confusion, although more commonly a sign than a symptom, is also a significant problem in people close to death, and is often undetected and poorly managed (Bruera & Neumann 1998).

Despite the high prevalence of distressing symptoms and the emphasis on their management in palliative care there is considerable evidence that symptoms are not well controlled (Higginson, Priest & McCarthy 1994), possibly because of inadequate assessment. As noted above, patient factors can influence identification of symptoms. These factors include a reluctance to disclose symptoms, or selectiveness about disclosure (such as people being more willing to disclose physical concerns than psychological concerns) (Heaven & Maguire 1997). However, professional factors are likely to be a major reason for symptoms not being identified. In one study, Heaven and Maguire (1996) found that nurses were able to identify fewer than 40% of their patients' concerns. This indicates significant problems in assessment skills and has provoked calls for an increase in skills training in communication and assessment (Wilkinson 1991; Wilkinson, Roberts & Aldridge 1998). Other work has found that community palliative-care nurses are reluctant to use systematic approaches (such as symptom-screening tools) to identify the presence of key patient symptoms, and that they commonly rely on patients to raise issues of concern (Aranda, Kissane & Long 2000).

Symptom assessment framework
Difference between occurrence and experience
The assessment of pain is well defined both in the literature and in practice, and thus provides a model that can usefully be applied to other symptoms. Although there are obvious differences between pain and other symptoms, the overall parameters of the assessment are similar. The discussion below is divided into two parts—assessing symptom *occurrence* and assessing symptom *distress*. This is an artificial distinction in practice because the two occur simultaneously, but presenting the framework in this way helps to highlight the difference in perspective. Practitioners have traditionally been more interested in the assessment of symptom occurrence, with less attention being given to the patient's distress. A clear example of this can be seen in the case of a young man who was receiving treatment for cancer and who hated the effects of the anti-

nausea medication. However, the nurses found it difficult to watch him making pizza while frequently reaching for the vomit bowl, and they therefore gave him the medication, even when it was clear that he would prefer not to receive it. Although most nurses are more sensitive to patient preferences than the nurses in this example, it remains true that it is often easier to focus on the *occurrence* of the symptom rather than the *experience* of the patient.

Although it is generally agreed that the authoritative source regarding a symptom is the person experiencing it, the practitioner assessing the symptom should be alert for evidence of incongruence between information gained from the patient (or family) and information obtained from his or her own clinical assessment. Clinical judgment is a critical element in symptom assessment. For example, if a person reported a pain score of 2 on a scale of 0–10 (in which 0 indicates 'no pain' and 10 represents 'the worst pain imaginable'), but was observed to be guarding a painful limb or refusing to mobilise, such an incongruous picture would require further investigation.

> 'It is often easier to focus on the *occurrence* of the symptom rather than the *experience* of the patient.'

The process of assessment must be seen as ongoing. Information from an initial assessment should be built upon and revised as knowledge of the person and his or her symptom experience develops (Roberts & Bird 2001). This is critical because the symptoms are likely to change over time and in response to interventions, and also because the person might be more willing to divulge important information as the relationship·with the care team develops.

Assessing symptom occurrence

The assessment of symptom occurrence involves two key components—(i) questioning related to the features of the symptom; and (ii) physical examination. The following discussion considers these two components in turn.

Assessing symptom occurrence by questioning

A useful model for questioning patients about symptoms is the 'PQRST' model developed by Estes (1998). As discussed below, the letters 'PQRST' stand for 'provoke', 'quality', 'regional', 'severity', and 'timing'.

Provoke
What provokes the symptoms? What makes them better or worse?
Asking questions that help to elicit the factors that make a symptom worse or

better is important for diagnosis and for the development of interventions. If it is not possible to avoid the factors that make a symptom worse, it might be possible to find ways of minimising these factors. For example, if the smell of cooking provokes nausea, an effective strategy might include avoiding the kitchen during cooking, or eating colder foods that have less aroma.

The identification of the things that help the symptom can reinforce self-care strategies that the person has already tried, or can open the way for trying new interventions that others have found useful.

Quality
What is the quality of the symptoms being experienced? What words does the person use to describe the symptom?

Assessment of symptom quality can be linked to clinical diagnosis—as in the case of pain when the words used by the person suffering the pain can offer important clinical information. The quality of a symptom can also be useful for diagnostic purposes for symptoms other than pain. For example, nausea might be described as 'a feeling of a lump in the throat' (thus indicating obstruction), or fatigue might be described in terms of localised weakness (thus indicating specific nerve damage).

'Words used by the person suffering the pain can offer important clinical information.'

Quality is also critical in providing an indication of the *experience* of the symptom through the use of such words as 'horrible', 'frightening', or 'intolerable'. (Assessment of symptom quality, in terms of patient distress, is discussed in more detail below; see 'Assessing symptom distress', page 96.)

Regional
Is the symptom regional, general, or local?

The region (or site) of a symptom refers to the part of the body affected. In the case of a symptom such as pain, location is obviously important in making a diagnosis. There might be multiple pain sites, or the pain might be localised. Even so, the localisation of pain can be difficult. For example, somatic pain is more easily localised than visceral pain, which tends to be more diffuse. Pain (both somatic and visceral) can also be experienced by the patient in a site distant from pathology (so-called 'referred pain').

Problems of location also occur with other symptoms. For example, a patient complaining of weakness might identify the weakness as being isolated to the legs, but this might indicate a diagnosis of spinal cord compression.

In assessing the region (location) of symptoms, it can be helpful to use a body chart on which the person marks the location of the symptoms.

Severity
On an agreed scale how does the person rate each symptom?
Symptom severity or intensity provides an indication of how problematic the symptom is for the person. The assessment of severity as recorded at the time of first assessment can be a useful indicator of the effectiveness of later interventions, or as an indicator of worsening symptoms. Severity assessments should always be accompanied by a temporal indication so that the patient response relates to a known time. For example, severity can be assessed as 'right now', 'worse today', or 'average severity over the past 24 hours'—and each of these provides a different perception of the situation. (For more on timing of symptoms, see 'Timing', below.)

Common methods of assessing severity include '0–10' visual and verbal analogue scales, faces scales, and word scales. Although '0–10' scales are used most commonly, some patients find these difficult, and such patients might relate more easily to 'fixed-point' word scales (for example, 'none', 'mild', 'moderate', 'severe'). If a '0–10' scale is difficult for a person to use, the nurse should try another type of scale. The most important thing is to find a scale that works for each individual, and then to use this consistently as the measure of severity over time.

Timing
What is the timing (or temporal nature) of the symptoms?
Timing includes the symptom's *onset*, *pattern*, and *frequency*. Each of these is discussed below.

Enquiring about *onset* helps to determine whether the symptom is long-standing, more recent, or new. This information can be important in assessing what interventions have previously been tried, whether symptoms are refractory, and the patient's response to past interventions. For example, if a person has a long-standing symptom and little has been of help in alleviating it, that person can feel hopeless about the likely success of any future interventions.

The *pattern* and *frequency* of the symptom can assist in diagnosis by relating the pattern and frequency to other aspects of the person's experience. For example, does the symptom occur more frequently at night than during the day? Does it relate to an empty or full stomach? Is it influenced by any medications or other treatments? Pattern and frequency are also useful in planning interventions. In such planning, a symptom of high severity occurring infrequently requires a different approach from that used for a symptom of less severity that is present continuously.

Assessing symptom occurrence by physical examination

The physical examination is a very important adjunct to assessment of any symptoms reported by a patient (either spontaneously or in response to questioning). The clinical picture can often change rapidly in advanced disease. For example, the development of a new metastatic site, cord compression, or pneumothorax can be manifested as new or altered symptoms that require further assessment of the patient by physical examination. The physical examination also assists in assessment of the person's ability to indicate symptoms. For example, physical examination is important in assessing a person's ability to move, breathe, respond to commands, and point to areas of altered sensation.

Physical examination, although usually performed primarily by medical staff, is a key nursing skill. Nurses in palliative care in particular must be able to undertake respiratory, gastrointestinal, cognitive, and basic neurological assessments to ensure timely medical involvement for symptoms (and associated signs) that might suggest the presence of bowel obstruction, infection, respiratory failure, or neurological impairment.

Components of the physical examination are:

▶ testing of movement and the person's capacity to perform daily activities;
▶ examination of skin turgor and hydration status;
▶ palpation to identify tender spots or altered sensation;
▶ percussion to assess bowel and respiratory problems;
▶ observation of behaviour;
▶ observation of responses to commands; and
▶ observation of non-verbal cues.

Assessing symptom distress

As described above, symptom *distress* refers to the impact of the symptom on the individual in terms of personal suffering and impairment of daily living. Symptoms affect what a person is able to do, and frequently limit social interaction, role function, and relationships. The key parameters of assessing distress are:

▶ the meaning that the symptom has for the person and those close to him or her;
▶ the impact it has on daily functioning; and
▶ the level of concern and distress that results.

Each of these is discussed below.

The meaning of a symptom

Understanding the *meaning* that a symptom holds for the person experiencing it is a critical aspect of assessing symptom distress. Does the symptom indicate to the person that the disease is advancing and that death is close? Is the person frightened of dying? Does the presence of the symptom mean that this person can no longer pick up a child, go out to work, or make love to a partner?

Sometimes the meaning of the symptom can be easily elicited by asking the person to relate what it is like to be fatigued, to have pain, or to live with constant diarrhoea. At certain times, eliciting the meaning of the symptom, without being invasive, is difficult or inappropriate. However, it is important to remember that the sense of isolation experienced by many patients can be heightened because a nurse is reluctant to ask questions about their personal experiences and the meaning of symptoms for them. Street and Kissane (2001) have offered a useful example of this. They related the story of a woman who was dying of cancer, and who had developed an offensive odour. The woman realised that all of her health professionals were pretending that the smell did not exist. This not only prevented her talking about what it was like to die while being aware of a dreadful odour, but also prevented her sharing the ideas that she had for reducing the smell in her room.

Effect on daily living

The meaning of a symptom is obviously related to the impact that the symptom has *on the person's life*. Although some of this impact is due to existential suffering, a far greater proportion results from the loss of the little things that make up daily life—being able to walk to the toilet, feed oneself, sit children on a knee, or read a book with mental clarity.

Assessing the impact of symptoms on daily life has emotional and practical benefits for the person involved. Such assessment not only gives 'voice' to the experience, but also opens up many opportunities for nurses, occupational therapists, physiotherapists, and others to make a difference through such practical assistance as volunteers reading a book, the provision of a commode, the assistance of feeding aids, advice about rest and activity, and so on.

Level of distress

Finally, assessment of symptom distress involves clarifying with the person experiencing the symptom *how distressing* it is for him or her. This can be undertaken formally (with scales similar to those described above in assessing severity) or informally (by asking the person to rank symptoms, beginning with those that bother him or her the most).

Symptom distress can also be used to measure the effect of nursing interventions with more accuracy than is possible by simply measuring severity. For example, a change in medication might not result in less pain than before the intervention. However, because the person is now up and about more than was previously possible, the *distress*

> 'Attention to symptom distress helps people to feel less isolated in their experience, and provides a sense of being "understood" as people.'

associated with the pain can be said to have been alleviated.

Apart from such practical therapeutic perspectives, attention to symptom distress helps people to feel less isolated in their experience, and provides a sense of being 'understood' as people.

Clarifying goals of treatment

When assessment is completed, before interventions are planned, discussion should take place about the person's expectations for improvement. This enables the setting of short-term and medium-term treatment goals. In the context of palliative care, decision-making must be influenced by the desires of the patient, and by an assessment of the balance between the likely benefits of the intervention and its negative aspects (including its invasiveness and the likelihood of side-effects). An open discussion of these issues needs to be handled sensitively to provide an opportunity for realistic goal-setting and honest discussion. Priorities at this time include recognition that:

◗ complete symptom relief is often unrealistic in advanced disease, and that alleviation of one symptom can cause undesirable effects (such as causing a new symptom);

◗ relief of symptoms needs to be balanced against other patient desires (such as a desire to stay alert);

◗ mobility and function might be a more appropriate focus than relief of the symptom itself; and

◗ trial-and-error approaches are important in palliative care because there is usually an opportunity to try something, but to withdraw the treatment if the side-effects compromise other aspects of quality of life.

If symptom management in palliative care is to be successful, it is essential that frequent reassessment is undertaken to ensure that the interventions being used are useful, that they do not cause unwanted side-effects, and that they are stopped as soon as possible if they are not of benefit to the patient.

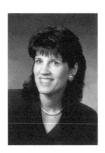

Jeannine Brant

Jeannine Brant is the oncology clinical nurse specialist and pain consultant at St Vincent Healthcare in Billings (Montana, USA). She is also an assistant adjunct professor at Montana State University College of Nursing. Jeannine is well recognised for her work in pain management and end-of-life care. She has presented more than 200 lectures and published more than 40 manuscripts, book chapters, and newsletters on pain management, palliative care, and cancer care issues. She was also the 1998 recipient of the ONS/Schering Clinical Lectureship Award and presented a lecture entitled 'The Art of Palliative Care: Living with Hope, Dying with Dignity'.

Chapter 8

Pain Management

Jeannine Brant

Introduction

Pain is a common symptom in patients at the end of life. Pain occurs in up to 90% of patients with advanced cancer, 80% of patients with acquired immune deficiency syndrome (AIDS), and 60% of patients with end-stage organ failure (AHCPR 1994; Britton & Miller 1984; Seale & Cartwright 1994). According to a survey by Ferrell et al. (2001), pain-management professionals ranked pain management at the end of life as the number one ethical dilemma in practice. Undertreatment of pain at the end of life was considered to be the most significant therapeutic problem. This survey, and other evidence in the literature, point to the need for more diligent management of pain at the end of life. Untreated pain causes unnecessary suffering and has significant effects on a patient's physical, psychological, social, and spiritual quality of life. Fortunately, pain can be effectively managed in more than 90% of patients (AHCPR 1994).

This chapter provides an overview of the assessment and management of pain at the end of life. Definitions of pain and barriers to adequate pain management are also addressed. Pain guidelines, developed internationally as a basis for evidence-based practice, are also discussed.

Nurses have a primary responsibility to recognise pain, to provide a comprehensive pain assessment, and to participate in the overall pain-management plan. Nurses should also act as advocates for patients and families, and reassure them that most pain can be adequately relieved.

What is pain?

The International Association for the Study of Pain (IASP) defines pain as 'an unpleasant sensory and emotional experience associated with actual or potential tissue damage or described in terms of such damage' (IASP 1979). The IASP definition is comprehensive in that it acknowledges that pain is both a physiological phenomenon and an emotional experience. The definition also notes that pain is a subjective experience, a perspective captured even more forcefully in McCaffery's (1968, p. 95) definition that pain is '. . . whatever the experiencing person says it is, existing whenever he/she says it does'.

> 'Pain is whatever the experiencing person says it is, existing whenever he or she says it does.'

Barriers to pain relief

Pain at the end of life is frequently undertreated. The barriers to adequate pain treatment can involve health-care professionals and patients, and, in some cases, the patients' families or carers.

Health-care professionals often lack knowledge about the assessment and management of pain. They are also frequently concerned about addiction, tolerance, and the side-effects of opioids (AHCPR 1994). In reality, the overall incidence of addiction is low (Porter & Jick 1980). This is especially true of patients taking opioids at the end of life. Nurses and other health-care professionals often misinterpret the meanings of the terms 'addiction', 'tolerance', and 'dependence'. The definitions of these terms, together with a clarifying comment on each, are presented in Table 8.1 (page 103).

The principle of 'double effect' is relevant to any discussion of the attitude of health professionals to the use of opioid medication. 'Double effect', a concept initiated by Roman Catholic moral theologians in the seventeenth century, justifies a potentially harmful effect when the intention is good. For example,

Table 8.1 Addiction, tolerance, and dependence

Addiction	**Definition**
	A neurobehavioural syndrome (with genetic and environmental influences) characterised by psychological dependence on the use of substances for their psychic effects, and by compulsive use despite harm.
	Comment
	Addiction is sometimes referred to by terms such as 'drug dependence' and 'psychological dependence', but physical dependence and tolerance are normal physiological consequences of extended opioid therapy for pain and should not be considered addiction.
Analgesic tolerance	**Definition**
	The need to increase the dose of an opioid to achieve the same level of analgesia.
	Comment
	Analgesic tolerance might or might not be evident during opioid treatment and is not to be equated with addiction.
Physical dependence	**Definition**
	A physiological state of neuro-adaptation characterised by a withdrawal syndrome if drug use is stopped or decreased abruptly, or if an antagonist is administered.
	Comment
	Physical dependence is an expected result of opioid use, and does not, in itself, equate with addiction.

Adapted from FSMBUS (1998)

some drugs used to relieve pain at the end of life, such as morphine and other strong opioids, and non-steroidal anti-inflammatory drugs, carry risk of serious adverse effects which may even result in death. However, their use is justified as the positive benefits of adequate pain relief outweigh the potentially harmful effects. The principle continues to be discussed by bioethicists today (Elliott 1997), and should be kept in mind when assessing the question of pain relief at the end of life.

Patients can present a barrier to their own pain relief. They can be reluctant to report pain for fear that their disease is getting worse, or that pain is inevitable and untreatable, and this can be especially common in patients who are nearing the end of life. Concern about not being a 'good' patient might result in some misleading the health-care professional by 'putting on a brave face'. In addition, patients can be reluctant to take pain medications as they may fear addiction, tolerance, and side-effects (AHCPR 1994). This can lead to non-compliance in the belief that nothing can prevent the pain from escalating; or the patient may stop the medication and fail to inform the health-care professional.

Assessment of pain
General approach to assessment
As noted above, a major barrier to pain management is inadequate pain assessment. Indeed, inadequate pain assessment might well be the single most important barrier to appropriate cancer pain management (Von Roenn et al. 1993).

> 'A major barrier to pain management is inadequate pain assessment.'

Adequate pain assessment begins with a global systematic approach that involves the person *and* the family. AHCPR (1994) has recommended an 'ABCDE' approach to pain assessment—an acronym formed by taking the first letters of the following steps.

▶ Ask about pain regularly and frequently. Assess pain systematically.
▶ Believe the patient and family in their reports of pain and what relieves it.
▶ Choose pain control options appropriate for the patient, family, and setting.
▶ Deliver interventions in a timely, logical, and coordinated fashion.
▶ Empower patients and their families. Enable them to control their course to the greatest extent possible.

An important element in assessing pain is to use a convenient assessment tool, and to use it consistently. The tool should include characteristics of the pain—including location, intensity, quality, and temporal factors. The person can point to the location of the pain, or a body diagram can be utilised to assist him or her in indicating the location. It is important that the nurse check for multiple pain sites. Each site should be evaluated separately because each pain might require a separate intervention.

Measuring pain intensity

When measuring intensity, a numerical scale of '0–10' (in which '0' indicates 'no pain' and '10' indicates 'the worst possible pain') is clinically useful. If the person is unable to use a numerical scale, verbal scales can also be used with descriptors such as 'no pain', 'slight pain', 'moderate pain', 'severe pain', or 'excruciating pain' (AHCPR 1994). Rating scales allow health-care professionals to assess and communicate pain intensity, and the response to pain interventions, on an ongoing basis.

Assessing the quality of pain

The quality of the pain is the person's description of how the pain feels. The quality of pain described can help to differentiate somatic, visceral, and neuropathic pain.

▶ *Somatic pain* is bodily pain in tissues other than viscera and neural tissues. Examples include bone metastases and soft-tissue inflammation. Somatic pain is usually well localised, and is usually described as 'constant', 'aching', or 'gnawing'.

▶ *Visceral pain* results from pathology in thoracic or abdominal organs. It is often poorly localised and can be experienced (or 'referred') elsewhere. Abdominal visceral pain often 'comes in waves', and might be described as 'cramping'.

▶ *Neuropathic pain* is pain emanating from the central and peripheral nervous systems. The pain might be described as 'numb', 'radiating', 'burning', or 'shock-like'.

Different types of pain respond to different medications. For example, inflammatory somatic pain is more likely to respond to nonsteroidal anti-inflammatory agents (NSAIDS), whereas centrally mediated neuropathic pain is more likely to respond to anticonvulsants. (For more detail on medications, see 'Analgesics at the end of life', this chapter, page 107.)

Temporal aspects of pain

The temporal assessment involves a description of how the pain feels over time. This includes a description of the onset, duration, and frequency of the pain. These should be considered in association with an assessment of factors that exacerbate or relieve the pain. Nurses should pay particular attention to the following temporal factors (Portenoy & Hagen 1989).

▶ *Incident pain:* This is pain that occurs with movement or activity. Incident pain is usually predictable and can be prevented with doses of analgesics administered at an appropriate interval before the painful activity.

▶ *Breakthrough pain:* This is an unpredictable exacerbation of pain that occurs against a background of constant pain that is otherwise controlled.

▶ *End-of-dose pain:* This is pain that occurs just before the next dose of analgesic is due. This indicates a need to increase the dose or to decrease the interval of administration.

Ongoing and consistent reassessment of pain is often a challenge. In 1995, the American Pain Society (APS) conducted a consensus study to develop quality guidelines on the assessment and management of pain (APSQCC 1995). One recommendation was that institutions make the assessment of pain highly visible so that it undergoes regular and frequent review. The adoption of pain as the '5th vital sign' (along with temperature, pulse, respiration, and blood pressure) is a useful strategy. At every consultation or visit, the clinician is thus encouraged to assess pain along with other vital signs.

> 'The assessment of pain should be highly visible so that it undergoes regular and frequent review.'

Studies also indicate that formal continuous quality-improvement programs help to ensure that pain is being measured and managed on an ongoing basis (Comley & DeMeyer 2001).

Behavioural assessment of pain

In addition to a physiological assessment, nurses should assess behavioural factors that affect the pain. This might be quite specific—such as limping or splinting (protection of the injured part). More generally, behavioural assessment of pain involves an awareness of whether pain is interfering with a person's social function. For example, the person might be unable to shop for groceries because walking for long periods of time exacerbates the pain.

Behavioural assessment provides information on how the person is functioning on a day-to-day basis and might lead to a modification in the plan of care. Adjusting the medication schedule and educating the person about the control of incident pain might assist him or her in optimal comfort and functioning.

Psychosocial and spiritual assessment of pain

Psychosocial and spiritual dimensions also play an important role in pain at the end of life. Psychosocial assessment includes the effect that pain has on mood, sleep, coping, goals, and finances (Elliott 1997). Spiritual assessment includes the effect of suffering on the person's understanding of meaning and purpose in life. Nurses can give people 'permission' to verbalise their personal feelings about pain and suffering (Spross & Wolff 1995).

A model for pain management

The World Health Organization (WHO 1990) has devised a structure to assist nurses and other health-care professionals in the management of cancer pain. The WHO principles for cancer can be used as a template for the management of other pain at the end of life. The recommendations include managing pain:

▶ 'by the ladder';
▶ 'by the clock'; and
▶ 'by the mouth'.

'By the ladder' refers to the WHO analgesic 'ladder'—a stepwise approach to effective pain management (Figure 8.1, page 108). On the first step of the ladder, when the patient describes the pain as mild, the usual choice of medication is the non-opioid class of analgesics. However, if pain is greater, persists or is increasing despite optimising the dose, weak opioids should be used (step two). If the pain persists or increases, move up the ladder to step three, strong opioids. It is important not to move sideways with analgesia in the same efficacy group. Adjuvant analgesics and non-opioids can be used on each step of the ladder to optimise patient comfort.

'By the clock' refers to the administration of analgesics around the clock, rather than on an 'as-needed' basis. Around the clock dosing produces a steady therapeutic blood level of analgesia, rather than a 'peak-and-trough' effect in which periods of relief alternate with painful peaks in pain. Additional doses should be used for breakthrough pain.

'By the mouth' refers to the administration of an analgesic by the oral route whenever possible. Other routes of administration, such as the rectal or transdermal routes can also be used.

Analgesics at the end of life
Non-opioid analgesics

The non-opioid analgesics include paracetamol and non-steroidal anti-inflammatory drugs (NSAIDs), such as aspirin.

Paracetamol is the drug of choice for mild pain and should be considered as a primary treatment or as an adjuvant for various types of mild musculoskeletal pain. Hepatotoxicity is the most significant potential side-effect of paracetamol, and the dose should not exceed 4000 mg in 24 hours. Patients with cirrhosis,

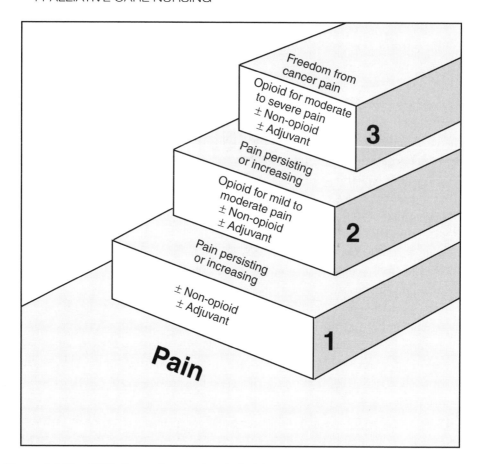

Figure 8.1 The WHO three-step analgesic ladder
World Health Organization (1990); published with permission

hepatitis, and liver metastases are especially sensitive to the hepatotoxic effects of the drug, even at daily doses of less than 4000 mg (Shiodt et al. 1997), and thus paracetamol must be prescribed with caution in patients with severe hepatic impairment.

The NSAIDs work by blocking the production of prostaglandins, thus inhibiting inflammation. The NSAIDs are categorised into two classes, each with distinctive side-effects. The older NSAIDs, including aspirin, block two types of enzymes and can therefore cause effects other than the desired anti-inflammatory effect. They can thus cause gastrointestinal ulceration, renal dysfunction, and platelet inhibition. Examples include ibuprofen, naproxen, diclofenac sodium, ketoprofen (Orudis), and indomethacin (Indocid). The newer NSAIDs, such as celecoxib and rofecoxib, are more selective and block only the enzyme responsible for inflammation and tissue injury, thus resulting in fewer episodes of gastrointestinal and renal dysfunction (Cryer & Feldman 1998). There is concern, however, that these 'COX-2 inhibitors', as they are known, might contribute to thrombo-embolism (and related cardiovascular events).

Opioid analgesics
Choice of opioids

Opioid analgesics are the mainstay of pain management at the end of life. In choosing an opioid, it is important to consider the efficacy of the agent, its half-life, its duration of action, the delivery and dosing options, and potential side-effects. In addition, the patient's age, comorbidity factors, and previous opioid use should be considered. It should also be noted that some opioids should not be used chronically because of their metabolites and ceiling doses (APS 1999). These include pethidine, buprenorphine, and pentazocine.

'Opioid analgesics are the mainstay of pain management at the end of life.'

Suitable weak opioids for mild to moderate pain include codeine and dihydrocodeine. For moderate to severe pain, morphine is the opioid of choice. Alternative opioids include hydromorphone, oxycodone, methadone and transdermal fentanyl (Hanks et al. 2001).

Dosage regimens

Because pain at the end of life is often constant, it is best to choose an opioid that is controlled-release or long-acting. A variety of suitable opioids (including some of those listed above) can be given by continuous intravenous infusion with bolus doses for breakthrough pain.

It is important to continue the opioid analgesics throughout the dying process, even when the patient is sedated or unresponsive. Restlessness and agitation can indicate increased pain, and doses might have to be increased to maintain adequate analgesia. If the patient can no longer take the prescribed opioid orally, an alternative route should be selected. If the opioid is stopped abruptly, the patient may experience withdrawal (Elliott 1997).

Side-effects of opioids

The most common side-effects of opioids include constipation, nausea and vomiting, sedation, confusion, and pruritus. Myoclonus (muscle spasm) can occur if opioids are used in high doses. Constipation is a major problem, and is the most common side-effect reported. Some patients even say that they would rather be in pain than suffer from severe constipation. Prophylactic bowel management can assist in managing this common problem. An overview of the most common opioid-related side-effects and management strategies is shown in Table 8.2 (below).

Table 8.2 Management of opioid side-effects

Side-effect	Management strategies
Constipation	Prevention is the key; advise patient to take prophylactic stool softeners and bowel stimulants. Assess bowel sounds frequently; assess bowel function daily through patient or family report.
Nausea and vomiting	Often mislabelled as an 'allergy'; question opioid 'allergy' symptoms and clarify information. Review other medications and conditions that might be contributing. If nausea and vomiting significant, use anti-emetics around the clock for 3–7 days (especially in high-risk patients); consider change in opioid.
Sedation, delirium, confustion, agitation, restlessness	Assess for sedation and confusion, especially with opioid initiation or titration of dosage. Ensure that patient is safe with bed rails up, and family or attendant in the room. Consider possible causes other than opioids; attempt to differentiate whether sedation and confusion is due to the dying process. Consider change in opioid; consider haloperidol, olanzapine or levomepromazine for restlessness or agitation; consider administration of psychostimulants to counteract sedation.
Pruritus	Morphine is opioid most commonly associated with pruritus; but consider causes other than the opioid. Consider antihistamines to counteract pruritus. *(Continued)*

Table 8.2 Management of opioid side-effects (*Continued*)

Side-effect	Management strategies
Pruritus (continued)	Might need to rotate opioids if pruritus intractable.
Myoclonus (jerking and twitching)	Assess for uncontrolled twitching and jerking movements. Consider rotating opioids. Consider benzodiazepines to counteract myoclonus.
Respiratory depression	Assess respirations per minute. Be aware that respiratory depression and sedation are separate phenomena. Attempt to determine if respiratory depression is due to opioid or the dying process; if due to opioid, consider nalaxone; do not administer naloxone too quickly as this can precipitate breakthrough pain and a pain crisis. Maintain patient comfort as a high priority.

Author's presentation based on material from Holdsworth et al. (1995); Ferris (1999); Rozan, Kahn & Warfield (1995); Bruera et al. (1989); Lichter (1993); Maddocks et al. (1996)

Adjuvant analgesics

Adjuvant analgesics are agents that: (i) have independent analgesic efficacy; or (ii) work synergistically with other agents to enhance comfort; or (iii) relieve symptoms associated with pain (such as anxiety). The adjuvants are used with each step of the WHO analgesic ladder (see page 108), and are often prescribed for specific somatic, visceral, and neuropathic pain symptoms.

The tricyclic antidepressants (amitriptyline, nortriptyline) are used as adjuvant therapy in the management of neuropathic pain, especially 'burning' pain associated with peripheral neuropathy. These drugs, which are usually administered orally, can produce anticholinergic side-effects (such as dry mouth). Anticonvulsants (clonazepam, carbamazepine, gabapentin) can also be used for neuropathic pain (especially shooting pain or radiating pain), but can produce sedation as an unwanted side-effect. Other drugs that can be used to assist in the management of neuropathic pain include local anaesthetics (mexiletine), drugs affecting bone metabolism (calcitonin), skeletal muscle relaxants (baclofen) and topical capsaicin, a naturally occurring alkaloid.

Corticosteroids (dexamethasone, prednisolone) are helpful as adjuvant therapy in the management of a range of problems, including cerebral oedema, spinal cord compression, bone pain, neuropathic pain, and visceral pain. These drugs can be administered orally, intravenously, or subcutaneously, depending on circumstances. Possible side-effects include 'steroid psychosis' and dyspepsia.

For the management of bone pain and hypercalcaemia related to metastatic bone disease, the bisphosphonates (pamidronate, zoledronic acid) are useful. However, these drugs can cause 'aches and pains' following administration. Calcitonin is also used to assist in the management of bone pain.

The bisphosphonates are especially noteworthy in pain management at the end of life. Initially indicated for the treatment of bone diseases such as osteoporosis and Paget's disease, they are now recognised for their role in the management of metastatic bone pain, although zoledronic acid is not currently licensed for this use. Disodium pamidronate and zoledronic acid work by inhibiting the osteoclastic activity of bone resorption and inflammation triggered by the tumour. Intravenous pamidronate reduces vertebral fracture, delays the onset of skeletal disease, and reduces radiation requirements. Moreover, patients have reported an improvement in quality of life while on the medication (Fulfaro et al. 1998).

Routes of administration

Approximately 75–85% of patients achieve pain control through simple routes of administration—such as oral, transdermal, or rectal administration. Another 5–20% require subcutaneous and intravenous drugs, and approximately 2–6% require intraspinal analgesics. It is important to begin with the simplest and least invasive method. A change in administration should be considered if the person has uncontrolled pain (despite aggressive titration) or unpleasant side-effects, or if the route is no longer intact (AHCPR 1994).

The transdermal route is an effective alternate to the oral and subcutaneous route but it is best reserved for patients whose analgesic requirements are stable. This route is now being used for fentanyl but consideration must be given to the latent period before the fentanyl starts working. After application of the transdermal fentanyl, serum levels rise after 1–2 hours with analgesic effects evident within 6–12 hours, with steady state achieved at 72 hours (Hanks et al, 2001).

The rectal route, although simple, is disliked by many patients. However, rectal administration should be considered if oral administration is difficult because the patient has become unresponsive close to death. When using the rectal route, it should be noted that absorption is highly variable, but can be faster than the oral route with some drugs (Warren 1996).

Parenteral administration of opioids includes the subcutaneous, intramuscular, and intravenous routes. The subcutaneous route is the preferred parenteral route, either for bolus injections or as a continuous subcutaneous infusion (CSCI) via a battery-driven portable syringe driver. The latter ensures constant analgesia and its use is less disturbing to the patient than repeated injections. Intramuscular administration is not recommended because it can be painful, inconvenient to use in the home situation, and can result in variable absorption (compared with subcutaneous or intravenous injection) (Elliott 1997). However, bolus doses of diamorphine and morphine when combined with an irritant additional drug, such as cyclizine, may be given intramuscularly. Intravenous administration provides rapid relief of pain, and most opioids peak within 10–15 minutes. This route is a possible alternate for those patients with venous access. For example, cancer patients who have a indwelling central venous catheter to administer chemotherapy and frequent blood sampling. These catheters can be used for both bolus injections and continuous infusions.

The intraspinal route (epidural and intrathecal) can be useful in patients whose pain does not respond to less-invasive measures. Local anaesthetics can be added to intraspinal opioids to produce additional analgesia. The route requires careful monitoring and expertise, and might not be suitable for home use without careful assessment (AHCPR 1994) and ready access to pain specialists.

Dosing and titration considerations

A decision on an initial opioid dose is based on the patient's prior exposure to opioids. Patients should start with the lowest dose, and this can be titrated to a higher doses until a satisfactory analgesic effect is achieved. The titration should be aggressive enough to provide optimal pain relief in a short time without causing profound side-effects. Some side-effects occur with initial dosing, but tolerance to side-effects usually develops over time.

Analgesics can be administered around the clock (ATC) or as required (prn). Patients with constant pain require ATC dosing to maintain a therapeutic blood level, and extra doses can be given between long-acting doses for breakthrough or incident pain.

'The titration of dose should be aggressive enough to provide optimal pain relief in a short time without causing profound side-effects.'

The breakthrough dose of opioids for both oral and parenteral should be ⅙ of the total 24-hour opioid dose (Hanks et al. 2001).

Invasive procedures

Approximately 1–5% of patients require invasive interventions to control their pain. These include nerve blocks, palliative surgery, and ablative surgery.

One of the most successful interventions for people suffering from visceral abdominal cancer pain is a neurolytic coeliac plexus block. This procedure is recommended by the WHO Cancer Pain Relief Program, and is considered to be the most suitable invasive procedure in the palliative-care setting (WHO 1990). The block is performed by injecting alcohol into the coeliac plexus (during laparotomy or percutaneously). Lillimoe et al. (1993) reported that some patients lived 3.5 times longer if a block was performed, perhaps due to improved function and pain control. Overall, a coeliac plexus block is well tolerated and provides optimal quality of life for patients suffering intractable abdominal pain (Eisenberg, Carr & Chalmers 1995; Yamamuro et al. 2000).

Non-pharmacological pain management

It is important to recognise that pain is an emotional experience, as well as being a physiological phenomenon. Cognitive-behavioural approaches can assist in modifying a person's perception of pain. Relaxation, distraction, music therapy, and hypnosis should be considered for incorporation in the plan of care. Although these are not the mainstay of therapy, they are complementary to pharmacological and procedural treatments.

Conclusion

Pain is one of the most feared symptoms that patients and families face at the end of life. Nurses have a primary responsibility to assess for pain diligently and to manage uncontrolled pain aggressively. By using opioid analgesics, adjuvants, and alternative methods of relief, comfort can be achieved in the majority of people. These people are then better able to focus on the psychological and spiritual issues that give meaning to their last days, thereby optimising their quality of life.

'Nurses have a responsibility to assess for pain diligently and to manage uncontrolled pain aggressively.'

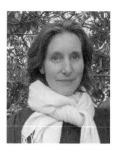

Mary Bredin

Mary Bredin is a registered general nurse with postgraduate qualifications in complementary health studies, and a background in cancer and palliative care nursing. Her specific interest in the subject of breathlessness began in 1996 when she became coordinator of a study to evaluate nursing intervention for breathlessness in patients with lung cancer at the Macmillan Practice Development Unit (MPDU) at the Centre for Cancer and Palliative Studies in London (UK). The MPDU was set up in May 1994 to provide information and to conduct research studies relevant to the needs of Macmillan Nurses. At the same time, she worked as a practitioner in a breathlessness clinic. She has now left the MDPU to be with her young daughter and to train as a counsellor at Sussex University (UK). Mary continues to teach and write about breathlessness and is interested in incorporating psychodynamic theory into her work on this subject.

Chapter 9

Breathlessness

Mary Bredin

Introduction

This chapter provides a broad overview of breathlessness in patients receiving palliative care. It draws on a variety of research studies and other literature on the subject, and outlines the most appropriate management strategies in the palliative-care setting.

Breathlessness is one of the most difficult and challenging of symptoms. To breathe is to be alive, and it is not surprising that any threat to breathing as a result of illness evokes profound physical and emotional discomfort and distress. Watching someone struggle to breathe can also induce feelings of helplessness and anxiety in nurses and other practitioners. Such feelings can trigger a need to act—to 'do something' to make things better. However, breathlessness is often resistant to palliative medical treatment. One of the important themes of this chapter is the enormous therapeutic value of simply 'being with' the patient in his or her distress and 'staying with' the discomfort this evokes in the practitioner.

It is hoped that this chapter will encourage nurses and other practitioners to develop their knowledge and confidence in addressing the problem of breathlessness, and that it will help them to trust in their own capacity to make a real difference for patients—even when this feels like an impossibly difficult task.

What is breathlessness?

> It is a frightened feeling where you don't think you'll get another breath, and because it is accompanied by fear and panic and feeling tight, you can actually feel that tightening feeling of fear in your chest and mind (O'Driscoll, Corner & Bailey 1999, p. 39).

Breathlessness is a subjective sensation that is hard to define. It is best understood as being more than merely a symptom of disordered breathing. Rather, it is a complex interplay among physical, psychological, emotional, and functional factors (O'Driscoll, Corner & Bailey 1999). Unlike the physical sensation of breathlessness experienced by healthy individuals during strenuous exercise, the sensation of 'pathological' breathlessness in patients with advanced disease can be frightening and devastating (Bredin 2001). Patients describe their experience of breathlessness in powerful and graphic images— 'steel bands around the chest'; 'breathing while drinking a glass of water'; or 'like a suffocation' (O'Driscoll, Corner & Bailey 1999).

'The sensation of "pathological" breathlessness in patients with advanced disease can be frightening and devastating.'

Prevalence of breathlessness in advanced disease

Because breathlessness is subjective, the degree of physical change in breathing might not necessarily reflect the patient's experience of breathlessness (Carrieri, Janson-Bjerklie & Jacobs 1984). For example, a patient can appear to be breathing relatively easily, yet complain of feeling severely short of breath. Therefore only the person who is experiencing the sensation of breathlessness can determine the severity of the problem. In published studies, the prevalence of breathlessness in advanced cancer has varied considerably, with estimates ranging from 15% to 79%. According to Vainio and Auvinen (1996), this variation reflects differences in:

▶ the definition of breathlessness;
▶ study designs;
▶ patient selection; and
▶ validated instruments used to measure the symptom.

In the United States, Reuben and Mor (1986) conducted a national study of 1754 cancer patients and found that the incidence of breathlessness in terminal cancer during the last six weeks of life was as high as 70.2%. Breathlessness was reported to be 'moderate to severe' in 28% of patients. In an international multicentre prospective study of 1640 palliative-care patients, with a whole

> 'Only the person who is experiencing the sensation of breathlessness can determine the severity of the problem.'

range of different types of disease, breathlessness was ranked as being among the top eight symptoms of advanced cancer (Vainio & Auvinen 1996). Breathlessness was commonest in lung cancer, occurring in 46% of patients. It was also common among patients with breast and oesophageal cancers but was reported as being less than 20% in patients with cancer in other primary sites. In a study conducted in England of 303 patients, 55.5% were breathless on admission to a hospice (Heyse-Moore, Ross & Mullee 1991). The prevalence of breathlessness was 78% for patients who survived less than a day after admission. Of the patients admitted, 11% were rated as severely breathless.

In short, breathlessness is not only a common symptom of advanced cancer but also one that is frequently severe.

Causes of breathlessness

Despite the many theories surrounding the causes of breathlessness, its pathophysiology remains incompletely understood. The process of breathing is mainly under involuntary control. However, it can be influenced by a variety of physiological and psychological factors. The actual experience of breathlessness by a patient results from a complex interaction between, on the one hand, abnormalities in breathing and physiology and, on the other, the *perception* of those abnormalities (Ripamonti & Bruera 1997). Effective nursing management depends on a basic knowledge and understanding of the physiology of breathing and the mechanisms of breathlessness. A useful explanation of the pathophysiology of breathlessness as it relates to patients in the palliative-care setting has been provided by Ahmedzai (1993). Other useful contributions have come from Ripamonti and Bruera (1997) and, in CD-ROM format, by Bredin (2001).

The sensation of breathlessness is inevitably affected by the patient's feelings and his or her interpretation of the underlying causes of breathlessness (Ahmedzai 1993). The longer a symptom continues, the more likely it is that psychological factors such as fear, depression, anxiety, and frustration will influence the perception and intensity of breathlessness. In addition, the causes of breathlessness in advanced disease can be complex. The sensation might be directly due to the disease, or its treatment, or other conditions (see Box, below). To a large extent, the underlying pathology will determine the most appropriate medical intervention. Nevertheless, the emotional and cognitive aspects cannot be ignored.

Causes of breathlessness in advanced disease

Causes due to the primary disease
- primary and/or metastatic tumour;
- airway obstruction (lower airway obstruction frequently accompanied by collapse or infection);
- effusions;
- obstruction of main bronchus;
- replacement of lung by cancer;
- lymphangitis carcinomatosis;
- tumour embolism;
- superior vena cava obstruction;
- pericardial effusion;
- vocal cord paralysis;
- ascites;
- hepatomegaly;
- aspiration pneumonia;
- chest wall pain;
- anaemia;
- generalised weakness (including respiratory muscle weakness).

Causes due to debility
- anaemia;
- atelectasis;
- pulmonary embolism;
- pneumonia;
- empyema.

Other conditions
- chronic obstructive airways disease (COAD);
- pneumothorax;
- asthma;

(Continued)

(Continued)
- heart failure;
- pulmonary fibrosis;
- acidosis;
- congestive cardiac failure;
- mitral or aortic valve disease;
- motor neurone disease;
- infection: bacterial, viral, fungal;
- psychological factors: anxiety, fear, panic, depression, anger.

Causes due to treatment
- surgery: pneumonectomy, lobectomy;
- radiotherapy or fibrosis;
- chemotherapy causing lung fibrosis;
- cardiomyopathy;
- myelosuppression causing anaemia or infection.

Adapted from Twycross & Lack (1990); Cowcher & Hanks (1990); Corner et al. (1997)

A model of breathlessness

Several models in the nursing literature provide a useful insight into breathlessness from the perspective of the patient (Gift 1990; Steele & Shaver 1992; Corner, Plant & Warner 1995). The Box on page 122 presents three models of breathlessness, culminating in the integrative model in which the problem of breathlessness, is understood 'holistically in the context of the individual's life, illness experience and its meaning' (Corner, Plant & Warner 1995, p. 6). This model assumes that the emotional experience of breathlessness is inseparable from the physical experience whatever its pathophysiological mechanisms. All of the factors that contribute to breathlessness (physical, emotional, and social) are considered to be important. Care is aimed at enabling individuals to manage breathlessness for themselves—helping them gain a sense of control—and, in addition, it addresses 'the existential impact of living and dying with breathlessness' (Krishnasmay et al. 2001, p. 105). This model is intended to augment medical care and is entirely compatible with approaches used by physiotherapists and occupational therapists.

Three models of breathlessness

1. Physiological/neural model
Description

Breathlessness has to do with neural pathways and biochemical processes and oxygen starvation.

Management implications

Treatment depends on the capacity of pharmacology to change these processes and responses.

2. Biopsychosocial model
Description

Breathlessness is not just about neural pathways and biochemical processes. The experience also has to do with the person's beliefs, attitudes, and ability to cope.

Management implications

Treatment includes ways to help make relevant behavioural and psychosocial changes.

3. Integrative model (incorporating models 1 and 2 above)
Description

A person's mental experience and bodily experience of breathlessness are viewed as inseparable. Since the two interact, they can potentially set up a vicious circle when the frightening feeling of breathlessness is reinforced by physiological changes and by experiences within the body that make breathing feel even more difficult.

Management implications

Breathlessness management aims to take into account both feelings and physiology; to increase a person's capacity to understand (and feel understood) and to cope better.

Adapted from Corner, Plant & Warner (1995)

Assessment and measurement of breathlessness

> Effective therapy can only be achieved once the nature and impact of breathlessness have been understood from the perspective of the individual experiencing it (Krishnasamy et al. 2001, p. 105).

Care of breathlessness aims to minimise the distress and disability associated with breathlessness, and this requires a thorough and accurate assessment of the problem (Corner & O'Driscoll 1999). The assessment should provide insight into the patient's experience—that is, what breathlessness means to the person, and how it affects every aspect of his or her life. Such an assessment takes time and can require several meetings, especially if the person is very breathless or exhausted.

It can be daunting to know where to start or how to approach someone who is gasping for breath. Corner and O'Driscoll's (1999) breathlessness assessment guide for use in palliative care is a useful first step. The guide was developed as a result of the research and experience of a group of nurses working in a nurse-led breathlessness clinic. It establishes a baseline record of a patient's breathlessness from which future interventions and care can be monitored and assessed.

> 'It can be daunting to know where to start or how to approach someone who is gasping for breath.'

Although the guide certainly takes time to complete, it provides a reliable framework for practitioners seeking a comprehensive assessment. It is more than just an exercise in collecting facts. The assessment is also an opportunity to develop relationships between the practitioner and the patient, and between the practitioner and the family—relationships in which all can feel safe, listened to, and understood. The areas that can be included in the assessment are outlined in the Box on page 124.

Management of breathlessness
Primary disease interventions
Ahmedzai (1993) has set out the general principles of palliation for breathlessness, and has recommended that, wherever possible, the underlying causes should be determined and treated without additional burden to the patient. Unfortunately, the results of studies examining palliative interventions suggest that they are often unsatisfactory (Corner et al. 1997). Medical and surgical interventions should therefore be evaluated on an individual basis and repeated only if they are clearly beneficial.

Therapies directed towards correcting the underlying cause of breathlessness as a result of the disease itself might include:
- chemotherapy;
- radiotherapy; and
- hormonal therapy.

Chemotherapy can have a limited role in the management and palliation of breathlessness—especially in small cell lung cancer. However, its effectiveness in other cancers is not established (Ahmedzai 1993). *Radiotherapy* can be a useful treatment for breathlessness in patients with carcinoma of the bronchus

Assessment of breathlessness

Areas that can be included in the assessment of breathlessness include;
- listening to the patient's story (how breathlessness began; how the person experiences breathlessness as a problem; how the person copes);
- obtaining information about the family's background, social circumstances, work, and domestic situation; how breathlessness has affected these areas of the patient's life;
- ascertaining the meaning of breathlessness for the patient and family; the emotions breathlessness arouses; thoughts and feelings about the future;
- assessing the degree to which breathlessness affects functional activity;
- identifying factors that ameliorate or exacerbate breathlessness;
- establishing the severity and pattern of breathlessness;
- identifying symptoms that might indicate hyperventilation (panic attacks, rapid changes in breathing patterns);
- identifying significant anxiety or depression;
- identifying personal goals;
- establishing the practical implications of managing breathlessness in the home or ward environment;
- identifying factors necessitating referral to other health-care professionals within the multidisciplinary team.

Adapted from Bredin (2001)

(Heyse-Moore 1993) and for endobronchial obstruction caused by primary and secondary tumours (Cowcher & Hanks 1990). In addition to radiotherapy, steroids might be necessary if tumour swelling causes tracheal compression or superior vena cava obstruction (Dunlop 1998). *Hormonal treatments* are used to shrink pulmonary secondaries from breast or prostate cancer, although the effects of chemotherapy and hormone therapy usually take several weeks (Dunlop 1998).

Other options aimed specifically at treating endobronchial lesions include laser ablation of tumours during bronchoscopy. This treatment is expensive and evidence for its efficacy is anecdotal. Stents are sometimes inserted to maintain patency of the bronchi, although complications due to haemorrhage and infections are high (Dunlop 1998). Pleural effusions commonly occur in tumours of the lung and breast and might have to be drained (Cowcher & Hanks 1990).

Symptomatic interventions
When the underlying causes of breathlessness cannot be reversed by medical or

surgical treatments, symptomatic measures (such as use of pharmacological substances) are the principal means of palliation (Ahmedzai 1993). Although pharmacological interventions have their place in the management of breathlessness, the majority of controlled clinical trials of drug therapies in patients with advanced disease have design weaknesses, involve small numbers of patients, and have shown equivocal results (Corner et al. 1997).

Opioids

Opioids, especially morphine, can benefit some patients reporting breathlessness on exertion. However they are more consistently of benefit to patients who are breathless at rest or in the last days of life (Corner et al. 1997). The mechanism by which opioids relieve breathlessness is unknown. In terminally ill cancer patients with breathlessness, morphine can reduce the perception of breathlessness (Bruera et al. 1990). Generally the dose of opioid is titrated in the same way as when used for pain control. However, lower doses and smaller increases are recommended (Davis 1997). Continuous infusion of morphine can help to relieve end-stage breathlessness (Cohen et al. 1991), although sedation is a major side-effect.

'Opioids, especially morphine, can benefit some patients . . . [especially] . . . in the last days of life. The mechanism by which opioids relieve breathlessness is unknown.'

Nebulised opioids have been used in the symptomatic management of breathlessness, but reported benefits are largely anecdotal and there is little scientific evidence to support their use (Davis 1997, Davis et al. 1996). The simultaneous use of both nebulised and oral (or subcutaneous) opioids carries a risk of cumulative toxicity (Ahmedzai & Davis 1997). Nebulised opioids can cause bronchospasm and can be problematic for patients when used at home (Ahmedzai & Davis 1997).

In summary, there appears to be no consensus as to the optimal dose, frequency, or method of administration of opiates (Davis 1997). Side-effects such as nausea, constipation, and sedation must be carefully monitored.

Benzodiazepines and phenothiazines

Benzodiazepines probably relieve breathlessness through their anxiolytic and sedative effects (Davis 1997), although there are no controlled studies evaluating their effects on breathlessness in advanced cancer. Anecdotally, it seems that benzodiazepines can help episodic breathlessness associated with anxiety and hyperventilation or severe unrelieved breathlessness in the last days of life, but unacceptable sedation can limit their use (Corner et al. 1997). Similarly, phenothiazines have been reported to reduce breathlessness in patients with chronic obstructive airways disease (COAD), but side-effects such as extra-pyramidal effects and hypotension restrict their use (Ahmedzai 1993).

Nebulised drugs, systemic corticosteroids, and bronchodilators

There is little scientific evidence to support the use of nebulised drugs in the symptomatic management of patients with breathlessness, and management regimens using these drugs have been derived mainly from experience in patients with COAD (Ahmedzai & Davis 1997). Anecdotal findings suggest that some patients can benefit, but nebulised drugs are usually ineffective in patients experiencing extreme breathlessness on minimal inspiratory effort (Ahmedzai & Davis 1997).

Bronchodilators are recommended when breathlessness is exacerbated by reversible airways obstruction, particularly for patients who have a history of smoking, asthma, or chronic bronchitis (Cowcher & Hanks 1990).

When patients with severe acute exacerbations of asthma or COAD fail to respond to bronchodilators, a short steroid course can be effective (Ahmedzai 1993). High-dose glucocorticosteroids can relieve breathlessness by reducing bronchospasm, by decreasing oedema around tumour masses, by exerting an anti-tumour effect, and by preventing lung oedema from pneumonitis during radiotherapy (Heyse-Moore 1993). Patients on steroids sometimes experience a heightened sense of wellbeing and an increased appetite. Steroids can also have an antiemetic effect.

Oxygen therapy

The place of oxygen in the relief of cancer-related breathlessness is unclear, although studies have shown it to be superior to placebo in advanced cancer (Dunlop 1998). Evidence exists for its use in specific situations, such as hypoxia or pulmonary hypertension as a result of chronic lung and heart disease (Davis 1997). Patients receiving oxygen therapy need to be assessed on an individual basis. An agreed trial period should be continued only when obvious benefit is obtained (Corner et al. 1997).

One of the drawbacks of oxygen therapy is that patients can become psychologically dependent—limiting their independence if they fear being without it. Paradoxically, because it can be given on demand, it offers some patients a degree of control over their treatment.

More research is needed to identify who might benefit from oxygen therapy. Alternatives such as a breeze from an open window or a bedside fan might be more beneficial (Davis 1997).

Nursing management of breathlessness

Given the current lack of clear research evidence, determining the most effective medical and surgical treatments for breathlessness in palliative care is problematic. Similarly, nursing research has, until recently, provided no evidence for selecting effective nursing strategies. Nurses and other health-care workers have consequently struggled with the problem of feeling helpless and ineffective (Roberts, Thorne & Pearson 1993). It has also been said that the impact of living with breathlessness, particularly in the context of a life-threatening illness, has largely remained hidden, or been overlooked (Krishnasmay et al. 2001).

In response to these difficulties, several recent nursing studies have highlighted the value of an integrated nursing approach for the management of breathlessness in lung cancer (Corner, Plant & Warner 1995, Corner et al. 1996, Bredin et al. 1999). Although the focus of this work has been breath-lessness in lung cancer, the strategies might be of value for other patients in the palliative-care setting—if breath-lessness is experienced in the context of a life-threatening illness; or if symptoms are complex and anxiety plays a large part in exacerbating problems.

'The impact of living with breathlessness, particularly in the context of a life-threatening illness, has largely remained hidden, or been overlooked.'

An integrated approach to managing breathlessness

An integrated approach to managing breathlessness uses a range of strategies to help patients and families to manage breathlessness. These strategies are outlined in Figure 9.1 (page 128). For ease of explanation the strategies have been divided into cognitive, behavioural, and psychotherapeutic (Bredin 2001) although, in reality, these areas overlap. The strategies are used simultaneously in practice, although though they appear to be separate in the illustration. For example, nurses and other practitioners offer practical advice and assistance with coping strategies alongside listening to fears, while also helping patients to adjust to the limitations breathlessness imposes.

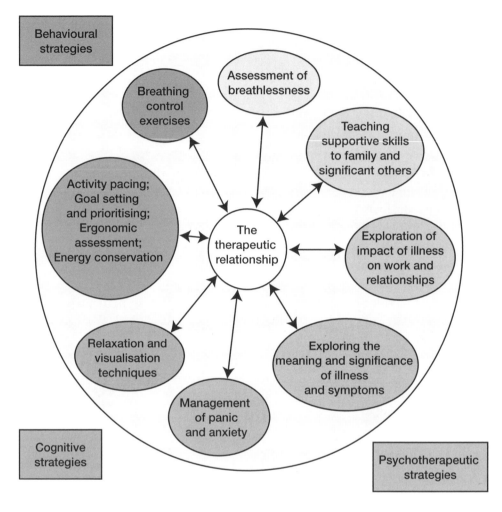

© Institute of Cancer Research

Figure 9.1

Copyright Institute of Cancer Research; published with permission

Developing a therapeutic relationship

As emphasised above, breathlessness can arouse great fear, especially in advanced disease. Patients quite often complain of feeling isolated and alone in their suffering (Roberts, Thorne & Pearson 1993). It follows that nurses working with people who are breathless must be able to respond therapeutically—that is, in ways that lessen anxiety and distress, and assist people to cope.

Responding therapeutically involves the nurse in listening to fears, and the nurse 'being with' his or her own uncomfortable feelings that breathlessness in others can evoke. It also involves what Bailey (1995) has called 'holding and containing' the patient's distress, so that it becomes more tolerable over time. Bailey's (1995) model for this therapeutic work draws on psychodynamic theory—in particular the work of Bion (1962). The nurse acts as a 'container' for the person's anxiety—rather in the way that a mother accepts her infant's distress, tolerates it, and tries to make sense of it (Bailey 1995). The process of understanding what is being 'contained' can be demanding for the nurse, because it requires him or her to accept and respond to whatever the patient brings (Bredin 2001). It is therefore important that nurses in this field have access to a framework of support that allows them to acknowledge and process their own feelings and reactions.

Cognitive strategies—understanding anxiety

How people behave and feel is intimately linked with what they believe about themselves and the world (Lanceley 2001). A person's beliefs about his or her illness and symptoms and the meaning attributed to feelings and sensations, influences how that person adjusts and copes (Bredin 2001). Cognitive approaches explore a person's beliefs and feelings, so that those feelings become more realistic and less overwhelming. For example, people frequently avoid activity for fear of becoming terminally breathless. Such fears are amplified by having a life-threatening illness. By explaining that breathlessness is, in itself, not damaging, and then suggesting ways of managing breathlessness attacks, the nurse can reduce anxiety, and patients can start to regain a sense of control.

Behavioural strategies—skills to control anxiety

> Patients often overlook improvement because their standard of comparison tends to be their old fully capable state. Therefore careful reflection of even the smallest increments of improvement offers hope and a sense of progress (Benner & Wruble 1989, p. 214).

People often compare their current condition with how they were before they were ill. Hopelessness and subsequent loss of motivation ensue, because they are unable to regain their old state. Behavioural strategies can then help to restore a sense of control by encouraging people to foster and mobilise a positive attitude to achieving personal goals, no matter how small (Bredin 2001).

'Careful reflection of even the smallest increments of improvement offers hope and a sense of progress.'

This approach involves teaching people coping strategies—specifically breathing retraining, relaxation and visualisation techniques, activity-pacing, and goal-setting. Much of the literature on the use of coping strategies in the management of breathlessness discusses the management of hyperventilation in people suffering with chronic obstructive pulmonary disease. However, these techniques are now recognised as legitimate aspects of the nursing management of breathlessness in many forms of terminal illness (Corner, Plant & Warner 1995; Gallo-Silver & Pollack 2000).

The specific techniques of (i) breathing retraining, (ii) relaxation and visualisation techniques, and (iii) activity-pacing and goal-setting are discussed below.

Breathing retraining

The practice of breathing techniques can modify the level of anxiety experienced by patients with breathing difficulties (Bass 1994). Breathing retraining (or breathing control) involves abdominal or diaphragmatic breathing. It entails relaxing the muscles of the upper chest and shoulders and using the diaphragm and lower ribs. Diaphragmatic breathing efficiently draws air into the lower part of the lungs (Lewis 1997). Typically, patients who are breathless tend to breathe with the upper chest and shoulders using rapid, shallow, and inefficient breaths. This type of breathing can be very tiring, and can trigger panic attacks. It increases tension in the upper body, eventually causing changes in body posture and making normal respiration even more difficult. In contrast, according to Bredin (2001), diaphragmatic breathing:

▶ promotes a relaxed and gentle breathing pattern;
▶ minimises the work of breathing;
▶ establishes a sense of control;
▶ improves ventilation at the base of the lungs;
▶ decreases breathlessness;
▶ improves exercise tolerance; and
▶ promotes a sense of wellbeing and improved quality of life.

Diaphragmatic breathing is a quick and simple exercise to use with patients and their families (see Box, page 131). The only way for a nurse to feel confident in teaching diaphragmatic breathing is if the nurse first practises it personally. Physiotherapist and occupational therapist colleagues can be a useful source of expert support and advice about breathing techniques.

Once patients can breathe diaphragmatically, they can be taught to use their breathing rhythmically to assist them to carry out activities such as walking, climbing stairs, dressing, and so on. It must be noted, however, that not all

Diaphragmatic breathing exercise

1. Start by making sure you are sitting or lying in a comfortable position with your back well supported.

2. Become aware of your body: feel your feet against the floor, drop your shoulders, soften the muscles around the stomach area. Allow yourself to relax into the chair for a few seconds.

3. Place your hand flat on your abdomen (just below your rib cage) and become aware of that part of your body.

4. Now become aware of your breathing. As you breathe in softly and slowly, feel your hand being pushed out gently by your belly as the diaphragm descends, drawing air into your chest.

5. Feel your hand move in as you breathe out and your diaphragm relaxes and rises up, pushing air out of your chest.

6. Continue to do this for a few minutes. Concentrate gently on breathing slowly in through your nose and out through your mouth, making your 'out-breath' slightly longer than your 'in-breath'.

patients will be able to practise diaphragmatic breathing. Working with the breath requires motivation and a willingness to practise. Patients who are very weak or who are in the terminal stages of their disease can still find it helpful to have a practitioner talk them through diaphragmatic breathing, even though they might be unable to use it effectively. They might, however, find it helpful to think about relaxing their upper bodies while imagining taking slower, gentle breaths. For these patients, simply stroking their backs with a downwards motion for a few minutes with one hand, while placing the other hand gently on their shoulders, can be very soothing and reassuring at times of extreme breathlessness.

Relaxation and visualisation

Relaxation is a valuable approach to helping patients cope with stress during illness (Ahmedzai 1993; Twycross & Lack 1990). If anxiety and breathlessness are viewed as being inseparable, strategies that break the vicious circle of tension (breathlessness leading to increased anxiety and panic states leading to increased breathlessness) will help restore physical and emotional calm and better breathing patterns. Literature that supports the benefits of relaxation comes mainly from work with patients who have breathlessness as a result of chronic respiratory diseases (Janson-Bjerklie & Clarke 1982; Renfroe 1988; Gift, Moore & Seoken 1992). Although there appear to be no studies reporting the specific use of relaxation for respiratory distress in cancer patients (with the exception of Corner, Moore & Seoken 1995; Bredin et al. 1999), relaxation and visualisation have been used quite widely in the management of pain.

It takes time to feel confident in using relaxation strategies with patients. However, it can be enjoyable for both giver and receiver, especially when the practitioner gets over that feeling that everyone else can do it better than they can. Relaxation techniques work even in the noisiest environments, as long as the patient is *properly prepared* for what he or she is being asked to do. Exercises need not take very long—five minutes can be enough time for a person to relax properly. Again, the best way to build up confidence in practising relaxation is for the nurse to try out it out personally—either by listening to a tape or reading through a script first, and then having a go. There are several self-help tapes that offer guided relaxations and it is worth experimenting to find the right one. Occupational therapy departments are usually a good source of information on how to obtain tapes of relaxation scripts. Scripts are also available in CD-ROM format (Bredin 2001).

> 'Using relaxation strategies with patients can be enjoyable for both giver and receiver, especially when the practitioner gets over that feeling that everyone else can do it better than they can.'

Visualisation, also referred to as 'guided imagery', can be used in a number of ways (Bredin 2001):

▶ for the relief of the symptom—for example, by helping the person to relax and then asking him or her to imagine the breath spreading through the body, all the way to the toes;

▶ taking the person through a guided visualisation, imagining being in a peaceful place, feeling calm and in control;

▶ helping the person to build up confidence in carrying out certain activities—for example, inviting him or her to rehearse a situation in the future mentally and imagining a positive outcome (such as getting into the shower and feeling calm, or climbing the stairs and getting to the top without difficulty).

Activity-pacing and goal-setting

Activity-pacing involves teaching the person to slow down, plan, and 'pace' (Bredin 2001). In late-stage terminal illness, the predominant strategy used by patients for controlling breathlessness is to reduce activity (Roberts, Thorne & Pearson 1993; Brown et al. 1986). Fear of failing or of becoming acutely breathless can result in loss of confidence and total withdrawal from activity. Therefore, an important part of managing breathlessness is helping people to plan their activities carefully, so that breathlessness does not become a total barrier to activity. Explaining that it is normal to be breathless on exertion and that breathlessness is, in itself, not harmful, can increase confidence.

The benefits of activity-pacing are decreased anxiety and increased activity, together with a feeling of control and wellbeing (Bredin 2001). Careful planning of activities should involve the person and the family, and might include discussion of the following:

▶ planning the best way to carry out an activity;

▶ consideration of the environment in which the activity is to take place (ergonomic assessment) and rearranging the environment to make tasks easier (for example, placing a chair at the top of the stairs to rest on);

> 'Fear of failing or of becoming acutely breathless can result in loss of confidence and total withdrawal from activity.'

▶ energy conservation—working out the times of day when people feel that they have the most energy, and planning activities around those times (looking at ways in which people can prioritise activities and conserve energy);

▶ offering advice on positioning and posture to assure maximum comfort and ease of breathing (for example, how to bend from the knees rather than the waist); and

▶ setting realistic goals to achieve a task or activity.

Summary of key points

The key points to be gained from this chapter include:

▶ the experience of being breathlessness is profoundly distressing for people, their families, and health-care professionals (Roberts, Thorne & Pearson 1993);

▶ although people receiving palliative care commonly experience breathlessness, the problem has been underacknowledged and remains difficult to manage (Higginson & McCarthy 1989);

▶ research suggests that medical palliation of breathlessness has an important, but limited, role in managing breathlessness;

▶ a more integrated approach is required—an approach that enables nurses to manage breathlessness holistically;

▶ relevant research and experience in managing chronic breathlessness exists in fields other than nursing—including physiotherapy, occupational therapy, psychology, and counselling;

▶ aspects of these approaches—especially those that address the functional and emotional aspects of breathlessness within a rehabilitative integrated model of care—might also be of value in managing breathlessness in a palliative setting; and

▶ research has shown that such an approach results in better patient experience and improvement in other outcomes—such as distress and functional capacity (Corner, Plant & Warner 1995; Corner et al. 1996; Bredin et al. 1999).

Conclusion

Breathlessness is an unpleasant and distressing symptom affecting every aspect of a person's life and wellbeing. Fears of being unable to breathe properly, or of dying during a panic attack, are common, and can be a source of perpetual anxiety for both patient and family.

Unlike pain (which, in the majority of cases, can be relieved), breathlessness in advanced cancer is unlikely to be reversed entirely. People therefore need support and encouragement to learn to develop ways of coping and living with the problem, while adjusting to the inevitable loss and change that such a symptom brings.

It is extremely distressing to observe a person fighting for breath, and it is therefore important to consider how practitioners' own fears and feelings might affect their caring. Peer supervision is essential, alongside careful evaluation of strategies used with patients.

Management of breathlessness requires a multidisciplinary approach. There is much that can be achieved—not only in terms of relieving the distress and anxiety caused by breathlessness, but also in terms of providing interventions that promote general wellbeing and enhance the quality of life.

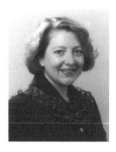

Davina Porock

Dr Davina Porock was a registered nurse and senior lecturer in Cancer Care Nursing, University of Hull (Yorkshire, UK). She has worked in cancer and palliative-care nursing since 1987 in both community and acute settings. Davina's interest in research grew through her master's degree at Curtin University and her doctoral studies at Edith Cowan University (both Perth, Western Australia). Since then, she has worked in Britain at the University of Hull as a senior lecturer in cancer-care nursing, and in the USA as an associate professor, Sinclair School of Nursing, University of Missouri-Columbia. Davina's research in cancer-related fatigue and its clinical management has developed through ongoing collaborative work with nurses in clinical practice, thus ensuring that theory development and research is grounded in the realities of nursing practice.

Chapter 10

Fatigue

Davina Porock

Introduction

The problem of fatigue is prevalent in all chronic and life-limiting illness, and this symptom and the way it affects people's wellbeing is therefore an important focus of palliative care. In particular, in people suffering from cancer, fatigue is the most prevalent symptom throughout the trajectory of the illness, and has been prominent in oncology nursing research and practice for many years (Mooney et al. 1991; Ropka et al. 2002; Stetz et al. 1995). To patients and their families, fatigue in the advanced stages

'In palliative care, fatigue is the most prevalent symptom.'

of chronic illness can be an overwhelming symptom impairing quality of life through its impact on:

- ▶ sense of wellbeing;
- ▶ daily performance;
- ▶ activities of daily living;
- ▶ relationships with family and friends;

▶ mood; and
▶ adherence to treatment.

Although this chapter focuses on patients with advanced cancer, the content is relevant to the care of people with other chronic and terminal conditions. The principal message of this chapter is that a single approach cannot manage fatigue. Fatigue is a total experience affecting a person physically, mentally, emotionally, and socially. Its aetiology is similarly multifactorial, and a comprehensive approach to nursing management is thus required.

What is fatigue?

Fatigue is a subjective feeling, and it is difficult to provide a succinct, undisputed definition. However, fatigue includes some or all of:
▶ *physical symptoms*: tiredness, weakness, malaise, lack of energy, lethargy, somnolence, exhaustion, aching body;
▶ *psychological symptoms*: boredom, lack of motivation, and depression; and
▶ *cognitive symptoms*: inability to concentrate.

Each of these groups of symptoms is considered in more detail later in the chapter.

The lack of a formal definition of fatigue in the literature means that it is difficult to compare research findings, and this hinders development of a theoretical understanding of fatigue as a clinical phenomenon. The lack of a definition also results in poor communication among members of the health team, and between researchers and practitioners, which creates difficulty for clinical decision-making. For example, it is difficult to judge an expected (or 'acceptable') level of fatigue at a particular stage in a terminal illness (Glaus et al. 1996).

Despite the difficulties in establishing a formally accepted definition, some useful descriptions and guidelines have been offered.

Piper (1993, p. 280) suggested that: '. . . in contrast to tiredness, subjective fatigue is perceived as unusual abnormal or excessive whole-body tiredness, disproportionate to, or unrelated to activity or exertion'.

And Carpenito (1995, p. 98) suggested that fatigue is: '. . . an overwhelming, sustained sense of exhaustion and decreased capacity for physical and mental work that is not relieved by rest'.

An important step forward in the recognition of fatigue as an important symptom deserving of attention was the inclusion of new diagnostic criteria for cancer-related fatigue in the International Classification of Disease (ICD-10) (see Box, page 139). The importance of this listing of diagnostic criteria is that fatigue can be more easily recorded for morbidity statistics.

Prevalence of fatigue

Due to variations in definitions and differences in methods of collecting statistics (in terms of demographics, disease stage, and treatment factors), reports in the literature of the prevalence of fatigue in the cancer population vary widely from 40% to 100%.

To determine the prevalence of fatigue in palliative-care patients (as distinct from the 'background' fatigue level in the general community), Stone et al. (1999) compared a group of palliative-care patients with a control group of volunteers without cancer. 'Severe fatigue' was defined as fatigue greater than that experienced by 95% of the 'normal' group. It was found that 75% of the palliative-care group had severe fatigue by this stringent criterion. Fatigue in the palliative-care group was not related to age, sex, diagnosis, presence or site of metastasis, anaemia, dose of opioid or steroid, most haematological and biochemical indices, nutritional status, or mood. In the palliative-care group,

---

ICD-10 criteria for cancer-related fatigue

Fatigue is said to be present if:

A. The following symptoms have been present every day or nearly every day during the same two-week period.

Significant fatigue, diminished energy, or increased need to rest disproportionate to any recent change in activity level; plus five or more of the following:

- complaints of generalised weakness or limb heaviness;
- diminished concentration or attention;
- decreased motivation or interest to engage in unusual activities;
- insomnia or hypersomnia;
- experience of sleep as unrefreshing or nonrestorative;
- perceived need to struggle to overcome inactivity;
- marked emotional reactivity (sadness, frustration, or irritability) to feeling fatigued;
- difficulty completing daily tasks attributed to feeling fatigued;
- perceived problems with short-term memory; and
- postexertional fatigue lasting several hours.

B. The symptoms cause clinically significant distress or impairment in social, occupational or other important areas of functioning.

C. There is evidence from the history, physical examination, or laboratory findings that the symptoms are a consequence of cancer or cancer therapy.

D. The symptoms are not primarily a consequence of comorbid psychiatric disorders such as major depression, somatisation disorder, somatoform disorder, or delirium.

Portenoy & Itri (1999)

severity of fatigue was associated with pain and dyspnoea, whereas, in the controls, it was associated with anxiety and depression. Fatigue in palliative-care patients was thus *more prevalent* and *more severe* than in the general community, and the *influencing factors differed.*

Physical sensations of fatigue

Although the physical sensations of fatigue in cancer patients are generally similar to those experienced by healthy people, weakness and a need for more sleep are much more severe (Glaus, Crow & Hammond 1996). These findings have been supported by many other studies (Ferrell et al. 1996; Smets et al. 1996; Stone et al. 1999; Winningham et al. 1994).

Other clinical manifestations of physical fatigue have been described. These include (Nail & Winningham 1993; Winningham et al. 1994):

- loss of physical performance;
- inability to complete tasks;
- decreased strength;
- tachycardia with exertion and anaemia; and
- increased shortness of breath.

Dyspnoea and fatigue are common coexisting symptoms in advanced cancer, with the intensity of dyspnoea being significantly related to fatigue, as well as to lung involvement, vital capacity, and anxiety (Bruera et al. 2000).

It is well known that advanced cancer patients are polysymptomatic, and research is confirming the interaction between physical and psychological symptoms.

Psychological and affective sensations of fatigue

Psychological or affective symptoms of fatigue include a lack of energy, loss of motivation, depression, sadness, and anxiety. There is often a sense that willpower and 'fighting spirit' are absent, and that personal resources that have kept a person going in the past are depleted (Juenger 2002).

Cancer patients often feel that 'there is no energy left'. Such patients have been shown to be more aware of the debilitating affective sensations of fatigue than healthy people experience with 'normal fatigue', thus highlighting the emotional and psychological burden that cancer adds to the perception of fatigue (Glaus, Crow & Hammond 1996). Patients can struggle to 'find meaning' in the fatigue experienced, and 'finding meaning' is an important aspect of psychological wellbeing (Krishnasamy 2000).

Reduced motivation and the inability to start a task are indicators of psychological fatigue (Juenger 2002), as well as being indicators of depression and anxiety (Richardson & Ream 1996; Smets et al. 1996). Studies have noted that approximately 47% of new admissions to a palliative-care service are diagnosed as depressed by the palliative-care team (Stromgren et al. 2002). The difficulty of separating fatigue from depression has led to the development of several research instruments to distinguish between the two. Although it is logical to propose that depression resulting from the stress of confronting life-threatening disease can cause feelings of fatigue, it is also logical to assert that depression can result from the lifestyle disruption caused by fatigue. From a theoretical point of view the distinction might seem irrelevant. However, from a practical perspective, it is sometimes necessary to make decisions about appropriate intervention for distressing symptoms. Clearly, the interaction between mood and fatigue complicates the diagnosis and treatment of cancer-related fatigue.

'The interaction between mood and fatigue complicates the diagnosis and treatment of cancer-related fatigue.'

Cognitive sensations of fatigue

The third major group of fatigue sensations relates to cognition. Examples of cognitive fatigue are an inability to think clearly and difficulty in making decisions. Such effects of fatigue on cognition were identified in 12% of inpatients with advanced cancer (Glaus, Crow & Hammond 1996). In that study, it was of interest that cognitive fatigue was actually reported more frequently by healthy subjects. However, for them, it was seen as a single issue that would be easily resolved, rather than as part of a whole-body experience.

Cognitive impairments and fatigue have been linked in many other studies with cancer patients, although the mechanism underlying the connection is unclear (Winningham et al. 1994).

What causes fatigue?

The factors that cause or promote fatigue are not yet well understood, and it is likely that many mechanisms play a role (Miaskowski & Portenoy 1998). The discussion that follows considers the possible roles of: (i) stress and the central nervous system; (ii) disease-related and treatment-related factors; and (iii) individual differences. This is followed by outlines of two comprehensive models of fatigue that draw the various theories together.

Stress and central nervous system factors

In 'normal' fatigue, energy is used up to meet the demands of activity and work. Sufficient rest and nourishment are usually sufficient to restore energy reserves and return the individual to normal activity. The early hypotheses about cancer-related fatigue were extensions of this simple understanding of 'normality'. It was suggested that prolonged, extreme stress (Aistars 1987; Selye 1974) and/or excessive demands on energy related to the tumour (Kaempfer & Lindsey 1986) explained fatigue in cancer patients. Rest and reduced stress were insufficient to alleviate fatigue in such people.

In the late 1980s, a neurophysiological model was incorporated into fatigue theory. The central nervous system regulates natural circadian rhythms, and this was thought to play a part in the cause and perception of fatigue. Funk, Tornquist and Champagne (1989) proposed that the brain, psyche, and spinal cord formed the central component of this model, and that the nerves and skeletal muscles comprised the peripheral component. The model proposed that impairment of the central component causes lack of motivation, impaired spinal cord transmission, and malfunction in the hypothalamic region. Disruption to sleep patterns and a feeling that sleep is not refreshing or restorative (Portenoy & Itri 1999) were taken as being manifestations of abnormal function in the central nervous system. However, the model had difficulties in palliative-care patients because the processes of the central nervous system, and problems with sleep and loss of motivation, are compounded by the concomitant use of analgesics, hypnotics, antiemetics, and anticonvulsants, all of which affect central nervous system function.

Disease-related and treatment-related factors

Imbalances in the intake, expenditure, distribution, and use of energy could be due to a competition between the tumour and the person for energy (Richardson 1995). Changes in energy availability and expenditure present as anorexia, ca-chexia, and alterations in metabolism (Kaempfer & Lindsey 1986; Lindsey 1986).

Different cancers have different patterns and severity of fatigue. Many studies have shown that lung cancer causes particularly severe and intense fatigue symptoms.

Conventional treatment for cancer includes surgery, radiation therapy, chemotherapy, and biotherapy in various combinations. All of these can cause fatigue.

Surgery makes many demands on the body through anaesthesia, pain, and narcotic and psychoactive drugs (Rhoten 1982), together with enforced bed rest, dehydration, and missed meals (Oberle, Allen & Lynkowski 1994). In addition, surgery is often the principal mode of diagnosis, and the anxiety and fear associated with the lead up to surgery also take a toll on energy resources. A cancer patient can undergo several episodes of surgery during the course of the illness, and this contributes to the total impact of fatigue.

The incidence of fatigue in the population of persons receiving *radiotherapy* has been reported as 65–100%, depending on cancer type and location of the tumour (Nail & Jones 1995). The prevalence and severity of fatigue can vary during and following courses of radiotherapy treatment. Fatigue is usually intermittent at the commencement of treatment and gradually increases as treatment progresses, with afternoon and evening being the most common times for patients to feel fatigued (Love et al. 1989; Nail & Jones 1995; Winningham et al. 1994). The subjective feelings of fatigue can continue for at least three months following the completion of treatment (Irvine et al. 1991; Irvine et al. 1994; Nail & Jones 1995).

Palliative radiotherapy is a common treatment. However, the benefits must be weighed against the potential side-effects, such as fatigue. A study of quality of life during palliative radiation for non-small cell lung cancer (Langendijk et al. 2001) showed a gradual increase in fatigue over the course of the treatment. Although palliative radiation produced improvement in a number of symptoms, there was a decline in measures of quality of life. Emotional function remained comparatively high during palliative radiation, perhaps due to the maintenance of hope, but this also declined following completion of radiation. It is apparent that tumour response alone is not an adequate indicator of quality of life.

A gradual decline in quality of life and an increase in symptom distress, particularly fatigue, also occurs with *chemotherapy* (Muers & Round 1993). Indeed, 80% of all cancer patients report moderate to severe fatigue during such treatment (Richardson & Ream 1996). The side-effects of nausea and anorexia certainly contribute to fatigue associated with chemotherapy, and the associated problems of nausea and vomiting and nutritional depletion add to the energy imbalance.

In addition to the factors noted above as contributing to fatigue in radiation therapy and chemotherapy, cell death and necrosis in the tumour releases metabolites. An accumulation of such metabolites has been established as a cause of fatigue (Simonson 1971).

Radiotherapy and chemotherapy often have a long-lasting effect on energy resources, and fatigue is therefore likely to be more severe in palliative-care patients due to the cumulative effects of treatment, disease progression, and the sedentary effects of other medication used for various distressing symptoms.

Biotherapy is also associated with fatigue. Biotherapy includes the use of interleukin-2, interferons, tumour necrosis factor, and colony-stimulating factors. Fatigue is such an important side-effect of biotherapy that it can be a dose-limiting factor. Physical and cognitive fatigue are particularly affected by biotherapy (Johnson et al. 1988), and is probably worse in older patients receiving a combination of biotherapy agents (Brophy & Sharp 1991; Wheeler 1997).

Personal and environmental factors

Different people react to, and cope with, the diagnosis, treatment, and terminal phase of illness in different ways. This reflects their different personalities, learned coping mechanisms, and domestic situations. Change is stressful, and can lead to sleep disruption and appetite loss, even in healthy individuals. Stress from family conflict and the making of life-changing decisions can contribute to feelings of fatigue, listlessness, and depression.

As previously noted, depression is associated with fatigue, and it has been estimated that 15–25% of cancer patients are affected by depression (Henriksson, Isometsa & Hietanen 1995). Although it is difficult to differentiate between fatigue causing depression and depression causing fatigue, there is anecdotal evidence that fatigued patients are less sad when treated with antidepressants, although no less tired. This has been supported by a large trial of the antidepressant paroxetine which showed that cancer patients on the antidepressant had significantly less depression than those who received a placebo, although there was little difference in levels of fatigue between the two groups (Morrow 2001).

Fatigue and depression are strong predictors of quality of life in cancer, and depression in the patient is more likely than fatigue to cause emotional distress in family caregivers (Hopwood & Stephens 2000). It is therefore important to manage depression, not only for the comfort of the patient, but also to reduce distress in the family.

'Fatigue and depression are strong predictors of quality of life in cancer.'

A strong association between fatigue and depression has also been revealed in cancer *survivors*, with those experiencing fatigue having higher levels of clinical depressive symptoms (Bower et al. 2000). Depression can thus be a disabling problem in cancer survivors as well as in cancer patients—eliciting anxiety, sadness, and fatigue. Nearly all patients with comorbid depression experience longer length of stay, higher hospital readmission rates, and higher medical costs than cancer patients experiencing no depression (Stoudemire, Bronheim & Wise 1998).

Antidepressants are not the only treatment for depression. If fatigue is treated with exercise, mood lifts and there is an improvement in the sense of wellbeing (Byrne & Byrne 1993; Cramer, Neiman & Lee 1991; Doyne et al. 1987; Berger & Owen 1992).

Nutrition is obviously an important aspect of energy production, and in palliative-care patients this is impaired by anorexia, nausea and vomiting, diarrhoea, and bowel obstruction. Furthermore, nutritional intake can be affected by malabsorption of nutrients as, for example, if there have been changes in gut mucosa following chemotherapy. In addition, the tumour competes for nutrients and energy, and patients often have a hypermetabolic state due to tumour growth, infection, fever, and dyspnoea (Watenabe & Bruera 1996).

Lethargy and apathy due to poor nutrition are often associated with cancer (Mays 1995). When weight loss exceeds 10% of normal body weight, mental performance begins to be affected, with disruption to cognitive function being manifested as lethargy, helplessness, hypochondria, and memory loss (Mays 1995; Shippee, Friedl & Kramer 1994).

Increasing nutritional intake increases body weight, increases respiratory and muscle strength, and can reduce breathlessness (Luce & Luce 2001). It would be logical to assume that this would also reduce fatigue and improve the ability to attend to the activities of daily living. Furthermore, it is well known that low levels of micronutrients—such as magnesium and iron—cause fatigue. Attention to supplementation of basic nutrients requires attention in addressing the problem of fatigue.

Theories of fatigue

Winningham (1999), an exercise physiologist and a registered nurse, focused her theory of fatigue on the 'deconditioning effect' of serious illness, its multiple symptoms, and its treatment. This 'deconditioning effect' was a result of patients reducing their activity levels when they became ill. Winningham suggested that a balance between rest and activity was needed to prevent spiralling loss of physical function in cancer patients. This model works particularly well when testing exercise and activity for prevention of fatigue (see Box, page 146).

Piper's integrated fatigue model (Piper, Lindsey & Dodd 1987) is probably the most comprehensive model to have been proposed. This model uses the notion of 'disruption' to the normal patterning of the individual, both internally and

Winningham's theory of fatigue

Winningham's theory of fatigue rests on ten principles:

1. Too much rest as well as too little rest contributes to increased feelings of fatigue.

2. Too little activity as well as too much activity contributes to increased feelings of fatigue.

3. A relative balance between activity and rest promotes restoration; an imbalance promotes fatigue and deconditioning.

4. Deconditioning is the adaptive energetic response whereby an organism's biological work potential is decreased over time.

5. Everyday energy expenditure in activity is the most potent known regulator of the body's energy systems ('use it or lose it').

6. Any symptom or condition that contributes to decreased activity will lead to deconditioning-increased fatigue and decreased functional status.

7. Any intervention that provides relief of a symptom or condition and that contributes to decreased activity can simultaneously serve to mitigate fatigue and promote functioning, provided that intervention does not have a sedating or catabolic effect.

8. The experience of fatigue potentiates distress associated with other symptoms and conditions.

9. The experience of other symptoms and conditions potentiates the feelings of fatigue.

10. Deconditioning and perceived fatigue interact to make every aspect of life more stressful and negatively affect quality of life, thus contributing to increased suffering.

Adapted from Winningham (1999)

externally. Piper's model integrates biochemical, physiological, and behavioural processes to suggest causes for the perception and impact of fatigue (see Figure 10.1, page 147).

How can nurses help effectively?

Ordinary fatigue or tiredness usually indicates overwork, stress or, perhaps, temporary illness. This kind of fatigue is acute and is usually relieved by a good night's sleep and a reduction in stress and tension or, at worst, a few days in bed. But rest alone does not relieve the fatigue experienced by people with advanced cancer. It is a chronic problem that leads to abstinence from activity and, often, a stress reaction (Piper, Lindsey & Dodd 1987). Although rest is the most

Integrated Fatigue Model©

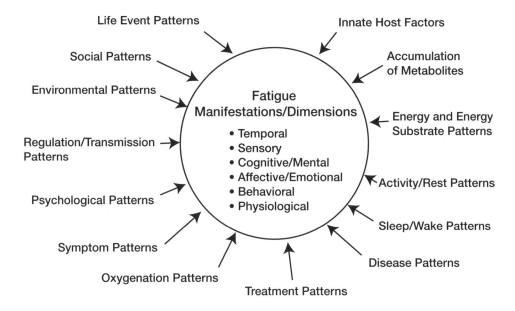

Figure 10.1 Piper's integrated fatigue model
Copyright 1997; reprinted with permission of Barbara Piper

frequently recommended intervention (Nail et al. 1991; Richardson & Ream 1996) it is now accepted that unnecessary bed rest can contribute significantly to the development of fatigue and weakness, resulting in rapid and potentially irreversible losses in energy and functioning (Winningham 1991). In fact, Winningham (1991) warns against the 'dangers of bed rest'.

Strategies to help patients manage their fatigue and obtain the most out of life are discussed below.

Communication and education

Talking about fatigue in very important for patients and family members. Fatigue is a real symptom, and is not the same as being lazy. People cannot just snap out of it! Fatigue might represent a very real fear of death or the dying process. It is important for the person to be able to express these concerns and to know that there are some positive steps to be taken, as well as difficult decisions to make as the end of life approaches. Nurses can help by:

▶ asking the person to describe how he or she feels, and how the fatigue is affecting daily life;

- encouraging the person to keep a diary to identify patterns in fatigue, noting when things are better or worse;
- teaching people to rate their fatigue (0–10 scale) so that they learn to plan activities and rest; and
- taking the time to discuss options for planning a change of focus as death approaches.

Cancer-related fatigue takes away the capacity to do the things that patients and families want to do or need to do. Control over life events diminishes, further affecting the person's quality of life. An essential part of nursing care for fatigue includes returning some of that control.

Fatigue often receives only fleeting mention in the standard cancer publications available to patients and families. Education can reduce anxiety because it minimises the fear associated with poor or no preparation (Porock 1995). Patients who are not aware that their treatment can cause fatigue might attribute the symptom to cancer progression, and such a misapprehension can cause unnecessary distress (Peck & Boland 1977). Providing strategies to manage fatigue returns control to patients and families.

Giving information is thus a positive way to return some control to the patient. Nurses can explain that fatigue is an expected occurrence in advanced cancer and that the afflicted person is not alone in the experience. Nurses can discuss the causes of fatigue—in particular the effects and side-effects of treatment, and the impact of stress and depression. This not only contributes to the nurse's professional assessment but also helps the person and his or her family understand why fatigue is worse at certain times.

> 'Giving information is thus a positive way to return some control to the patient.'

It is important for the person and his or her family to understand the reasons for the fatigue being experienced because this will help them to manage the fatigue more effectively. An important part of the education strategy is to determine the variations in fatigue during the course of a day and with particular activities.

Topics for educational materials should include:
- What is fatigue?
- What causes fatigue?
- How can fatigue be controlled?
- What are the dangers of bed rest or a sedentary lifestyle?
- How can time be managed with fatigue?
- What exercise or activity should be undertaken?

▶ What is the best nutritional advice?
▶ How can breathlessness be managed?
▶ How can pain and other symptoms be managed?
▶ What is anaemia and how can it affect fatigue?

There is a great deal of information on the Internet for patients with cancer. Although the focus of this information is usually on fatigue during curative treatment, the ideas can be modified and adapted easily as the patient's abilities and desire for intervention change. Two particularly useful websites are maintained by the Oncology Nursing Society (ONS 2002).

Balancing activity and rest

Given the type of information presented above, the patient and family will probably be able to think of some strategies for planning rest and activity that are in line with the things they think are important. The nurse plays an important role in helping the family find that balance.

Rest alone cannot fix fatigue, but it is a part of the solution. Finding a balance between activity and rest ensures that the energy that is available is used most effectively. Patients have things that must be done, such as keeping medical and nursing appointments, undertaking the activities of daily living, attending to dressings, and organising family matters. Individual people also have particular things they want to do. Things have varying importance depending on time and circumstances. Prioritising is essential, as is the art of compromise. But when all the things that need to be done use up the limited energy available, a plan is required. Skalla and Lacasse (1992) refer to such a plan as an 'energy bank'. The idea is that 'deposits' can be made through rest, extra nutrition, or exercise, whereas 'debits' are drawn out for activities that require energy.

Exercise and activity are vital aspects of fatigue management, and these should be encouraged, allowing for the capacity of the patient. This can vary from bed or chair exercises to fitness training. One study found that patients

'Rest alone cannot fix fatigue, but it is a part of the solution.'

with advanced cancer who volunteered for a month-long exercise program were able to achieve more, and felt happier and more hopeful (Porock et al. 2000).

Exercise programs should consider the following (Winningham 1999):

▶ *status of the individual*: exercise should be tailored to age, gender, condition, risk factors, disease, and treatment;
▶ *type of exercise*: rhythmic, repetitive movement of large muscle groups is helpful—walking, swimming, cycling, dancing, stretching;

▶ *intensity*: exercise should never be so strenuous that the person is out of breath;

▶ *frequency*: for a walking program or some other moderate activity, several days per week is sufficient; for very gentle exercise, such as stretching, a few minutes two or three times a day is beneficial; and

▶ *duration*: start with what the person can do comfortably and work up *very* gradually from there.

Sleep is essential to health and restoration. The physical and emotional distress of illness frequently disturbs sleep, and hospitalisation alters the usual bedtime rituals (such as locking-up the house or having a bedtime drink). Medications might have altered natural sleep patterns. All of these things can mean that it is difficult to get to sleep, and that the sleep that is taken is not restorative.

'Sleep is essential to health and restoration. The physical and emotional distress of illness frequently disturbs sleep.'

Many patients nap during the day. However, this can further disrupt the circadian rhythms and interfere with night-time sleep. Winningham (1999) has suggested 'power-naps' only. These should be approximately 20 minutes long. The timing of naps is also important, with naps taken late in the day causing the most disruption to night-time sleep. Another barrier to good sleep can be polypharmacy (see below, page 151).

Some suggestions to promote sleep include the following:

▶ determine usual sleep patterns and re-establish bed-time rituals;

▶ encourage only short 'power naps' of about 20 minutes; have an alarm clock or someone to wake the person;

▶ find alternatives to naps (such as an energy-boosting snack, guided imagery, exercise or activity, or a change of activity); and

▶ try complementary therapies at bedtime (for example, aromatherapy, massage, or acupuncture).

The pharmacological approach to fatigue management is limited. The stimulant drugs that have been used are commonly associated with the management of attention-deficit and hyperactivity disorders. They can elevate mood, promote wellbeing, and improve concentration. However the side-effects can include anxiety, insomnia, agitation, and feelings of nervousness. High doses have been known to cause nightmares, paranoia, and cardiac complications. Caffeine can be used as a stimulant, and corticosteroids can improve a sense of wellbeing, although none of these drugs is without side-effects. Possible pharmacological options for managing fatigue include:

▶ methylphenidate (Ritalin);
▶ dextro-amphetamine (Dexedrine);
▶ caffeine; and
▶ corticosteroids.

Polypharmacy can also be a problem, particularly in the elderly and those who have multiple symptoms. One of the most beneficial interventions that can be undertaken with a patient with cancer is to take the time to sort out the medication regimen, with a view to reducing medications that overlap or clash, and introducing an administration regimen that fits with meals and other activities of daily living. This takes time, and requires consultation with the doctors (and possibly a pharmacist), but it is time well spent. In such a review, nurses can:

▶ assess all medication use and check for drug actions (and interactions) that could exacerbate fatigue or related symptoms (nausea, constipation, anorexia, sedation);
▶ develop a medication administration plan to encourage adherence to medication regimen; and
▶ consider complementary approaches to pain management (relaxation, massage, imagery) to reduce the need for sedating analgesics.

Time management is another important aspect of balancing activity and rest. At first, delegating tasks to other family members seems like the easiest aspect of fatigue management. However, many people find that loss of tasks represents their decline, and find this distressing. Rearranging activities requires an understanding of the individual's fatigue pattern and emphasises the need for good assessment and patient understanding of the problem. Useful approaches include:

▶ using a diary to identify appropriate fatigue patterns; trying to schedule activities for times of higher energy;
▶ taking time to set and prioritise goals; compromising on the time spent in an activity might be better than not participating at all;
▶ saving energy for desirable activities;
▶ reducing the time and frequency of health-related physical interventions (for example, ensuring adequate home equipment for showering; using dressing materials that can be left for several days rather than those that require daily dressings);
▶ managing health-related appointments (for example, assessing whether appointments are necessary, and whether a telephone consultation be sufficient; coordinating appointments so that the minimum amount of time is spent in travelling); and

▶ anticipating that nausea or anxiety may be associated with treatment or other visits, thus increasing fatigue.

Fatigue at the end of life

Increasing fatigue and sleepiness is often a sign that the end of life is near. If fatigue has been actively managed with exercise, nutrition, hydration, and balanced stimulation and rest, there comes a time when a decision to stop active treatment must be made and the focus shifted to supporting the patient through the natural decline towards death. A decision to discontinue active fatigue management must be made with the patient, and comes most easily when nurses listen to what the patient and family want. The desire for intervention, and the priorities that patients and families place on particular symptoms requiring intervention, will change. Nurses must remain sensitive to such changes in desires as part of being skilled in fatigue management.

> 'Increasing fatigue and sleepiness is often a sign that the end of life is near.'

Conclusion

Cancer-related fatigue is a whole-person experience. Management of fatigue, like symptom management in general, cannot be achieved if fatigue is addressed as an isolated symptom. The fundamental principle of holistic management must remain foremost in all symptom management. The effects and side-effects of all interventions—nursing, medical, and allied health—must be weighed before proceeding, and their various impacts require regular and frequent review. Assessing and prioritising all distressing symptoms is therefore of paramount importance in managing fatigue in people receiving palliative care.

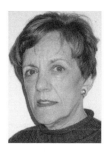

Beth Bailey

Beth Bailey is a registered nurse and midwife with postgraduate qualifications in rehabilitation studies. During her postgraduate studies, Beth developed a strong interest in using clinically based research to improve nursing practice and patient outcomes. She has extensive experience in palliative care at Caritas Christi Hospice, Kew (Victoria, Australia) as a clinical teacher and project officer. More recently, Beth has been involved in palliative-care research at the School of Postgraduate Nursing, University of Melbourne (Victoria, Australia).

Chapter 11

Constipation

Beth Bailey

Introduction

Constipation is a common and distressing condition for people living with advanced cancer and end-stage disease. Nursing practice in managing this problem varies across and within settings of care. This chapter focuses on a best practice approach to the management of constipation in palliative care, and provides an overview of constipation management in the context of caring for adults at the end of life.

Definition and prevalence of constipation

There are many definitions of constipation available, most of which include a reference to infrequent, difficult or incomplete bowel evacuation. Constipation is essentially a change from the frequency of bowel movements that is normal for the individual concerned with an associated more difficult passage of stool. Constipation is more common in patients with advanced cancer than in those with other terminal diseases (Fallon & O'Neill, 2000). Of patients admitted to

British hospices about 50% complain of being constipated (Sykes, 1993; Fallon and Walsh, 1998).

Causes of constipation

Constipation can be caused by a number of factors including decreased mobility, poor nutrition, medications, and bowel obstruction. Ageing is also a predisposing factor, and many patients receiving palliative care are elderly. Studies (Miaskowski, 1995; Robinson et al, 2000) have identified constipation as the most troublesome side effect of pain management, and it is especially associated with opioid medication.

Constipation can be classified as *primary* (which is associated with lifestyle factors such as age, diet, and mobility), *secondary* (due to anatomical abnormalities, metabolic or endocrine disturbances or pathological processes) or *iatrogenically induced* (a consequence of the administration of pharmacological agents). In the palliative-care setting constipation is usually associated with a multiplicity of factors: as, for example, an elderly patient with a poor appetite taking opioid analgesia has at least three risk factors for becoming constipated. An extensive list of causes of constipation is given in the Box (page 157), and these should be considered in any assessment to establish the level of risk for constipation for individual patients.

As noted above, opioids are a major cause of constipation. Opioids cause constipation through a variety of mechanisms (O'Mahoney, Coyle & Payne 2001):

◗ by direct action on opioid receptors in the bowel (as well as in the central nervous system);
◗ by decreasing peristalsis in the ileum and colon;
◗ by decreasing intra-intestinal fluid volume as a result of increased fluid absorption;
◗ by increasing sphincter tone; and
◗ by increasing non-propulsive segmental movements of the gut.

Although constipation is a common problem in patients receiving opioids, medical and nursing staff consistently underdiagnose the condition, in both outpatient and inpatient palliative-care settings (Bruera et al. 1994; Bruera 2001).

Consequences of constipation

Constipation is not simply an uncomfortable or distressing symptom. It is a significant condition with a number of potential complications. If undetected and untreated, constipation can have important consequences, especially for

Causes of constipation in palliative care

Malignancy
- directly due to tumour
- intestinal obstruction due to (1) tumour in the bowel wall, (2) external compression by abdominal or pelvic tumour
- spinal cord compression
- hypercalcaemia

Due to secondary effects of disease
- anorexia leading to inadequate food intake
- low fibre diet
- dehydration (due to poor fluid intake, vomiting, sweating, or polyuria)
- confusion (perhaps due to sedation)
- depression
- impaired cognitive function
- cerebral tumour
- decreased abdominal muscle tone

Concurrent disease
- diabetes
- hypokalaemia
- hypothyroidism
- painful ano-rectal conditions
- hernia
- diverticular disease
- colitis

General factors
- inconvenient toilet access and/or suboptimal posture
- fear of incontinence
- lack of privacy (shared accomodation)
- distress through loss of independence (reliance on others for assistance)
- adverse past experiences (inability to access or use toilet facility; past effects of laxative use)

Drugs
- opioids, non steroidal anti-inflammatory drugs (NSAIDS)
- drugs with anticholinergic effects – hyoscine, tricyclic antidepressants, phenothiazines, haloperidol, antiparkinsonian agents
- diuretics
- iron
- anticonvulsants
- antacids (calcium and aluminium compounds)
- antihypertensive agents
- vincristine

Adapted from Sykes (1993)

people receiving palliative care. These complications can be psychological and cognitive (including distress and confusion) or physical (affecting the gastro-

Consequences of constipation

Psychological and cognitive
- distress, anxiety;
- confusion.

Perianal problems
- anal fissure;
- haemorrhoids.

Faecal impaction
- spurious diarrhoea;
- faecal incontinence.

Gastrointestinal symptoms
- anorexia, nausea, vomiting;
- abdominal distension;
- abdominal pain;
- bowel obstruction.

Urinary
- urinary retention;
- urinary tract infections.

Adapted from Burke (1994)

intestinal and urinary systems in particular). A list of some of the potential consequences of constipation is provided in the Box above.

Assessment of constipation

In view of the potential consequences of constipation it is important that the condition be detected and properly assessed. Assessment and planning for optimum bowel care should be an integral part of the initial and ongoing assessment for all palliative care patients in whichever setting they are receiving care.

History and examination

Assessment should not be confined to enquiries about bowel habit. Assessment includes identification of risk factors and symptoms associated with constipation. These risk factors include decreased mobility, anorexia, and certain medications (see above), and symptoms that might indicate constipation including nausea, vomiting, flatulence, abdominal distension, and pain. In a person who is close to death, restlessness might indicate the presence of a full rectum.

A full clinical assessment of constipation includes the following (after Woodruff 1999):

- the pattern of recent bowel movements;
- the pattern of pre-illness bowel movements;
- past history of use of laxatives;
- the use of potentially constipating drugs;
- food intake (especially fibre content);
- fluid intake;
- presence or absence of faeces in the rectum;
- consistency of faeces—soft or hard;
- presence of anal tone and reflex;
- evidence of normal or abnormal sacral nerve root sensation;
- presence of predisposing factors for constipation;
- overall disease status and prognosis.

To avoid excessive demands on the patient, medical and nursing assessment of constipation should be coordinated, including clear and shared documentation. Lack of coordination can mean unnecessary over-questioning and examination of the patient—including invasive assessments such as rectal examination. Indeed, rectal examination should be in response to findings from history and examination, rather than being a routine procedure.

'To avoid excessive demands on the person, medical and nursing assessment of constipation should be coordinated, including clear and shared documentation.'

If constipation is suspected, a more thorough physical examination is required. This will usually include:

- assessment of the mouth for possible causes of reduced intake of food and fluids (such as ulceration or ill-fitting dentures);
- inspection of the abdomen for distension;
- abdominal palpation, which might reveal a palpable colon and faecal mass;
- assessment of bowel sounds, which might be diminished, slow, or absent;
- inspection of the anus for haemorrhoids, fissure, or faecal fluid leakage (bearing in mind that patients with faecal impaction sometimes complain of 'diarrhoea' as a result of passing faecal fluid as an overflow phenomenon); and
- rectal examination, which might reveal hard stools in the rectum, or an empty rectum if impaction is higher in the bowel.

An abdominal x-ray might be required to aid diagnosis, especially if high impaction is suspected.

An important issue in relation to bowel assessment in persons suffering from a terminal illness is the high incidence of cognitive impairment in such patients (Breitbart et al. 1995). This is of importance in two respects.

▶ In this group of people, diagnosis and treatment of constipation is very important because it has been recognised as a cause of cognitive failure, particularly in the elderly. Relief of constipation might therefore assist in cognitive function.

▶ Impaired cognitive function might, however, make diagnosis of constipation more difficult. In the community, members of the family or other carers might be able to assist with the history. However, in a residential-care or hospice setting, obtaining an adequate history of constipation may be dependent on accurate observation and documentation using appropriate assessment tools.

Assessment tools

In addition to clinical assessment of constipation as part of general history-taking and examination, specialised assessment tools have been developed. These facilitate an individualised scientific approach to the assessment and prevention of constipation using relevant assessment data (McMillan & Williams 1989; Burke 1994).

In palliative care all patients will be at risk of becoming constipated and any assessment tool used must reflect this. It is essential that assessment tools are valid and reliable, and are quick and easy to use in a range of care settings. The aim will always be to achieve an accurate and consistent record of an individual's bowel status.

Assessment documentation should be suitable for patient self-completion whilst enabling health-care professionals to differentiate easily between the severity of the constipation symptoms being described and recorded.

The documentation must include record of:

▶ frequency of bowel movements
▶ size and consistency of stool
▶ alteration in the amount of gas passed rectally
▶ abdominal distension or bloating
▶ urge but inability to pass stool
▶ rectal pain or fullness

The addition of the Bristol stool-form scale to an assessment tool may facilitate an accurate and consistent recording of bowel status, especially when different carers are completing documentation. Ideally the same assessment documentation will be used for each individual across all care settings.

The Bristol Stool Form Scale

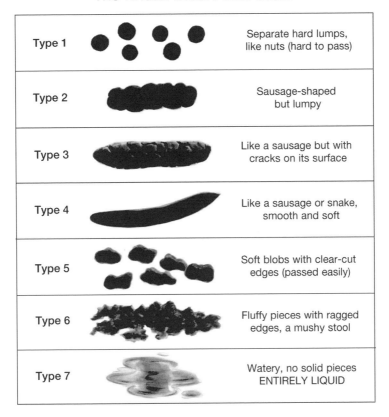

Type 1	Separate hard lumps, like nuts (hard to pass)
Type 2	Sausage-shaped but lumpy
Type 3	Like a sausage but with cracks on its surface
Type 4	Like a sausage or snake, smooth and soft
Type 5	Soft blobs with clear-cut edges (passed easily)
Type 6	Fluffy pieces with ragged edges, a mushy stool
Type 7	Watery, no solid pieces ENTIRELY LIQUID

Figure 11.1 The Bristol stool form scale
Reproduced by kind permission of Dr KW Heaton, Reader in Medicine at the University of Bristol. © 2000 Norgine Ltd.

Summary of assessment

An effective bowel care plan is based on a thorough assessment which includes:

- obtaining a comprehensive history including the person's preferences for bowel management;
- assessment of the impact of constipation on quality of life;
- physical assessment;
- identification of risk factors;
- accurate documentation; and
- ongoing assessment and evaluation of intervention and personal comfort.

If constipation is absent but risk factors are present, a preventive regimen is commenced. When constipation is present, the findings of the assessment will determine appropriate interventions.

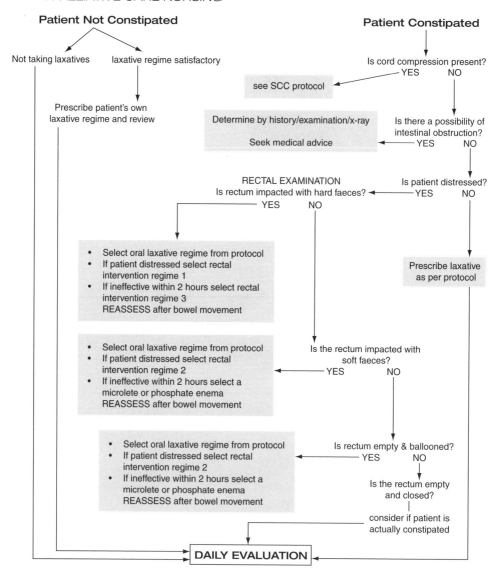

Figure 11.2 Bowel Assessment Flow Chart

Nursing management of constipation
General principles of management

Effective palliative care is essentially the provision of comfort, and includes a preventive approach to symptom management. In the case of constipation, such a preventive regimen will usually involve the dose of laxatives being titrated against the clinical effect. This is primarily because palliative care patients will be taking constipating medications and are unlikely to be able to modify their lifestyle to reduce the risk of becoming constipated. An accurate descriptive bowel record is essential for determining an effective regimen. In addition, an effective plan requires an understanding of the disease process and the resulting changes which occur in the individual. For example, if weakness increases and mobility decreases, and if the person is unable to swallow laxatives, bowel management should not be ignored. It is imperative that the person's bowel needs are continually monitored and the plan adjusted accordingly.

Consultative approach to nursing management

An effective individualised approach to bowel care depends primarily upon the competence of the nursing and medical staff. However, other members of the team have important roles to play. For example, the physiotherapist can advise on positioning to assist defaecation and strategies to increase exercise potential. The occupational therapist can advise on the provision of aids such as rails, commodes, and raised toilet seats. The pharmacist can advise on pharmacological interventions and possible side-effects. The dietician may be able to give advice to help encourage fluid and food intake. Consultation with family and carers is essential if they are to understand the prevention plan.

Diet, fluids, and exercise

The usual preventive measures of increasing fluid intake, dietary fibre, and exercise require extra thought and care in persons receiving palliative care. Nurses should take extra care to:

▶ ensure that fluids are left within easy reach and replenished frequently;
▶ ensure that the food and fluids offered are acceptable and attractive (such as not offering supplements made with milk to a person who does not like milk);
▶ offer fibre in acceptable forms (such as fruit purées and soups);
▶ encourage visitors to assist with meals and fluids;
▶ ensure good control of pain to maximise the person's activity, mobility, eating, and drinking;
▶ ensure that nausea and vomiting are controlled to maximise the opportunities the patient has to eat and drink;
▶ provide a range of activities that encourage mobility (e.g. a walk in the garden).

Above all there should be realistic expectations of the degree to which alterations can be made to fluid and fibre intake and mobility for each individual and hence the effect non-pharmacological measures can have in preventing constipation for palliative care patients.

Privacy and positioning

The plan should also include the removal of factors that might inhibit defaecation, such as lack of privacy or poor positioning. Some important points to remember include the following.

▶ The provision of a private environment allows the patient to be able to talk more easily about sensitive and embarrassing subjects.

▶ Shared inpatient facilities can cause delayed toileting. Facilitating the use of the bathroom (rather than pan or commode) can assist in providing an environment more conducive to bowel use.

▶ Whenever possible, the person should be assisted to sit on the toilet rather than a raised seat (because the lower position is more suited to bowel emptying).

▶ Whenever possible, timing of visits to the bathroom should coincide with the person's usual bowel habit.

▶ Whenever possible, the patient should be left undisturbed for as long as s/he requires to achieve a satisfactory bowel movement.

Other non-pharmacological measures

Abdominal massage can be useful when combined with pharmacological therapy, particularly in people who have a neurogenic bowel. However, there is a lack of research into the use of massage in bowel management for palliative-care patients.

Laxatives

It is imperative that nurses have a good working knowledge of the action and side-effects of laxatives.

The aim of laxative therapy is to achieve comfortable defaecation rather than a particular frequency of evacuation (Fallon & O'Neill 2000). To achieve this, the dose of laxatives is titrated against the clinical effect by adding or subtracting an osmotic (for example, macrogols) or a stimulant (for example, senna) until a desirable consistency and frequency of bowel movement is achieved. If the person is receiving opioids, the situation is reassessed each time the dose is increased or decreased to ensure that the laxative dose is adjusted accordingly (see Box, page 165).

It is important that nurses understand the action time of laxatives commonly used in palliative care. Some examples are:

▶ a stimulant laxative such as dantron (co-danthramer standard preparation) as 2 capsules or 10mls suspension at night takes 6–12 hours for onset;
Note: use is restricted to terminally-ill patients and there is a risk for skin irritation and excoriation if stool is in prolonged contact (as in incontinent patients);

Guidelines for bowel management for patients taking opioids or other constipating drugs

- To select the correct laxative, a knowledge is required of the nature of the stools, cause of (or potential cause such as opioid medication) constipation and an understanding of how the different laxatives work. Oral laxatives should be reviewed every 3–4 days using stool consistency and ease of defaecation as guides to *dose titration*. Prescribing outside regimes should be documented in patient notes with reasons.
- Routine practice when ordering opiate medications (including codeine) is to order appropriate laxatives simultaneously.

The most commonly ordered laxatives are:

A. Codanthramer*

Initial dose

1. 10mls Codanthramer at night **or** 2 caps Codanthramer at night

Increasing incrementally to:

2. 10mls Codanthramer twice daily **or** 2 caps Codanthramer twice daily
3. 5mls Codanthramer **strong** twice daily or 2 caps Codanthramer **strong** twice daily.
4. 10mls Codanthramer **strong** twice daily or 4 caps Codanthramer **strong** twice daily.

* due to risk or perianal irritation do not use for patients at risk of urinary or faecal incontinence.

B. Senna tablets plus Lactulose
- senna** (Senokot) 7.5 mg 2–4 tablets; plus
- Lactulose 10 ml at night–30 ml thrice daily

** if colic presents related to senna stop or reduce dose of senna.

C. Movicol
- 1 sachet dissolved in 125ml water daily; increase to 2–3 sachets daily if required.
- Up to 8 sachets daily for up to 3 days for faecal impaction
- Can also be used in conjunction with Codanthramer **or** senna

D. Alternatives
- Bisacodyl 5 mg at night–20 mg twice daily (alternative to Senna)
- Magnesium Hydroxide mixture 25–50ml up to twice daily (alternative to Lactulose)
- Docusate up to 5 capsules daily in divided doses (stimulant and softener)
- Codanthrusate (Codanthramer with docusate) 1–3 caps at night

E. Rectal measures (if necessary):

1. Glycerine suppository $4g \times 2$
2. Bisacodyl suppository $10mg \times 2$ **or** micro-enema
3. Arachis oil enema*** (retained as able) followed by micro-enema or phosphate enema

**** patients with nut allergy should not be given an arachis oil enema*

N.B . All doses should be titrated to patient response to laxative and patients encouraged to self manage their regime.

Based on findings from A Study of the Management of Constipation in Palliative Care Across the Marie Curie Cancer Care Centres (Goodman, 2003a)

- a stimulant laxative such as senna (Senokot) in 7.5 mg tablets or 5.5 mg granules or 10–20 mls at night takes 6–12 hours for onset;
- osmotic laxatives such as macrogols (Movicol 2–3 sachets daily, 4–8 hours for onset).

A useful reference for detailed information about laxatives is *Therapeutic Guidelines: Palliative Care Version 1* (see References, page 364).

> 'It is important for nurses to have an understanding of the mechanism of action and the potential complications of each laxative.'

It is important for nurses to have an understanding of the mechanism of action and the potential complications of each laxative. For example, bulk-forming agents, such as Ispaghula Husk (Fybogel) require a concomitant fluid intake of 1.5–2.0 litres of fluid daily. For patients with terminal illness, it is often very difficult to drink this quantity of liquid, meaning that bulk-forming agents actually exacerbate constipation in such circumstances.

There is significant variation among patients with respect to the acceptability of different laxatives, depending on:
- palatability of the product;
- frequency of cramps or colic experienced as a result of taking the product;
- flatulence and diarrhoea experienced as a result of taking the product.

Issues that need to be considered by nursing staff in the prevention and management of symptoms include:
- Is there a link between certain laxatives and pain?
- Is such pain due to constipation or to side-effects of the laxative?
- Is it advisable to switch to a different opioid less likely to cause constipation?

Patients often prefer preparations in the form of dietary supplements, finding them to be more palatable than even more pills. A mixture of prune, apple, and bran (PAB) (see Box, page 167) is often suitable for people who are able to tolerate a fluid intake of 1500 mL in 24 hours. Other alternatives suggested by patients include syrup of figs and licorice.

Rectal laxatives

Rectal suppositories and enemas are undignified and uncomfortable for many patients, and should therefore not be used routinely. However, they are sometimes necessary for treating faecal impaction and for conditions such as spinal cord compression (Fallon & O'Neill 2001). If faecal impaction can be relieved only by disimpaction, patients should be given appropriate analgesia cover.

Prune, apple, and bran mixture (PAB)

Ingredients:
pitted prunes: 12 tablespoons
apple purée: 9 tablespoons
bran (unprocessed): 15 tablespoons
boiling water: 2 cups

Method and administration:
Purée all together.
Give 2 tablespoons daily on porridge or cereal.

Macrogols (Movicol) have been demonstrated to be effective in the relief of impacation in the elderly (Thacker, 2001) and should be considered as an alternative before manual disimpacation. Rectal intervention is contraindicated in patients with neutropaenia or thrombocytopaenia.

Summary of laxatives

The choice of laxative depends on:
▶ the consistency of the stools;
▶ the underlying cause of constipation;
▶ fluid intake; and
▶ acceptability to the patient.
Categories of laxatives are:
▶ bulk-forming laxatives;
▶ predominantly osmotic agents;
▶ predominantly faecal-softening agents;
▶ predominantly stimulant laxatives;
▶ a combination of the last two.

Assessment should occur after each intervention to maintain symptom control and to assess side-effects of laxatives. A bowel protocol in which assessment relies on 'intervention on the third day if no action' is not acceptable. It does not constitute an individualised approach to symptom management. There is little research evidence to support the use of any specific laxative or combination of laxatives (Goodman 2003b) in palliative care. Protocols and laxative regimes therefore tend to be based on local experience (which may or may not be research/audit based) together with individual patient preferences. It is however essential that laxative prescribing follows an identified protocol with very regular monitoring of the patient's bowel status to ensure management is effective and the prevention of constipation.

Management of neurogenic bowel

A neurogenic bowel can be due to: (i) a spinal cord lesion; or (ii) sacral nerve root lesion. The Box on page 168 lists the signs that can help to differentiate the two.

The aim of bowel care in people with a neurogenic bowel is to evacuate the bowel every one or two days, depending on the person's previous bowel habit. Evacuating the bowel on a regular and frequent basis prevents both constipation and incontinence. The bowel-care plan for people with a neurogenic bowel includes identifying whether the person prefers intervention in the morning or the evening. More details on the appropriate nursing care plan can be found in the Box below.

Management in the patient close to death

In the end stages of a patient's illness, it can be difficult to decide when to cease bowel treatment. If treatment is withdrawn too early, this can result in the person

---

Neurogenic bowel

Spinal cord lesion

Signs
- spastic bowel;
- hypertonic anal sphincter;
- sacral reflexes intact.

Nursing care plan
- adequate fluid intake;
- oral laxatives (avoid laxatives that cause excessive softening);
- rectal suppositories or stimulation leads to increased peristalsis and sphincter relaxation.

Sacral nerve root lesion

Signs
- reduced peristalsis;
- flaccid sphincter;
- sacral reflexes absent.

Nursing care plan
- adequate fluid and fibre intake;
- oral laxatives;
- rectal suppositories (or stimulation can lead to evacuation);
- straining and abdominal massage;
- cholinergic drugs (for example, bethanechol 10 mg, orally, every 8 hours).

Adapted from Woodruff (1999)

experiencing extreme discomfort, distress, and restlessness from a full rectum. Conversely, if a routine bowel regimen is continued for too long, this can cause unnecessary distress to the person and his or her family. A balanced decision has to be made in each individual case. If the person has an urge to defaecate, but is too weak to do so, suppositories or microenemas can be used to evacuate the bowel.

Management in patients with stomas
The general principles of bowel care apply as outlined above. Because no sphincter exists, suppositories need to be held in place with a gloved finger.

Case study
The following case study provides an opportunity to review the principles of a holistic approach to the management of constipation, as outlined in this chapter.

Mrs Ahmed

Presentation
Mrs Ahmed, a 44-year-old Muslim has a diagnosis of ovarian tumour with boney metastases. This has previously required debulking laparotomy and chemotherapy. She has experienced a number of spontaneous fractures that have made her very reluctant to undertake all except the very gentlest of activities. This fear of mobility means that she is virtually confined to a wheelchair or bed. Her family is very supportive and they provide care for her children aged 21, 19, 15, 12, and 10 years.

The purpose of her admission to hospice is to review and implement symptom management for pain, nausea, and constipation whilst attempting to increase her mobility. Mrs Ahmed is able to communicate her fear and embarrassment at the prospect of bowel treatment. In the past she has experienced incontinence following laxatives that were too strong. Her family provides most of her diet which consists mainly of meat, a few vegetables, and rich cakes. They are reluctant to encourage fluids because 'she has never really liked a lot of fluid'. Her medications include analgesics, an antiemetic, an antispasmodic, an anticonvulsant, an antidepressant. and laxatives (combined tablets of Lactulose 10ml and senna 7.5mg, two tablets, twice per day). On the day that Mrs Ahmed is admitted, the only available bed is in a shared room.

Risk-factor assessment
The assessment of Mrs Ahmed in terms of bowel management revealed the following risk factors for constipation:
• the disease process and effects of surgery;

(Continued)

(Continued)

- medications (various);
- psychological and emotional issues;
- sociocultural factors; and
- environmental factors.

Bowel management plan

Using an individualised, evidence-based practice approach to the prevention and management of constipation, the following were included in Mrs Ahmed's plan.

- A private area was provided to take the history, jointly by nurse and doctor. Mrs Ahmed's views and preferences were identified.
- Mrs Ahmed's concerns were taken seriously, and explanations and reassurance were offered to reduce fear and anxiety.
- A female doctor performed the physical assessment, which included abdominal and rectal examination because of the possibility of intestinal obstruction.
- Rectal examination demonstrated a rectum packed with hard faeces. She was distressed at the prospect of rectal laxatives, so was given 2 sachets of Movicol dissolved in 250ml of water initially followed by a further 2 sachets 4 hours later resulting in a satisfactory bowel movement in the early evening.
- She was then started on a laxative regime in accordance with hospice bowel management protocol.
- Dietary risk factors were assessed. She was reassured that she could eat and drink what she wished, and the benefit of increasing her fluid intake was explained. The family members were not criticised for the food they gave to Mrs Ahmed— because they are fulfilling important family responsibilities and cultural practices. An education plan was implemented to help them understand how they could help to alleviate the problem of constipation.
- Immobility risk factors were identified. The physiotherapist and occupational therapist were consulted for strategies to increase positioning for comfort and to facilitate good bowel evacuation. These measures were introduced alongside an activity plan to support a stepped increase in her mobility.
- Accurate descriptive bowel records were maintained using appropriate tools, and these were used to titrate the laxative dose to achieve the right stool consistency.
- Care was taken to reduce laxative dose when her stools were loose rather than stopping laxative completely in order to avoid alternating between constipation and diarrhoea.
- Once Mrs Ahmed became able to use the bathroom without minimal assistance she used the Bristol stool-form scale to show the nurses the consistency of her stools and discuss with them how many laxatives she needed each day.

(Continued)

(Continued)

- Mrs Ahmed was reassured and supported in varying the dose of laxatives she needed on a daily basis to prevent a recurrence of her constipation.
- Mrs Ahmed's medications were reviewed in consultation with the medical staff because most of her medications had the potential to cause constipation.
- Good symptom control was implemented to relieve pain and nausea.

Mrs Ahmed's psychological, emotional, social, and spiritual needs were considered to ensure that the team responded appropriately when Mrs Ahmed and her family indicated that they wanted assistance and support.

- Information and education was provided for the family and carers in response to their expressed fears and anxieties relating to Mrs Ahmed's terminal illness.
- When complex situations arose, the appropriate steps were taken as a result of: (i) nurses using reflective practice; (ii) nurses searching the literature; (iii) nurses holding nursing case conferences; and (iv) discussions in the multidisciplinary team meetings.

Conclusion

This chapter has presented an approach to the management of constipation based on the limited available evidence that can be applied to clinical practice in the palliative-care setting. Constipation is a frequent and distressing problem for patients receiving palliative care, and a successful individualised approach depends upon the competence of the nurse. If management of constipation is based on comprehensive knowledge and directed towards the provision of comfort, the potential to improve quality of life cannot be overestimated.

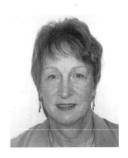

Robyn Millership

Robyn Millership is a registered nurse and midwife with qualifications in intensive care, ward management, and nursing education. Robyn has worked in palliative care as a nurse consultant for many years. Her background is diverse, including clinical practice, administration, and education. Robyn's current position is that of nurse consultant in palliative care at the Peter MacCallum Cancer Institute, Melbourne (Victoria, Australia), and at Caritas Christi Hospice, Melbourne. Robyn is passionately committed to providing excellence in symptom control for patients with a terminal illness. She was a recipient of a Victorian Nurses Care Award in 1994 as recognition of her work in putting into effect her belief that most people can achieve apparently impossible goals if they are provided with optimal symptom control, knowledge, encouragement, and support.

Chapter 12

Nausea and Vomiting

Robyn Millership

Introduction

The palliative-care nurse has a pivotal role as a team member in the alleviation of nausea and vomiting and associated symptoms. The nurse's role in the management of nausea and vomiting requires excellent assessment skills and contemporary knowledge of physiology, current pharmacology, and appropriate non-pharmacological interventions.

It is estimated that 50–60% of patients with advanced cancer suffer from nausea and/or vomiting (Baines 1997). These are distressing symptoms, and the feeling of wretchedness can severely diminish the quality of life of the patient and severely stretch the resources of the family and caregivers, both physically and emotionally.

> 'It is estimated that 50–60% of patients with advanced cancer suffer from nausea and/or vomiting.'

Nausea needs to be addressed whether or not it is associated with vomiting.

Persistent nausea, with or without vomiting, can lead to a multitude of physical, psychological, and social problems (Jenns 1994).

Definitions

It is appropriate to begin the discussion by establishing some accepted definitions of the terms that will be used in this chapter.

Vomiting is the forceful expulsion of gastric contents through the mouth. (Twycross 1995). It involves coordinated contraction of the diaphragm, chest wall, and abdominal muscles (Fessele 1996), and causes distress and fatigue, especially for an already debilitated patient.

Nausea is a subjective sensation that is often described as an unpleasant feeling of 'the need to vomit'. It is frequently accompanied by autonomic symptoms, including pallor, cold sweats, salivation, tachycardia, and diarrhoea. Nausea can be associated with gastric stasis, or can be mediated through taste or smell. It is often experienced in situations of anxiety or fear.

Retching is a rhythmic, laboured, spasmodic movement of the diaphragm and abdominal muscles, usually occurring in the presence of nausea and often culminating in vomiting.

Regurgitation is the effortless expulsion of undigested or partly digested food, often associated with obstruction of the oesophagus.

Physiology

Knowledge of the physiology of nausea and vomiting is necessary for an accurate diagnosis and the choice of the most appropriate antiemetic. Most antiemetics act primarily by blocking neurotransmitters (Baines 1997).

Mechanisms of vomiting

Vomiting is a complex reflex process controlled by the vomiting centre, which is located in the medullary reticular formation of the brain. The vomiting centre is stimulated by a variety of pathways that originate from the chemoreceptor trigger zone, the vestibular apparatus, the cerebral cortex, and the abdominal viscera (see Figure 12.1).

Causes of vomiting

The causes of nausea and vomiting can be divided into four categories (Fessele 1996):

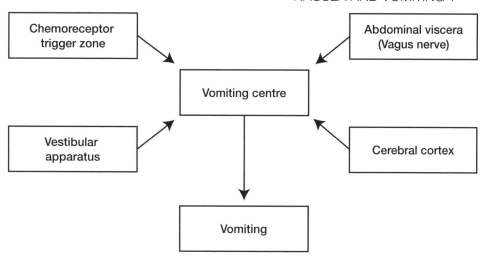

Figure 12.1 Mechanisms of vomiting
Author's presentation

▶ chemical;
▶ visceral;
▶ central nervous system; and
▶ vestibular dysfunction.
  See the Box on page 176 for a list of causes under each category.

Assessment
The person's story
The key to getting useful information from patients is to allow them to tell their stories in their own terms. Asking closed questions that seek specific responses can result in the omission of some relevant information, whereas asking more open questions that call for the person's own account of the symptoms widens the information.

'The key to getting useful information from patients is to allow them to tell their stories in their own terms.'

In hearing the story the key is to listen for (or specifically ask about) symptoms that might point to a cause of the nausea and vomiting (see Box, page 176).

Causes of nausea and vomiting

Chemical
- direct stimulus of the chemoreceptor trigger zone by a wide variety of drugs including opioid drugs, chemotherapy, some anaesthetic agents;
- metabolic disturbances (various, such as hypercalcaemia and uraemia);
- toxic states.
- radiotherapy can be a cause, depending on the site irradiated.

Visceral
- inflammation (appendicitis, peritonitis, cholecystitis, etc.);
- obstruction and mechanical disturbances (constipation, tumour, outlet obstruction, ascites);
- gastric stasis and irritation (drugs such as NSAIDs and anticholinergics; gastric irritation due to blood or alcohol; increased gastric secretions associated with stress);
- pharyngeal irritation (sputum, cough, candidiasis).

Central nervous system
- physical and psychological stimuli (including fear and distress);
- physical changes in the brain (including meningitis and brain tumours);
- olfactory stimuli;
- anticipatory vomiting (often associated with chemotherapy).

Vestibular dysfunction
- motion sickness;
- labyrinthitis;
- migraine;
- infection;
- raised intracranial pressure (tumour, infection);
- VIII cranial nerve damage.

Nausea and vomiting: clues from history

When taking a history, certain associated symptoms point to possible causes of nausea and vomiting:
- epigastric pain—gastritis; ulcer
- pain on swallowing—thrush, stomatitis
- hiccups—uraemia
- vomiting without nausea—raised intracranial pressure
- nausea without vomiting—associated fear and anxiety; offensive smells
- small-volume vomiting—'squashed stomach' syndrome
- large-volume vomiting—bowel obstruction
- drowsiness and confusion—hypercalcaemia
- sore mouth—thrush; stomatitis
- exacerbated by movement—brain tumour
- dysuria—urinary tract infection

Apart from being alert to the symptoms listed in the Box, issues to consider in taking a history include:

▶ other symptoms of gastrointestinal dysfunction (for example, abdominal pain, constipation, diarrhoea, or rectal bleeding);
▶ dietary changes (intolerance of specific foods; nausea and vomiting immediately before or after eating);
▶ cancer diagnosis and known metastases; and
▶ medications (relationship of symptoms to medications; review of all medications, especially as the patient deteriorates because decreasing renal function can cause nausea and vomiting through drug toxicity).

Physical examination

After noting the person's story about the symptoms, a physical examination is performed. Because the patient might be feeling uncomfortable, the extent of physical examination should be limited to that which provides useful information in determining the cause of nausea and vomiting. Certain physical signs are especially relevant (see Box, below).

Investigations

Decisions on relevant investigations are based on the history, the clinical examination, the illness trajectory, and the intention to intervene. It is of no value to the person, and can cause further discomfort, if investigations are carried out without a definite view to improving patient comfort.

The following should be considered:

▶ if biochemical imbalance is suspected, serum creatinine, calcium, and albumin levels might assist in diagnosis; and
▶ if relevant, the blood levels of specific drugs such as digoxin or carbamazepine might provide useful information.

Nausea and vomiting: clues from examination

When performing an examination, certain signs are significant in assessing nausea and vomiting:

- mouth—oral thrush, stomatitis, tumour;
- skin—dehydration;
- abdomen—hepatomegaly, rigidity, tenderness ascites; gastric or bowel distension; auscultation for bowel motility; loaded colon;
- rectal examination (if necessary)—constipation;
- neurological examination—papilloedema, nystagmus.

At the end stage of the illness, when death is imminent, investigations are unlikely to add to the management and can be counterproductive in the provision of good palliative care.

Documentation

Documentation is important as a communication tool and as a guide to therapeutic intervention. It can also provide a basis for research.

The systematic documentation of the symptoms of nausea and vomiting is the foundation for the adjustment of antiemetic drugs and other therapy to allow optimal control of these distressing symptoms (Jenns 1994). Too often medication is altered without adequate documentation regarding the positive and negative effects of the therapy.

'Too often medication is altered without adequate documentation regarding the positive and negative effects of the therapy.'

Observers can assess and document the level of nausea only indirectly by expressions of discomfort from the patient, and by the monitoring of vital signs, appetite, and food intake. The involvement of the patient in documentation is essential for an accurate record. The use of a diary might help the person keep a record of the feeling of nausea and the number of episodes of vomiting. It is important to distinguish between nausea and vomiting, and it should be remembered that persistent nausea is often more debilitating and distressing for the patient than a single episode of vomiting.

In the management of nausea and vomiting associated with chemotherapy, a once-daily assessment (at the same time each day, representing the situation over the past 24 hours) is an effective mode of assessment (Jenns 1994). This once-daily method avoids the person focusing too intensely on the distressing side-effects of the treatment. The same principle can be applied to people in the terminal phase of illness. Minimising discussion about the symptom might limit the distress experienced by the patient.

Specific assessment tools have been developed. For example, Rhodes and McDaniel (1999) have tested the reliability of their index of nausea, vomiting, and retching (INVR)—a self-reporting instrument that allows patients to quantify their own symptom experiences. The development of such tools and their integration into palliative-care practice will improve the quality of information collected and form a scientific basis on which to decide the most appropriate interventions.

Intervention

A multidisciplinary team approach is most effective for optimal symptom control. The person, family, nurse, doctor, pharmacist, dietitian, chaplain, and other therapists can all contribute to the management plan and its execution. Obviously the doctor and pharmacist have the major role in the prescription of drugs, but the administration of the drugs and patient compliance is the responsibility of the nurse in the hospital, and of the nurse, patient, and family in the home. Education and information regarding the reason for the drugs and other aspects of the management regimen is essential. Encouraging the patient to take control of symptom management is important for an effective care plan.

Management of nausea and vomiting can be separated into:

◗ immediate non-drug measures;
◗ the use of antiemetics or other pharmacological agents;
◗ mechanical and surgical intervention; and
◗ complementary measures.

Each of these is discussed below.

Immediate non-drug measures
Food preparation and environmental measures
Measures to reduce nausea and vomiting include planning and presenting meals in accordance with the likes of the person. Careful selection of food to avoid those that are fatty, fried, or overly sweet can reduce feelings of nausea. Cooler foods are more palatable, and the addition of salt can stimulate the appetite.

Small meals and restricted fluid intake at mealtime can assist in avoiding over-distension of the stomach. Reducing adverse stimuli (such as cooking smells and unpleasant odours) can also be helpful. Preparing food away from the person helps to reduce odours that precipitate nausea and or vomiting.

If the person is partial to alcohol, a small sherry or wine before the meal can help stimulate the appetite.

Distressing procedures should not be undertaken near meal times. It can also be helpful to avoid exercise or other activities at these times—such as bathing or showering which can cause fatigue.

Gastrointestinal factors
Taste can be altered by a number of factors, including damage to the taste buds due to radiotherapy or chemotherapy, poor oral hygiene, stomatitis, or the effect of drugs.

Attention to oral hygiene is particularly important if the person is mouth-breathing or if oral intake is reduced. If vomiting is ongoing, fasting might be necessary. A small amount of fluid in the form of ice chips or sips of a clear, cool fluid help to maintain patient comfort.

Attention to bowel function is important because constipation can contribute to nausea and vomiting. Analgesics or iron supplements can cause constipation.

Review of the person's routine medications should be carried out frequently. As the patient deteriorates, weight loss or impaired renal or hepatic function can alter the absorption and excretion of drugs. Some drugs that might have been taken for many years can cause toxicity in this situation.

Drug therapy

The list of antiemetic drugs is expanding rapidly. However, because the causes of nausea and vomiting are so varied, there is no specific agent that is effective in all situations. Nurses require a basic understanding of the available drugs, their types, duration of effects, dosages, and side-effects.

The route of administration depends on the ability of the patient to absorb the medication. If appropriate, oral medication should be used. However, alternative routes (such as rectal or parenteral administration) will be necessary in cases of severe vomiting or persistent nausea which reduce gastric emptying (Baines 1997).

The choice of antiemetic depends on a range of factors, and combination regimens can be effective. Table 12.1 lists some antiemetics, their use, actions, side-effects, and dosage regimens.

If possible, drug therapy should be started early to have maximum effect and to prevent the onset of a conditioned response.

If other drug therapies used in the overall management might cause nausea and vomiting, prophylactic drug treatment should be considered. For example, antiemetics can be considered with the introduction of opiate therapy, and aperients with the commencement of analgesics.

Most orally administered medications require 20–30 minutes after ingestion to achieve an effect. Most reach peak levels in 1–2 hours. If nausea or vomiting is associated with food intake, medication should be taken at least half an hour before the meal.

If the symptoms persist despite the regular use of oral antiemetics the subcutaneous route is recommended. A butterfly needle left *in situ* allows regular administration and provides for optimal absorption.

A syringe driver can be used for continuous subcutaneous delivery of medication. In general, all drugs (except cyclizine) should be diluted with normal saline for continuous subcutaneous administration. In the UK some centres use

Table 12.1 Antiemetics

metoclopramide (Maxolon)

Type	dopamine antagonist
Indication	gastric stasis; gastric irritation; chemotherapy; opiate-related vomiting (contraindicated in complete bowel obstruction)
Mode of action	increased lower oesophageal sphincter tone; promotes gastric emptying; stimulates gastric motility; blocking effect on CNS receptors
Side-effects	mild sedation; dystonia; extra-pyramidal reactions; diarrhoea
Dosage regimen	10–20 mg, 6 hrly, orally, IV, IM, SC; 20–100 mg/24 hours SC infusion

haloperidol (Serenace; Haldol)

Type	dopamine antagonist
Indication	uraemia; hypercalcaemia; opiate-induced vomiting
Mode of action	potent antagonist at CNS receptors
Side-effects	extra-pyramidal reactions; dry mouth; drowsiness
Dosage regimen	1.5–5 mg, 6–8 hrly, orally; 2–10 mg, 8–12 hrly SC infusion

prochlorperazine (Stemetil)

Type	dopamine, histamine antagonist
Indication	cerebral metastasis
Mode of action	antidopamine effect in CNS receptors
Side-effects	extrapyramidal reactions
Dosage regimen	5–20 mg, 6 hrly, orally; 12.5 mg, 6 hrly, IM or rectal

cyclizine

Type	histamine antagonist
Indication	motion sickness; vertigo; raised intracranial pressure; radiotherapy and chemotherapy
Mode of action	vomiting centre and vestibular afferents
Side-effects	drowsiness; sedation; dry mouth
Dosage regimen	50 mg three times daily during the day; 50 mg repeated during the night if necessary.

lorazepam (Ativan)

Type	benzodiazepine
Indication	chemotherapy-induced vomiting; refractory anticipatory vomiting; anxiety states
Mode of action	at the cortical level
Side-effects	drowsiness; confusion
Dosage regimen	0.5–2 mg, 8–12 hourly, orally; 1–4 mg, 8–12 hourly, IV

(Continued)

Table 12.1 Antiemetics (*Continued*)

---

dexamethasone (Decadron)

Type	steroidal anti-inflammatory
Indication	raised intracranial pressure; hepatic metastases; intra-abdominal tumour
Mode of action	reduction of inflammation and oedema around the tumour
Side-effects	short-term: restlessness (if given at night); long-term: Cushingoid symptoms
Dosage regimen	Tailored to individual–24 hour regime if given by infusion. Oral medication 24 hour dose given in one to two doses 4–6 hours apart in the morning.

---

chlorpromazine (Largactil)

Type	major tranquilliser
Indication	fear, anxiety, anticipatory vomiting; uraemia; hiccups; opiate-induced vomiting
Mode of action	antidopamine effect in CNS receptors
Side-effects	drowsiness; dry mouth; postural hypotension
Dosage regimen	25–100 mg, 6 hrly, oral, IM, rectal

---

ondansetron (Zofran), granisetron (Kytril), tropisetron (Navoban)

Type	serotonin receptor antagonist
Indication	persistent vomiting; chemotherapy- and radiotherapy-induced vomiting
Mode of action	prevents vagal stimulation in the gastrointestinal tract; serotonin antagonist
Side-effects	constipation; headache
Dosage regimen	8 mg, 8–12 hrly oral, IV

---

cisapride (Propulsid)

Type	pro-kinetic agent
Indication	opiate-induced vomiting; pseudo-obstruction
Mode of action	increases peristalsis from the oesophagus to the rectum
Side-effects	colic, diarrhoea
Dosage regimen	5–20 mg, 8 hrly, orally

---

olanzapine (Zyprexa)

Type	antipsychotic
Indication	intractable nausea and vomiting
Mode of action	blocks serotonin receptors
Side-effects	dizziness, drowsiness, dry mouth, constipation
Dosage regimen	2.5–5 mg, nightly, orally

---

water as the standard dilutant for drug mixtures whilst others use saline in syringe drivers. Back (2001) indicates that there is no strong evidence to support the use of one over another. Primary care trusts are developing palliative care formularies and these, along with BNF and PCF2, should be consulted to determine local procedures. Cyclizine must be diluted with sterile water. Care should be taken in mixing any two drugs in the same syringe. If in doubt, consult a pharmacist for advice.

'If used appropriately, the medications available today can have a significant impact on the quality of life for those who experience nausea and vomiting.'

If used according to appropriate dosing schedules, the medications available today can have a significant impact on the quality of life for those who experience nausea and vomiting (Walsh et al. 2000).

Mechanical and surgical intervention

In the palliative setting it is imperative to give careful consideration to the benefits and the consequences of any surgical intervention, particularly if the prolongation of life might lead to even more distressing symptoms as the disease progresses. Intervention of a mechanical or surgical nature requires careful discussion with the patient to ensure that the intervention will lighten the burden of symptom control and not cause other distressing side-effects. The following procedures can be considered.

Nasogastric tube

The insertion of a nasogastric tube can reduce gastric distension if there is total obstruction to gastric outflow, and if conservative medical management is inadequate in reducing discomfort or restlessness.

General guidelines for antiemetic therapy

- If possible, the cause should be determined.
- Identified contributing factors should be reduced or reversed.
- The mechanism of action is important in the selection of drugs.
- The possibility of overlapping toxicity must be considered.
- Drugs must be used at the optimal dose and route.
- Patient compliance must be ensured.
- Regular re-evaluation is necessary to optimise treatment.

Twycross (1995)

Percutaneous gastrostomy

Percutaneous gastrostomy might be appropriate for persistent nausea and vomiting related to bowel obstruction (Ashby 1991). The simplicity of the technique 'allows this procedure to be performed safely with minimal morbidity in seriously ill patients under endoscopic control' (Ashby 1991).

Complementary therapy

Complementary therapy has been defined as 'the diagnostic and therapeutic practices, which are separate from and in contrast to, conventional scientific medicine. The term complementary infers use of these therapies in conjunction with orthodox medicine' (Fulder 1988).

Acupressure is a non-invasive technique involving the application of pressure by finger massage to an acupuncture site. The relevant point for the control of vomiting is the P6 or the Neiguan point (situated approximately 5 cm from the wrist on the anterior aspect of the forearm). The literature is inconclusive about the value of this technique in the hospice setting (Brown et al. 1992; Maxwell 1997; Dibble 2000).

The application of *transcutaneous electrical nerve stimulation* (TENS) as an adjunct to antiemetic therapy has been reported by McMillan and Dundee (1991). It offers an option of a safe, easily administered, and inexpensive treatment for persistent nausea and vomiting.

Relaxation therapy is a major technique for reducing anxiety, and anxiety is known to be a contributing factor in nausea and vomiting. Relaxation can be taught on an individual basis (using audiotapes according to the particular needs of the patient) or can be taught in group therapy sessions.

It is worth investigating whether anxiety can be reduced by lifestyle changes that help to produce a calm environment.

> 'It is worth investigating whether anxiety can be reduced by lifestyle changes that help to produce a calm environment.'

Aromatherapy has been reported as useful complementary therapy. For example, peppermint oils have been administered in electric burners to reduce nausea in cancer patients receiving high-dose chemotherapy, and has been cited as reducing the incidence of nausea (Hudson 1998). A study of massage aromatherapy was carried out in a palliative-care setting comparing the effect of 1% roman chamomile essential oil with that of plain almond oil. The study demonstrated that the aromatherapy had a persistent effect on nausea and vomiting for one week after the cessation of the treatment (Wilkinson 1995).

Therapeutic touch and massage can be helpful. This can range from a gentle placing of a hand on the patient to convey comfort or understanding to intentional massage designed to relieve muscle tension, improve circulation, or reduce lymphoedema. Touch helps many people to relax and can be a means of facilitating open communication. However, although touch can be a very powerful tool in caring, it must be remembered that this simple act can be interpreted differently by various individuals. It might be acceptable in a structured process of massage, but less welcome in a more informal setting. The mechanism of effect on nausea and vomiting is likely to be indirect—that is, by a reduction of distress and anxiety, rather than a direct effect on the physiological causes of vomiting.

Management in the last hours of life

Recognition of impending death and consideration of the most appropriate intervention is essential for optimal symptom control and support for those caring for the patient. In the last hours of life, discontinuing many routine medications and procedures can increase comfort. Essential medications can be delivered continuously by syringe driver.

Nursing activities, such as routine turning or pressure care, should be minimised because they can create further discomfort and distress.

A possible source of considerable distress for the family and carers at the time of death is the expulsion of a large volume of gastric contents. Insertion of a nasogastric tube can prevent this (Chan & McConigley 2001).

In general this can be avoided but where felt necessary the thoughts and feelings of the patient and carers should be elicited to ensure full understanding of the procedure and to avoid raising unrealistic expectations.

Conclusion

Symptom control in palliative care aims to alleviate physical and emotional distress for the patient, and emotional distress for the family and other loved ones. A less obvious but equally important benefit is allowing the patient to pursue end-of-life issues. The effect of nausea and vomiting over a prolonged period decreases the likelihood of 'wholeness of being'.

Careful analysis of the causes of nausea and vomiting combined with appropriately applied therapeutic intervention can usually improve these symptoms to an acceptable level for the patient. This contributes to a quality of life, a peaceful death, and positive memories for those who live on.

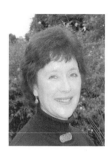

Margaret O'Connor

Dr Margaret O'Connor lectures in cancer and palliative care at La Trobe University, Melbourne (Victoria, Australia), within a unit that is dedicated to academic and clinical studies of cancer and palliative care, in association with a tertiary referral hospital. Margaret's doctoral thesis in nursing explored discourses about care of the dying in residential aged care. Her ethical interests have evolved from the work of her first degree in theology. Margaret is board member of Eastern Palliative Care, a large domiciliary service in Melbourne, and she chairs the Clinical Standards Committee and the Ethics Committee of that organisation. The combination of her academic and clinical roles has contributed to Margaret's thinking about the provision of hydration and nutrition as a key clinical issue in caring for the terminally ill.

Chapter 13

Nutrition and Hydration

Margaret O'Connor

Introduction

The presenting picture of someone requiring palliative care is often one of frailty and general cachexia. During assessment, difficulties with appetite, diet, and fluid intake might be described. Readily observable changes in the person's appearance might be evident—for example, loose-fitting clothes or a dry mouth that makes talking difficult. In addition, the nurse might observe that the caregiver is experiencing difficulties in providing a varied, nutritious, and appetising diet. These difficulties might be due to various factors—including the effects of treatment and the advance of disease. In providing appropriate nutritional support for a terminally ill person, an important part of the assessment process is to delineate these aetiological factors as clearly as possible.

Because the person is in the final stages of life, there can sometimes be a view that there is no need to address nutritional and hydration needs in any comprehensive way. However, in this chapter, it is assumed that nutritional care is given to alleviate symptoms and not to seek a prolongation of life. Nutritional and hydration decisions are usually taken to satisfy daily comfort needs. Even if a person has limited life expectancy as a result of a terminal or chronic illness, people can, and do, access the support of palliative-care services at various stages of their illnesses, and it should not be assumed that everyone receiving palliative care is necessarily nearing death.

Decisions in relation to the nutritional and hydration needs of a person with a terminal illness should be taken within a holistic framework and should therefore encompass a range of views from the multidisciplinary team of health professionals, as well as the terminally ill person, his or her family, and significant others. It is becoming much more common for a person to have a 'managed death'—that is, a death involving some sort of technology, such as artificial hydration and nutrition. Such 'managed deaths' involve ethical and legal questions in the decision-making processes.

> 'Nutritional care is given to alleviate symptoms and not to seek a prolongation of life.'

A balance between the benefits and burdens to the person, and to his or her family and loved ones, needs to be uppermost in the minds of those making such decisions.

This chapter thus addresses the nutritional and hydration needs of people receiving palliative care with an awareness that the major tenet of palliative care is the comfort of the individual. For the purposes of clarity, the broad nutritional needs of the terminally ill person will be addressed first. The chapter then discusses specific hydration needs—a subject that becomes more important than diet as the person nears death.

The food ritual

Dying can be regarded as a 'social' event. The confusion of families and health professionals about the desirability of the provision of food is, perhaps, part of a general social confusion about the process of dying itself.

An inability to eat is just one of myriad losses for a person dealing with a life-threatening illness. The symbolic importance of food and fluids is central within most cultures (Byrock 1995). The preparation and presentation of food for family and friends are parts of the rituals and celebrations of our community. They are also regarded as tangible expressions of love and care for another. Lack of involvement in food rituals can therefore be a poignant reminder that life has changed forever. This loss can be experienced with emotional overtones that might be overlooked, misunderstood, and unacknowledged by health professionals.

Because of these emotional connections, families and other carers need particular consideration when they are involved with the support of a loved one at this stage of life. Reassurance is needed that an inability to eat, or a lack of interest in food, are parts of the dying process. Support of family members and carers is vital as they endeavour to meet the altered needs of the ill person. Creativity with shopping, preparation, cooking, and presentation of food is often needed to encourage the person to eat.

Prevalence and causes

In a study of those receiving palliative care, Bruera and MacDonald (1988) found that malnutrition was a major problem for 51% of people with advanced disease and for 80% of those in the terminal stages of disease. Feelings of weakness because of weight loss can be overwhelming, and these feelings can be accentuated by frustration resulting from increasing physical limitations

There are three main causes of malnutrition—decreased intake, increased caloric needs (if suffering from a malignancy), and malabsorption (Bruera & MacDonald 1988). Most people with advanced disease experience some form of disruption in normal eating, and the resulting malnutrition is almost always irreversible (Arbolino & Sacchet 2000). Indeed, Meares (2000, p. 136) has described a 'cancer anorexia–cachexia syndrome' with a clinical picture of 'anorexia, tissue wasting, poor functional status, and eventual death'. This syndrome is usually irreversible.

Assessment

The role of the nurse in assessment of eating difficulties is vital. The assessment includes symptoms of illness that can contribute to the person's disinterest in eating—such as nausea, vomiting, pain, or constipation—experienced singly or in combination.

Medications that are frequently used in palliative care, such as morphine and paracetamol, can have side-effects that are relevant in a nutritional assessment— such as reduced appetite, nausea, and constipation. Ascites, a condition commonly experienced by terminally ill people, can interfere with appetite, the ability to eat, and the absorption of food.

'The role of the nurse in assessment of eating difficulties is vital.'

When a nutritional assessment is undertaken, the nurse might observe signs of a lack of nourishment. Weight loss, as evidenced by loose clothing, might be obvious, but other signs and symptoms to note include a loss of interest in food, difficulty in swallowing, dry mouth and skin, mucosal inflammation (perhaps caused by thrush), and other signs of generalised and localised mouth and gum soreness. The carers, be they family members or significant others, are essential if the nurse is to develop a picture of the person's eating pattern—likes and dislikes, and the amounts that can be tolerated. In the home setting, if the person has few family or social supports and is not able to leave the house, the nurse might question the source of food. The ability of the carer to provide a variety of appetising food might also be explored, especially if the carer is elderly, not used to cooking, or displays frustration or anxiety about providing the range of needs required by the person.

It is also helpful if the nurse gently questions the person about such things as how he or she feels about dependence on others for shopping or feeding, what different ways have been tried to provide nourishment (for example, high-kilojoule food supplements such as Sustagen), and whether there has been discussion about what might happen when the person can no longer eat or drink.

Advice and management

Nurses are often asked for advice about diet, particularly if the terminally ill person is feeling the limitations of what he or she is able to tolerate. Arbolino and Sacchet (2000, p. 16) have noted that, in their experience, breakfast is the 'best' meal of the day for such people, because:

> . . . energy levels are often highest in the morning. There has also been sufficient time for gastric emptying so that the patient may experience 'an appetite'. Traditionally breakfast foods are usually easily ingested and well tolerated.

Some practical suggestions for nurses can be found in the Box on page 191.

Some people with an obstruction find that pressure builds up during the day. It is recommended that such people be encouraged to eat early in the day. Many people in this situation do want to eat, even though they know that vomiting will occur.

If the terminally ill person, or the family, are expressing concern about nutritional intake, this needs to be viewed in a holistic context. If the person is able to be involved in the activities of daily living, but is inhibited by a lack of nutrition, percutaneous enterostomy gastrostomy (PEG) feeding can be

Practical advice for the nurse on general management

Before a meal:
- If the person is anorexic, give 'permission' to eat less.
- Anticipate and treat nausea with appropriate medication. If the symptom is chronic, this can involve trying different medications (depending on the cause of the nausea; see Chapter 12), and the nurse should discuss these matters with the prescriber on the patient's behalf.
- To maximise the effectiveness of antiemetic medication, it should be given at least half an hour before a meal.
- The presence of pain will cause loss of appetite. Ensure that the analgesic regimen is effective in relieving the person's pain.
- Constipation can dull the appetite. If the person is on any medication that might cause constipation, the introduction of a regular aperient should be routine to avoid this occurring.
- Regular mouth care is vital to prevent soreness and to keep the mouth clean. If thrush is present it should be treated with appropriate medication. A piece of pineapple or paw-paw can assist with cleansing the mouth after a meal. Appropriate topical medications and mouth rinses should be used if the mouth is sore.
- If possible, meals should be taken at a table to maintain normality and socialisation.

Fluids for dryness:
- An alcoholic drink with a meal can stimulate the appetite, reduce any anxiety that might be associated with eating, and reinforce the social nature of eating.
- Encourage regular sipping of fluids during the day by keeping a glass of fluid at hand, or by frequent presentation of a variety of fluids.
- Crushed ice or ice-blocks made of cordial, fruit juice, or Coca-Cola can also relieve dryness.
- Chewing gum can stimulate the production of saliva, and can relieve nausea.
- Sour sweets (such as 'lemon drops') will stimulate saliva.
- Use gravies, sauces, or ice-cream to moisten food.

Serving meals:
- The best appetite stimulant is providing the food that the person likes! (Arbolino & Sacchet 2000).
- Fizzy drinks are often preferred to tea or coffee. Small bottles are preferred to ensure that drinks do not go flat.
- Frequent small meals are often more easily digested, and should be offered when the person feels like eating.
- Meals served on a smaller plate (such as a 'bread-and-butter' plate) can look less daunting to a person with little appetite.
- Salty foods are less likely to induce nausea.
- For a sore mouth, try using a straw for some foods (to direct them away from the painful areas).

(Continued)

(Continued)
- Variations in the temperature of food can stimulate the taste buds (for example, a small amount of meat with salad, or fruit with warm custard).
- Meals at room temperature have fewer odours, and serving cooler meals can thus reduce nausea.
- Dietary supplements such as Sustagen are only of use if the person likes them. Otherwise a milkshake might be just as nutritious.
- Meals at home can now be provided through various private services, as well as through the government-funded 'Meals on Wheels'.

considered. This possibility should be carefully addressed with the person, the family, and carers, because gastrostomy feeding will be instituted in hospital and continued at home. All those involved must be able to cope with a procedure that can be burdensome and invasive. The benefits and burdens of the procedure need to be weighed against one another. However, it is inappropriate that a terminally ill person die of malnutrition. The decision therefore needs to be taken after an assessment of the likely prognosis of the person, his or her nutritional needs over time, and the prevention of starvation.

'It is inappropriate that a terminally ill person die of malnutrition.'

In some situations, for example in bowel obstruction for which surgery is not considered appropriate, the person can have fluids provided subcutaneously. This is referred to as 'hypodermoclysis', and it can be of benefit in the home setting or in residential aged care, where a registered nurse might not be readily available 24 hours a day. Fluids can be administered in this way as a bolus, continuously, or during the night while the person is sleeping (at a rate of about 1 litre over an 8-hour period) (Jackson 2000). This means of hydration can be effective when other avenues are not available (Malone 1994; Steiner & Bruera 1998; Noble-Adams 1995; Worrobee & Brown 1997). This method of hydration can be readily and safely used in the home setting (with the support of a nurse), and there is no need for hospitalisation.

At all stages of the illness, it is most important to remember that the goal of care is to promote the best quality of life. Even though it is possible to sustain life in many artificial ways, the end point is inevitably the death of the person, and artificial nutrition might serve only to delay this in ways that are often not dignified. The holistic management of all symptoms is the key, because a person who is free of pain and nausea is more likely to feel like eating at his or her own pace.

Medical Treatment Acts

Legislation covering the legal requirements for care of those with shortened life expectancy is in place in most states of Australia, and in many other jurisdictions throughout the world. For example, in the State of Victoria (Australia), the law distinguishes between the right of a person to refuse treatment and the duty of care of a carer to provide reasonable food and fluids. Because the precise details of such laws vary among jurisdictions, it is recommended that nurses become familiar with the requirements of the law in their local jurisdiction.

The dying process
Management dilemmas

There comes a stage in the dying process when the person begins to lose interest in everyday events and activities that surround him or her. This typically includes a loss of desire for food and fluids and, at this stage of life, it gradually becomes clear that eating is burdensome.

In this situation, the nurse needs to be clear about the goals of care. In particular, an important distinction needs to be made—that malnutrition and dehydration are different from hunger and thirst. The Hastings Center of New York (1987, pp 59–60) has expressed the distinction in the following terms:

> Medical procedures for supplying nutrition and hydration treat malnutrition and dehydration; they may or may not relieve hunger and thirst. Conversely hunger and thirst can be treated without necessarily using medical nutrition and hydration techniques and without necessarily correcting dehydration or malnourishment.

The reactions of family and friends need to be closely monitored to ensure that the process of dying is understood and that they have every opportunity to be involved as they wish in decision-making about care. It should be made clear that the provision of fluids will only hydrate the person, without pro-viding sustenance or prolonging life.

'Malnutrition and dehydration are different from hunger and thirst.'

For the nurse, a multidisciplinary assessment is of the utmost importance in determining the stage of the person's illness. An inappropriate assessment of hydration needs can mean that unnecessarily burdensome attempts are made to provide such support when the person is near death.

Signs and symptoms of imminent death

There are many distinctive symptoms and signs that occur as life nears its end. The goal of providing optimal quality for the person is no less important as life eases away. Twycross and Lack (1990) have described what occurs for the person who is nearing death. The person becomes:

▶ profoundly weak;
▶ essentially bedbound;
▶ drowsy for extended periods;
▶ disorientated in time, with a limited attention span;
▶ increasingly uninterested in food and fluids; and
▶ increasingly unable to swallow medication.

Those who are experienced in the care of people as death approaches, report such signs and symptoms as:

▶ decreased urinary output;
▶ decreased need for bedpans;
▶ discomfort from incontinence or a catheter;
▶ a reduction in pulmonary secretions (and therefore less coughing and congestion); and
▶ less vomiting (because of decreased gastro-intestinal fluid).

Even though a dry mouth can be reported, there seems to be a distinction between this and a sensation of thirst. What is observed is a natural state of 'anaesthesia', induced by electrolyte imbalance (Andrews & Levine 1992).

There are certain disadvantages that might be attributed to dehydration, including depression, thirst, nausea, vomiting, headaches, and cramps (Andrews & Levine 1992). However, these symptoms might not be entirely attributable to dehydration, and are far outweighed by the potential burdens of hydrating an imminently dying person.

The debate in the literature

There is some debate in the literature about the value of hydrating a person at this stage of life (Dunlop et al. 1995; Wilkes 1994; Craig 1994). However, on balance, there is more evidence for the benefits of allowing a natural state of dehydration to occur as part of the dying process (Wade 1998; Zerwekh 1983; Andrews & Levine 1989). In palliative-care settings in which nurses are experienced in the care of the terminally ill, terminal dehydration is viewed as beneficial when death is imminent (Andrews & Levine 1989). There is a need for these nurses to impart this knowledge to those who work in other health-care settings where people die.

In an attempt to define this difficult issue of whether to treat terminal dehydration, Viola, Wells and Peterson (1997) undertook a systematic review of the literature. They concluded that it was impossible to enunciate firm conclusions regarding this matter, and suggested that each person needs to be individually assessed, including a careful consideration of the person's wishes and those of his or her loved ones.

Practical suggestions for nurses

The central role for the nurse at this stage of the person's life calls for many practical skills on the part of the nurse, as well as a skilled eye that will detect the signs of potential problems. The Box on pages 195 and 196 summarises some useful practical advice.

Practical advice for the nurse on the dying process

Management of symptoms that are reversible

To manage symptoms that are reversible, such as vomiting and sore mouth, fluids should always be offered and creativity is often required. Suggestions include:

- a clean moistened cloth for the person to suck;
- a fine-mist spray bottle; or
- a small syringe to squirt fluids into the side of the mouth.

Lips should always be kept moist with lanoline or peppermint cream. Regular mouth care will also keep the mouth comfortable. Loved ones can often perform these tasks under direction.

Nurse's ready availability and presence

The nurse's ready availability and presence at this stage is vital in assisting family and loved ones as they come to terms with the dying person's inability to eat or drink.

A failure to answer questions at this stage can lead to an inordinate emphasis on the need for nutrition, at the risk of not seeing other needs.

Support of families

Support of families and loved ones extends to simple education about what is occurring for the dying person, and reassurance that dehydration is a normal part of the dying process and is probably not painful.

The nurse can perform a key role in listening to concerns of family members. The constant presence of the nurse provides reassurance and removes unnecessary fear.

Families who wish to be involved in care should always be encouraged to do so— to feed ice chips, offer sips of fluid, or undertake mouth care.

Answering questions

If questions arise about hydration, processes for addressing these questions are required.

(Continued)

(*Continued*)

A family meeting might be appropriate, particularly if family perceptions differ from those of the health professionals. Such a meeting should be undertaken as soon as questions begin to arise.

Support and consistent communication with families is essential because families with a simplistic understanding of the dying process can be left with feelings of guilt (such as a mistaken belief that they contributed to the death because they failed to feed the person).

Policy support for nurses

Significant work has been undertaken in providing policy support for health professionals who grapple with these difficult issues. Statements include:

- the European Association for Palliative Care: 'Guidelines on Artificial Nutrition versus Hydration' (see Bozzetti et al. 1996);
- the Association for Palliative Medicine of Great Britain and Ireland: statement on artificial hydration (see NCHSPCS 1997); and
- position papers from the American Nurses Association (1992), the American Medical Association (1986), and the American Dietetic Association (1992).

Conclusion

Nurses need to recognise that the provision of food is more than the physiological feeding of the body to provide nutrition. Even when nutrition is no longer part of the goal of care, food meets other holistic needs for the person in terms of the social, psychological, and emotional aspects of his or her life (Arbolino & Sacchet 2000)

Decisions about the nutrition and hydration needs of a person with a terminal illness must therefore be taken within a holistic framework and should encompass a range of views from the team of health professionals, as well as the family and other carers. Ethical and legal opinion might be required from time to time. A balance of the risks and burdens to the person and his or her family must be uppermost in the minds of decision-makers.

'Nurses need to recognise that the provision of food is more than the physiological feeding of the body to provide nutrition.'

At any stage of the journey of a person facing the end of life, issues of hydration and nutrition are essential in seeking to provide the best quality of life. Familiarity with what happens for someone on this journey is essential in achieving a holistic understanding of the experience. Knowledge of the variety of non-invasive interventions that have been described in this chapter will assist in achieving comfort for the person—which should always be the goal of care.

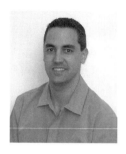

Wayne Naylor

Wayne Naylor is a registered nurse who first worked as a staff nurse in New Zealand with a forensic psychiatry unit before moving into general surgery, and then into reconstructive plastic surgery and burns. While working at the Royal Marsden Hospital in London (UK), Wayne gained further qualifications in cancer nursing, and was involved in research, clinical patient care, education, and quality-assurance wound care in cancer patients. Wayne has published several journal articles, and was lead editor for the *Royal Marsden Hospital Handbook of Wound Management in Cancer Care*. Wayne now works as a clinical nurse specialist at the Wellington Cancer Centre in New Zealand. He has a special interest in the management of wounds related to cancer and cancer therapies, including malignant wounds, radiotherapy skin reactions, and cutaneous graft versus host disease.

Chapter 14

Malignant Wounds

Wayne Naylor

Introduction

Many cancer patients live with the knowledge that their disease is progressing and incurable. For a significant minority of these people this reality can be present in the form of a malodorous, exuding, necrotic skin lesion that is a constant physical reminder of disease progression (Mortimer 1998; Englund 1993). These lesions are often referred to as 'fungating' or malignant wounds.

In general, malignant wounds occur more frequently in people with advanced cancer. However, it is possible for people to live many years with such wounds if their cancers are localised (Grocott 1999; Collier 1997b; Goodman, Hilderley & Purl 1997; Haisfield-Wolfe & Rund 1997). For the majority of these people, healing of their wounds is not a realistic goal. In fact their wounds are likely to continue to deteriorate over time (Bale & Jones 1997; Collier 1997b; Hallett 1995; Haughton & Young 1995). The problems associated with a malignant wound can have a devastating effect on a person's physical, psychological, and social wellbeing, and can cause a marked decline in quality of life.

Clarifying the terminology

There is some uncertainty in the use of terminology to describe these wounds, with the terms 'fungating' or 'ulcerating malignant' being the most commonly used. Other descriptions such as 'malignant cutaneous' have also been used (Haisfield-Wolfe & Rund 1997). The term 'fungating' usually refers to a malignant process involving both ulceration and proliferative growth (Grocott 1995a; Bycroft 1994). Lesions that predominantly have a proliferative growth pattern can develop into a nodular 'fungus-shaped' or 'cauliflower-shaped' lesion, whereas a lesion that is ulcerating produces a wound with a crater-like appearance (Grocott 1999; Collier 1997a). It is possible for a lesion to present with a mixed appearance of both proliferating and ulcerating areas (Young 1997; Carville 1995). This creates some confusion when describing and discussing these lesions (Bycroft 1994) and, for nurses, the term 'fungating wound' is often associated with breast cancer only. The definition used throughout this chapter is, simply, 'malignant wound'. This term does not differentiate between wound appearances and is also more appropriate when considering the various ways in which these lesions can develop.

Malignant wound development

A malignant wound can develop through three main mechanisms:

▶ a primary skin tumour (such as squamous cell carcinoma, basal cell carcinoma, or malignant melanoma);

▶ direct invasion of the structures of the skin by an underlying tumour (for example, breast cancer or soft-tissue sarcoma); this can be from a locally advanced primary tumour or from recurrent disease; or

▶ metastatic spread from a distant tumour.

Metastasis can occur along tissue planes, capillaries, or lymph vessels (Bryan 1994). Spread to the skin can also occur through implantation or 'seeding'— for example in the abdominal wall during surgery for ovarian and colorectal tumours (Manning 1998). Tumours commonly associated with the development of malignant wounds include tumours of the breast, head and neck, kidney, lung, ovary, colon, penis, and bladder, as well as lymphoma and leukaemia (Gallagher 1995).

In the early stages the patient usually develops discrete, non-tender skin nodules (Manning 1998). As the nodules enlarge, they cause disruption of skin capillaries and lymph vessels which, along with altered coagulation and disorganised microcirculation within the tumour, leads to tissue hypoxia and subsequent skin necrosis (Mortimer 1998; Young 1997). The development of a sinus or fistula is also possible, especially in the case of abdominal or perineal wounds (Collier 1997a).

Less commonly, a malignant wound can develop as a result of malignant changes in a chronic wound—such as a burn scar ulcer, a pressure ulcer, or a venous leg ulcer (Malheiro et al. 2001; Esther, Lamps & Schwartz 1999). Known as a 'Marjolin's ulcer', the type of malignancy in such lesions is usually an aggressive squamous cell carcinoma with a high rate of local recurrence and metastatic spread. The average time that an ulcer is present before such a malignant change occurs is 25–40 years (Hill et al. 1996). The signs of malignant change in a chronic wound include:

▶ the appearance of a mass in the wound;
▶ the onset of wound pain not previously present;
▶ a change in odour of the drainage from the wound; and
▶ a change in the character, volume, or appearance of drainage.

Although these changes can indicate the presence of malignant change, a definitive diagnosis of Marjolin's ulcer can be confirmed only through biopsy of the wound (Malheiro et al. 2001).

Incidence of malignant wounds

The exact incidence of malignant wounds has not been established, but it is estimated that 5–10% of people with metastatic cancer develop such a wound (Haisfield-Wolfe & Rund 1997). Malignant wounds tend to occur in older patients (60–70 years old) with advanced cancer, and usually occur during the last six months of life (Haisfield-Wolfe & Rund 1997; Ivetić & Lyne 1990). In a survey conducted by Thomas (1992) approximately 62% of malignant wounds developed in the area of the breast, 24% in the area of the head and neck, 3% in the groin and genital area, and 3% on the back.

'Malignant wounds tend to occur in older patients with advanced cancer, and usually occur during the last six months of life.'

Wound-related signs and symptoms

An understanding of the main signs and symptoms of malignant wounds, and their causes, is of assistance in planning patient care and in anticipating the potential needs of patients. See Box, page 202, for a list of the main signs and symptoms.

Signs and symptoms of malignant wounds

The most frequently reported wound-related signs and symptoms are:
- bleeding (superficial or large vessel);
- presence of necrotic tissue;
- heavy exudate;
- wound infection;
- malodour;
- pain;
- pruritus in skin around wound;
- damage to surrounding skin by exudate; and
- tunnelling, undermining, fistula, and sinus.

The most frequently reported of these wound-related signs and symptoms are odour, exudate, pain, and bleeding. These are discussed below.

Malodour

Malodour is most commonly caused by anaerobic bacterial infection of the hypoxic, devitalised tissue present within the wound. The odour produced by a malignant wound is often constantly detectable, and can trigger gagging and vomiting reflexes (Collier 1997b; Van Toller 1993). Malodour can also be due to stale exudate in dressings that have been in place for a number of days.

Exudate

Exudate is frequently produced in significant volumes by malignant wounds. The increased permeability of blood vessels within the tumour and the secretion of vascular permeability factor by tumour cells are the most likely causes of the high exudate levels encountered with malignant wounds (Haisfield-Wolfe & Rund 1997). Exudate production can also be increased if infection is present, as a result of inflammation and tissue breakdown by bacterial proteases (Collier 2000).

Pain

Pain from a malignant wound might be due to tumour pressing on nerves and blood vessels, or exposure of the dermis (Manning 1998). The type of pain most often described in relation to malignant wounds is a superficial stinging or a persistent deeper ache due to painful ulceration (Grocott 1999). If there is nerve damage, patients can experience neuropathic pain. In some instances pain can be due to the choice of dressing product used, or the dressing procedure employed (Jones, Davey & Champion 1998). For example, pain can be caused by dressing adherence to the wound bed or by an inappropriate cleansing technique.

Bleeding

Bleeding can occur from the wound spontaneously or as a result of trauma during dressing changes (Jones, Davey & Champion 1998; Hallett 1995). Profuse spontaneous bleeding can occur if the tumour erodes a major blood vessel, and this can be a distressing event for both the patient and his or her family carers (Haisfield-Wolfe & Rund 1997). Bleeding can be exacerbated by decreased platelet function within the tumour.

Dressing-related problems

As the above discussion has suggested, because of these signs and symptoms the dressing of malignant wounds can cause particular problems. The Box on page 203 summarises these.

Assessment of malignant wounds

General assessment

The assessment of malignant wounds should be a holistic process that includes the gathering of information on the person's psychological and social state, as well as local wound factors. The management of the symptoms of malignant wounds should always be focused on the person's quality of life, and priorities should therefore be based on problems that are identified by the patient as being the most troublesome, combined with the clinical concerns of health professionals (Grocott 1995b; Jones, Davey & Champion 1998; Pudner 1998; Collier 1997a). In discussions with the person, it is important to discuss the acceptability of various wound-management strategies (Price 1996). This information can best be gained by using patient self-report—for example, assessing pain using a pain scale (visual or descriptive), or asking the patient to rate the severity of wound odour (Collier 1997a).

It is very important that all relevant areas of the assessment be properly documented to fulfil all legal and professional requirements.

Dressing-related problems

The dressing of malignant wounds can cause difficulties due to:
- the frequency of dressing changes;
- the location of wound;
- pain related to dressing changes; and
- the size and shape of the lesion being dressed.

Symptom assessment

Patient self-ratings are generally considered the 'gold standard' for symptom reporting. These should be brief, reliable, and easily administered. However, with very ill persons with advanced disease, self-reporting can be problematic. If the person has cognitive impairments or communication difficulties, self-reporting can be unrealistic (Sneeuw et al. 1999). Difficulty can also occur if the patient is experiencing severe symptom distress or if the burden of self-assessment is physically or emotionally demanding. However, it is at this point, when the person is most unwell, that accurate assessment becomes most important (Grassi et al. 1996).

Summary of assessment

The Box below outlines some general criteria that should be included in the assessment of a malignant wound.

Assessment criteria for malignant wounds

Patient
- past health history and disease status;
- impact of wound on activities of daily living;
- self-care ability;
- psychosocial issues (depression, body image, stress, sexuality);
- social support and resources;
- nutritional status;
- information needs;
- patient strengths and coping abilities;
- sleep and rest; and
- spiritual and cultural needs.

Wound
- aetiology of wound;
- location of wound;
- size, depth, and shape of wound (photography can be useful in recording);
- amount and nature of exudate;
- presence and extent of malodour;
- type of tissue present (necrotic, sloughy, granulating, epithelialising);
- signs of infection (heat, redness, swelling, pain; increases in odour and exudate);
- nature and type of pain;
- pain related to dressing changes and wound cleansing;
- condition of surrounding skin; and
- episodes of bleeding.

Adapted from Naylor, Laverty & Mallett (2001)

Management of malignant wounds

Principles of management

The overall goals of nursing care for a person with a malignant wound are to promote comfort, confidence, and a sense of wellbeing, to prevent isolation, and to maintain or improve the patient's quality of life (Laverty, Cooper & Soady 2000; Ingham & Portenoy 1998). Management is focused on controlling the symptoms associated with the wound, and on addressing the psychosocial needs of the person and his or her carers.

Elements of management

The important elements of treatment for a malignant wound as derived from the above principles are outlined in the Box below.

Role of cancer therapies

Although malignant wounds are generally a sign of advanced disease, the palliative use of anticancer therapies can be beneficial in symptom control, so long as a balance is maintained between benefits and potential negative effects on the person's quality of life.

Radiotherapy is the most commonly used treatment, and often reduces the size of the wound, thereby decreasing exudate, bleeding, and pain. The side-effects

---

Elements of wound management

General management
- identification of realistic treatment objectives that promote the patient's quality of life;
- effective symptom control to promote patient comfort;
- prevention of any further wound deterioration or complications;
- application of aesthetically acceptable dressings; and
- provision of psychological and spiritual support to promote self-esteem and patient acceptance.

Specific management
- control of malodour;
- management of excessive exudate production;
- prevention and control of haemorrhage;
- control of pain related to the wound or dressing procedures;
- care of the skin surrounding the wound, including management of itching and irritation; and
- prevention and control of wound infection.

of radiotherapy include tiredness and skin reactions (such as erythaema and desquamation).

Cytotoxic chemotherapy can also be effective in reducing wound size and relieving symptoms. Single agents or low-dose combinations are less likely to cause side-effects. The response rates to palliative chemotherapy can be low. *Hormone therapy* can be employed if the primary tumour is hormone sensitive (for example, breast cancer). Hormone therapy can reduce the size and progression of the wound, but the response time is long, and can take 4–6 weeks.

Surgery is rarely used as a palliative measure for malignant wounds. It can be useful in some cases to debulk a large fungating tumour or to debride a wound, but problems with bleeding and underlying disease limit the general usefulness of surgery. In selected cases, plastic surgery should be considered as a useful method of symptom control. The excision of a malignant wound, with reconstruction of the defect using flaps or skin grafts, can provide an extended symptom-free period, and can improve cosmesis (Offer, Perks & Wilcock 2000).

Dressings and other measures

General

During therapy with any of the above treatments, or when they are no longer effective, wound dressings and topical or systemic treatments must be utilised for the control of wound-related symptoms. Table 14.1 (page 207) provides a summary of treatment options for the most common physical symptoms experienced.

Wound-cleansing

Gentle irrigation with warm 0.9% sodium chloride or water is the recommended method of wound-cleansing (Hollinworth 1997). The use of gauze or cotton balls can damage delicate new tissue and cause pain, and using cold irrigation fluid or high-pressure irrigation can also be painful and unpleasant for the patient. Using a sterile gloved hand, rather than forceps, can help reduce wound trauma (Hollinworth 1997).

'The use of topical antiseptics . . . is not recommended because these agents can exacerbate tissue damage and cause pain.'

The use of topical antiseptics—such as chlorhexidine, povidine-iodine, hydrogen peroxide, and sodium hypo-chlorite—is not recommended because these agents can exacerbate tissue damage and cause pain (Gould 1999; Thomas 1989). The use of these products in wound care should be restricted, if not

Table 14.1 Treatment strategies for malignant wounds

Physical problem	Treatment options
Malodour	debridement of necrotic tissue topical metronidazole (Flagyl) gel activated charcoal dressings sugar paste sterile honey (from leptospermum species plants) occlusive dressings (wound/stoma drainage bags) deodorisers essential oils (aromatherapy)

Exudate
  light
 	
  heavy
	
	hydrocolloids
	semi-permeable films
	low-adherent absorbent dressings
	alginates (light to moderate exudate)
	hydrofibre dressings (Aquacel)
	foam dressings
	non-adherent wound contact layers with a secondary
	  absorbent pad
	stoma appliance or wound manager bag

Bleeding
  preventive
 	
  light
  heavy
	
	non-adherent dressings
	maintain a moist environment
	cleansing by irrigation
	oral antifibrinolytics
	sucralfate pastealginate
	haemostatic surgical products
	topical adrenaline
	topical tranexamic acid
	cautery or ligation

Pain	regular analgesics (opioid/non-opioid/adjuvant) premedication or booster predressing change nitrous oxide (Entonox) topical opioids
Pain at dressing change	use non-adherent dressings maintain a moist wound environment change to a product that can be left in place longer irrigation of the wound with warm saline complementary therapies

(Continued)

Table 14.1 Treatment strategies for malignant wounds (*Continued*)

Itching and irritation of skin	hydrogel sheets (cooled) menthol in aqueous cream transcutaneous electrical nerve stimulation (TENS)
Protection of surrounding skin	alcohol-free skin barrier films 'frame' the wound with a thin hydrocolloid sheet

abandoned, due to their toxic effects on healthy tissue and the fact that they are rapidly inactivated on contact with organic matter (Gilchrist 1999; Fletcher 1997; Oliver 1997; Trevelyn 1996; Leaper 1996).

Malodour

The primary treatment for malodour is debridement of necrotic tissue, which removes the medium for bacterial growth. However, surgical or sharp debridement is not recommended due to the tendency of these wounds to bleed. Hence autolytic or enzymatic debridement is recommended, so long as the chosen method does not significantly increase exudate production (Grocott 2001).

Antibiotic therapy can be effective, as this will kill the bacteria thought to be responsible for odour production (Newman, Allwood & Oakes 1989). The most commonly used treatment is metronidazole. It can be given systemically, but side-effects such as nausea, neuropathy, and alcohol intolerance can diminish patient acceptability (Hampton 1996). In addition, a lack of blood supply to the malignant wound can reduce the antibiotic's effectiveness (Thomas et al. 1998a). It is more practical and effective to use a topical preparation of metronidazole gel (Metrotop, Anabact) (Gilchrist 1999; Cutting 1998; Bower et al. 1992; Ashford et al. 1984). This gel is applied directly onto the wound once daily for 5–7 days, but might need to be repeated often to keep odour under control. The gel should be spread over the whole of the wound bed if the wound is flat, or it can be used to fill shallow cavities. For deeper cavities the gel can be used to coat a cavity-filling dressing (Moody 1998).

Another option is the use of an activated charcoal dressing. These dressings are available in a number of forms including plain activated charcoal cloth (CliniSorb), combined with other dressing materials (CarboFlex, Lyofoam C) or impregnated with silver (Actisorb Silver 220). Activated charcoal attracts and binds the volatile odour-causing molecules, thus preventing their escape from the local wound area (Williams 1999; Miller 1998).

Sugar paste and honey have recently come back into use, mainly due to the emergence of many antibiotic-resistant strains of bacteria. Both of these agents have antibacterial and debriding properties. Because of their high sugar content, both of these products produce a hyperosmotic wound environment that inhibits bacterial growth and assists in wound debridement (Edwards 2000; Morgan 2000; Cooper & Molan 1999). Honey also contains bacteriocidal hydrogen peroxide, which is slowly released as the honey is diluted in wound exudate. Specific types of honey have plant-derived antibacterial properties (Molan 1999; Dunford 2000).

Occlusive dressings can help to contain wound odour. Daily dressing changes, together with the correct disposal of soiled dressings, prevents a build-up of stale exudate. Deodorisers can help to mask the odour, and products such as essential oils, environmental air filters, and commercial deodorisers can be useful (Naylor, Laverty & Mallett 2001). However, these products, especially commercial deodorisers, can make the odour worse or can cause unpleasant associations with certain smells.

Exudate

Malignant wounds with only small amounts of exudate should be managed with dressings that have a low absorbency, so as not to dry out the wound. Examples of dressings that can be used include hydrocolloids, semi-permeable films, and low-adherent absorbent dressings (Jones, Davey & Champion 1998). Care should be taken with low-adherent absorbent dressings because they can stick to the wound if it dries out too much.

More commonly, malignant wounds produce moderate-to-high amounts of exudate, and it is important to choose a dressing that will absorb the excess exudate but still maintain a moist wound environment. Suitable dressings for moderate-to-high exudate wounds include alginate and hydrofibre dressings, foam dressings, and non-adherent wound contact layers, such as Mepitel or NA Ultra, with a secondary absorbent pad (Grocott 1999; Pudner 1998). For wounds with a small opening and large amounts of exudate, a stoma appliance or wound manager can be used (Boon, Brophy & Lee 2000; Jones, Davey & Champion 1998).

It is also important to consider protection of the skin around the wound, which can become damaged from contact with excess exudate and the repeated application and removal of dressing products. Alcohol-free skin-barrier films offer an effective method of skin protection that is easy to use. These products are applied to the skin as a liquid and dry rapidly to form a very thin protective film on the skin. Examples include Cavilon No-Sting Barrier Film and SuperSkin (Hampton & Collins 2001; Williams 1998). An alternative method of skin protection is the use of a thin hydrocolloid sheet to 'frame' the wound

(Hollinworth 2000). This protects the skin because it can be left in place for a number of days while the main dressing is changed as necessary. If tape or adhesive dressings are used, they can be fixed to the hydrocolloid sheet, rather than to the patient's skin.

Bleeding

Preventive measures are important to reduce the possibility of bleeding occurring. Using non-adherent dressings that maintain the wound in a moist environment, and cleansing by irrigation rather than swabbing, will prevent bleeding due to trauma. Oral antifibrinolytics, such as tranexamic acid, can also help by reducing the tendency of the wound to bleed (Pudner 1998).

There are several strategies available to help with actively bleeding wounds. For slow oozing, sucralfate paste or an alginate can be applied (Thomas, Vowden & Newton 1998b; Emflorgo 1998). Caution is advised in using alginates. There is evidence that these dressings can actually cause bleeding in fragile tumours (Grocott 1998). In wounds with moderate-to-heavy bleeding, the use of a haemostatic surgical sponge (such as Spongostan or Oxycell) will promote rapid haemostasis. However, these dressing can be expensive and are not usually available in the community. Alternatively, topical adrenaline or tranexamic acid can be applied, but they should be used only under medical supervision. Caution is advised because adrenaline can cause ischaemic necrosis by local vasoconstriction (Grocott 2000). Excessive bleeding that refuses to stop might need referral to a surgeon for cautery or ligation.

Pain

Accurate and appropriate assessment is the key to successful pain management. It is important to identify the nature, severity, frequency, and duration of pain to ensure that the most appropriate treatment is selected (Naylor 2001). Any analgesic drugs should be prescribed following the World Health Organization guidelines for the control of cancer pain (WHO 1996), and in accordance with local prescribing policy. It can be useful to give the patient a premedication before the dressing change, or a booster dose of his or her usual opiate. Also consider using nitrous oxide (Entonox) gas during the procedure (Travis 2000).

'Accurate and appropriate assessment is the key to successful pain management.'

To prevent pain during dressing changes, non-adherent dressings should be used. Maintaining the wound in a moist environment not only reduces dressing adherence but also protects exposed nerve endings (Hallett 1995; Emflorgo 1999). If pain is unavoidable at dressing changes, changing to a product that can be left in place longer reduces the frequency of pain. Complementary therapies can play an important part in pain management. Therapies such as relaxation, distraction, or visualisation can help anxious and stressed patients who have a heightened response to pain (Ryman & Rankin-Box 2001; Downing 1999).

Topical opioids represent an interesting alternative form of pain control that can be useful for painful ulcerating wounds. There has been limited research on the use of topical opioids, but several published case studies and theoretical papers support its use and attest to its ability to reduce wound pain significantly (Grocott 2000; Twillman 1999; Krajnik & Zylicz 1997; Back & Finlay 1995; Stein 1995). Morphine and diamorphine are most commonly used, mixed with a hydrogel to produce a 0.1% w/w solution (for example, 1 mg of morphine to 1 gram of hydrogel). Metronidazole gel has also been used as a carrier for the opioid to provide combined pain and odour control (Flock, Gibbs & Sykes 2000; Grocott 2000). The mixture is usually applied to the wound once a day, although some patients have used it on an 'as required' basis.

Itching and skin irritation

Itching can be a chronic problem when new tumour nodules are beginning to emerge in surrounding skin. The stretching of the skin irritates nerve endings and can cause a biochemical reaction leading to local inflammation. Relief can be achieved through the application of hydrogel sheets, which have a cooling effect when applied to itching skin. This effect can be enhanced if the dressing is stored in a non-food refrigerator. The dressing should be covered with a semi-permeable film, to prevent dehydration of the dressing. Another option is menthol in aqueous cream, which can usually be supplied by a pharmacy. This cream does not dry out on the skin and the menthol has a cooling effect. The cream can be applied to itchy areas 2–3 times a day, or as necessary, although it should not be applied to open wounds (Naylor, Laverty & Mallett 2001). Transcutaneous electrical nerve stimulation (TENS) can also be effective in relieving itching associated with a malignant wound (Grocott 2000).

Psychosocial problems

Malignant wounds can have a significant impact on the psychological and social welleing of people. It should also be remembered that these people will have advanced cancer with its associated symptoms and problems. The Box on page 212

Psychological and social problems associated with malignant wounds

Psychological
- body image concerns; cosmetic effect of dressing;
- embarrassment and shame;
- denial;
- depression;
- fear;
- guilt;
- revulsion and disgust;
- self-esteem problems;
- sexual problems.

Social
- communication difficulties;
- impact on family;
- information needs;
- restrictions due to dressings changes;
- social isolation;
- problems with social support and resources.

presents a list of problems that can be encountered by a person with a malignant lesion.

Wound malodour is probably the most distressing symptom for patients (Young 1997; Price 1996; Haughton & Young 1995; Fairbairn 1994). Malodour can also be a severe problem for the patient's family and caregivers (Gallagher 1995). The presence of a pervasive odour can lead to embarrassment, disgust, depression, and social isolation (Jones, Davey & Champion 1998; Van Toller 1994). The social stigma, guilt, and shame associated with a malodorous wound can also have a detrimental effect on sexual expression leading to relationship problems (Hallett 1995; Haughton & Young 1995).

Patients have reported that the main problem with leakage of exudate from dressings is staining of their clothes and bedding (Davis 1995; Boardman, Mellor & Neville 1993; Grocott 1993, 1995a), and the presence of malodour can cause embarrassment, depression, and social isolation. The effective management of wound exudate will increase patient confidence and comfort.

The position of the wound can be a source of embarrassment for the person, especially if it is in an area that is considered private and personal, such as the breast or genitals (Pudner 1998).

The aesthetics of a cosmetically acceptable dressing are important to enable people to continue an active social life, and to maintain a sense of normality for the family (Grocott 1993; Carville 1995). Nurses should strive to devise cosmetically acceptable dressings that restore body symmetry and boost confidence and socialisation. Other strategies that can be useful in helping the patient to cope with the psychosocial distress caused by the presence of a malignant wound include:

‣ providing 'bedside' counselling or referring the person for professional counselling;

‣ ensuring that patient and their families have appropriate social support to reduce stress around the home;

‣ offering appropriate spiritual care according to the patient's beliefs;

‣ involving patients and families in any decisions about care;

‣ encouraging open and honest communication so that all parties are aware of goals and decisions;

‣ using touch to let the person know that the nurse is 'there' and that the patient is seen as a 'whole' person; and

‣ providing access to complementary therapies (such as massage, aromatherapy, and acupuncture) to improve the person's quality of life (Haisfield-Wolfe & Rund 1997; Fairbairn 1994; Neal 1991; Ivetić & Lyne 1990).

Conclusion

A malignant wound can be very distressing. Apart from the extra burden of the wound and its management, the wound is a constant reminder to the person that he or she has progressive and incurable cancer. This alone is enough to cause considerable psychological and social distress, but many patients also suffer, often unnecessarily, from poorly controlled wound symptoms and the unsightly cosmetic appearance of the wound.

'Many patients suffer, often unnecessarily, from poorly controlled wound symptoms and the unsightly appearance of the wound.'

By using a holistic assessment that incorporates patient self-reporting it is possible to identify those areas most in need of intervention to improve the patient's quality of life. This information, along with an indepth knowledge of treatment options, allows the nurse to develop an appropriate management plan that addresses the patient's needs.

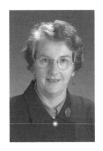 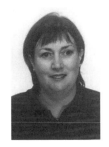

Eleanor Flynn

Dr Eleanor Flynn graduated in medicine from the University of Melbourne (Victoria, Australia) and in education from LaTrobe University, Melbourne, and is a fellow of the colleges of General Practice and Medical Administration. She is a consultant in palliative care at Caritas Christi Hospice, Melbourne, and a senior lecturer in medical education at the University of Melbourne, where she is also coordinator of palliative-care input into the new medical curriculum. Eleanor has an active interest in all aspects of clinical education in palliative care. For many years, she has been involved in medical education at undergraduate and postgraduate levels, and in continuing professional education. Eleanor's publications include papers on the incidence of psychiatric disease in older people in hospitals and services for sufferers of dementia. She has presented papers at conferences in Australia and overseas on health service management, education of medical students and junior doctors, and delirium in palliative-care patients. Her particular clinical research interest is the recognition and management of delirium in palliative-care settings.

Karen Quinn

Karen Quinn is a registered nurse with a background in various medical, surgical, and midwifery specialties, and graduate qualifications in palliative care. Before commencing full-time research study at the University of Melbourne (Victoria, Australia) in 2001, she had worked on an inpatient palliative-care unit for seven years. While working in palliative care, Karen developed an interest in evidence-based practice and later undertook a research project aimed at identifying appropriate screening for acute confusion in palliative care. Her current research involves a systematic review of screening for psychosocial distress in adult patients with cancer. Karen has recently been appointed clinical nurse educator at Caritas Christi Hospice, Melbourne.

Chapter 15

Confusion and Terminal Restlessness

Eleanor Flynn and Karen Quinn

Introduction

Acute confusion is a common problem in end-of-life care. The likelihood of the problem increases in patients with advanced disease, in those who are elderly, and in people with multiple morbidities. Moreover, improved cancer treatments are resulting in patients living longer, sometimes with complications involving organic mental states and potential for the development of confusion. Unrecognised and untreated confusion is a distressing experience for both the person and the family. It can interfere with valuable communication opportunities and can leave family members with unpleasant memories of their loved one's final hours. A further challenge in managing these patients is

> 'Unrecognised and untreated confusion is a distressing experience for both the person and the family. It can leave family members with unpleasant memories of their loved ones.'

the threat to patient safety—if confusion causes restlessness and agitation, with a risk of falls and injury.

This chapter explores the phenomena of acute confusion and terminal restlessness. Optimising quality of life within the limitations of the disease process is a key factor in measuring clinical outcomes in all aspects of palliative care. The current evidence regarding assessment and management is discussed, and practical strategies are provided for nurses caring for confused patients.

Definition of terms

The terms 'delirium', 'acute brain syndrome', and 'acute confusion' are used interchangeably in the literature. Most of the research literature uses the term 'delirium'. The definition is guided by the diagnostic criteria provided by the *Diagnostic and Statistical Manual of Mental Disorders* (DSM) developed by the American Psychiatric Association. The important criteria are that acute confusion presents as a significant alteration in cognitive functioning, with the change fluctuating over time (even several times a day), and with the presence of a known cause. *Delirium* is defined as a changed mental state characterised by (APA 1994):

▶ acute onset;
▶ fluctuations over time;
▶ association with reduced awareness, attention deficit, and cognitive and perceptual disturbances; and
▶ the presence of a known cause.

Other observed features include: disturbed sleep/wake patterns (with the person awake and confused at night, but somnolent during the day); uncoordinated muscle twitching involving one or more limbs; and labile emotions (McCaffery Boyle et al. 1998). The person can be very distressed and teary, without understanding why he or she feels that way, and can experience nightmares (Barraclough 1997). Perceptual disturbances can include misinterpretations, hallucinations, and illusions (Breitbart and Cohen 2001).

Acute confusion presents differently from chronic confusion associated with dementia, and therefore requires assessment and management specific to the problem (see Table 15.1, page 217).

Hypoactive delirium is often misinterpreted as depression or dementia. This form of confusion is associated with drowsiness, social withdrawal, and generalised lethargy (McCaffery Boyle et al. 1998). There is far less in the literature in relation to this form of confusion. Because they are quiet, these people are more likely not to be diagnosed and appropriately managed. They are

Table 15.1 Acute and chronic confusion

Feature	Acute confusion (delirium)	Chronic confusion (dementia)
Onset	acute	insidious
Course	fluctuating	steadily progressive
Consciousness/orientation	clouded; disorientated	clear until late stage
Memory/attention	poor short-term memory; inattention	poor short-term memory; attention usually normal
Psychotic features (for example, hallucinations)	common	less common

Adapted from Meagher (2001)

therefore at risk of a poorer outcome (Lindesay 1999). The assessment and management is the same as for hyperactive delirium.

Terminal restlessness is variously termed 'terminal agitation', 'agitated confusion', or 'agitated delirium'. It is arguably one of the least-understood conditions in palliative care, as is evidenced by the lack of specific literature on the subject before the 1990s. Terminal restlessness is marked by: (i) behavioural signs; and (ii) mental agitation. The *behavioural signs* associated with the physical restlessness include: (i) pulling at the bedclothes; (ii) frequent changes of position; and (iii) being unable to relax physically. The *mental agitation* is manifested by: (i) twitching; (ii) moaning; and (iii) calling out—often incoherently. Myoclonus (generalised involuntary muscle twitching) is common in terminal restlessness (Burke 1997). There is overwhelming anxiety, not amenable to reassurance (Barraclough 1997). Families find this agitated behaviour very distressing to witness. Unfortunately, the diagnosis is sometimes made retrospectively, following the death of the person.

Prevalence of confusion and terminal restlessness

Estimates of the prevalence of confusion vary, but up to 88% of palliative-care patients can become confused in the last days or hours of their lives (Lawlor, Fainsinger & Bruera 2000), compared with 15–20% of general medical patients (Meagher 2001). A study by Caraceni et al. (2000) found that in a sample of

393 palliative-care patients, 109 had an episode of confusion, and that these people had an average survival time of 21 days, compared with 39 days for non-confused patients. This suggests that acute confusion might be a predictor of death in palliative-care patients.

Scope of the problem

Clinicians caring for confused persons often feel inadequate, and sometimes frustrated, in their efforts to manage their problems adequately. Nurses often express concerns about not being able to provide relief and comfort for those in their care. These people often have some awareness of being confused, and this compounds their distress (Lindesay, MacDonald & Starke 1990). Families and friends seek advice and support from nurses in understanding the changed behaviour of their loved one. They might even feel that it might be best if they do not visit because it seems to them that their visits cause further distress.

'People often have some awareness of being confused, and this compounds their distress.'

All of this compromises the quality of life of both the person and the family. Confused patients have an increased risk of falls and injury, and this can cause further distress to the person, family, and staff.

Clinical presentations

The common presentations of delirium include:

▶ agitated or restless behaviour;
▶ paranoid thoughts or speech;
▶ disturbed sleep/wake pattern;
▶ aggressive or inappropriate behaviour;
▶ withdrawn behaviour;
▶ hallucinations or delusions; or
▶ distracted or inattentive behaviour.

These clinical presentations might lead admission to hospital for assessment because an acutely confused and agitated person presents extra challenges for the family and other carers in the home.

The Box on page 219 describes three presentations of acute confusion due to reversible causes.

Clinical presentations of confusion

Case 1

Mr WF was an 86-year-old widower with locally spreading prostate cancer admitted for assessment and possible terminal care. Before his admission he required an indwelling catheter. Not long after this he became aggressive and his daughter was not able to care for him at home. On admission he was found to have a urinary tract infection and this was treated. Within a few days the ward staff discovered that Mr WF was a quiet man with a wry sense of humour who was interested in discussing his hobbies. He was keen to return home. During his admission he suffered another two urinary tract infections and each time his behaviour changed radically. He became aggressive, refused to be helped, and used colourful language to describe staff members and their care of him. Although the behaviour change alerted the staff to diagnose and treat the infection quickly, his delirium took some days to settle each time. He was then tried on permanent antibiotics, which were successful, and allowed him to return home.

Case 2

Mrs EB was a 94-year-old Greek widow, who spoke no English. She had been recently diagnosed with bowel cancer and had been admitted for terminal care. Her only complaint was abdominal pain which was sometimes, but not always, colicky. She was started on a very small dose of oral morphine, which helped the pain but caused distressing delirious misperceptions. These were brought to the attention of nurses by her daughter because Mrs EB remained quiet and uncomplaining. She was convinced that the cords hanging from the ward televisions were snakes, and that there were mice and other animals under her bed. Soon after the morphine was stopped the misperceptions stopped, but the pain returned. After some trials, a small dose of another opioid relieved the pain without Mrs EB seeing snakes and other beasts in the room.

Case 3

Mr AL was a 39-year-old man with head and neck cancer admitted for symptom management. He had severe face and neck pain, both localised and neuropathic, and any movement caused great discomfort. To minimise movement, he was nursed in bed with special pillows and gadgets to enable him to reach his writing equipment, radio, TV control, and drinks. In spite of large doses of appropriate analgesia his pain was still not optimally controlled, and the opioid was changed. Over the next few days he became so agitated and confused that he got out of bed and threatened the staff. He required sedation to settle and returned to his normal quiet self only after the original opioid was reinstituted.

Causes of delirium

The causes of acute confusion can be understood in terms of: (i) predisposing factors; and (ii) precipitating factors. *Predisposing* factors are present before a new clinical challenge produces *precipitating* factors that push people into acute confusion. It is important to be aware that one episode of delirium increases the risk of the occurrence of future episodes.

Predisposing factors

The most common predisposing factors are (Meagher 2001; Inouye 1990):

▶ advanced age;
▶ pre-existing cognitive deficit;
▶ sensory deficits (such as sight and hearing deficits);
▶ other serious illnesses;
▶ advanced metastatic disease;
▶ severe depression;
▶ dehydration; and
▶ malnutrition.

The more severe the predisposing factors, the less serious the noxious insult needs to be to cause acute confusion. This can be understood in terms of 'the straw that broke the camel's back'—one more straw might be enough to break the back of a camel with an already onerous load. In a similar way, a relatively trivial event, such as a lower urinary tract infection, might be enough to tip a palliative-care patient into a confused and agitated state.

Precipitating factors

The range of potential precipitating factors is very wide indeed. They include medications, disease processes, metabolic disturbances, environmental issues, and so on. Table 15.2 (page 221) lists some of the more significant types of predisposing factors and examples of each.

The pathophysiology of delirium in palliative care is rarely mentioned in any detail in the literature. However, it is likely that delirium is due to a multifactorial interruption in the usual activity of several areas of the brain (Breitbart & Cohen 2001). Assessment and treatment strategies must take account of this multifactorial causation.

Assessment
General

Assessment of acute confusion in persons receiving palliative care presents a difficult nursing challenge. The diagnosis of delirium requires careful observation of the person and a clear history of recent events. There is no single diagnostic test to prove that someone has delirium. Diagnostic tests can help to determine

Table 15.2 Precipitating causes of delirium and restlessness in palliative care

Type of cause	Example
Medications (commencement or withdrawal)	opioids, over-the-counter medications, psychotropics, anti-Parkinsonian agents, chemotherapeutic agents, benzodiazepines, anticonvulsants, digoxin, steroids, anticholinergics (for example, atropine, hyoscine), antidepressants, NSAIDs
Disease-related	cerebral disease (metastases or cerebral oedema); advanced disease (of many kinds)
Metabolic	hypercalcaemia, hypoglycaemia, hyponatraemia, liver failure, renal failure, dehydration
Physical signs and symptoms	constipation, urinary retention, uncontrolled symptoms (pain, nausea), hypothermia
Infections	respiratory infections, urinary infections
Hypoxia	respiratory failure, cardiac failure, pulmonary emboli
Withdrawal from drugs of dependence	alcohol, nicotine, other drugs
Environmental issues	unfamiliar place or people
Existential issues	unresolved issues, life regrets, fear of dying, anger, denial of illness and death, sadness, sense of losing control, spiritual pain/issues

Adapted from Back (1992)

the *conditions that might be causing* the delirium, but the diagnosis of delirium itself is clinical.

The onset of acute confusion frequently signals a worsening of the primary illness. It is important that any decisions about investigations and management are discussed with the person and his or her family, while respecting personal, cultural, and spiritual beliefs.

History
Because the patient is often not able to communicate clearly and because the family might also be distressed, it is important to obtain information about the person's recent clinical state from his or her doctor or other carers. This especially applies to the medication history.

Examination

A thorough physical examination is essential. This should include assessment of the person's mental state and cognitive function.

Various instruments have been designed to aid in the assessment and documentation of mental state. One of the most widely used and well-validated instruments to assess cognitive function is the 'Mini-Mental State Examination' (MMSE) (Folstein, Folstein & McHugh 1975).

Early recognition of acute confusion

Alert nursing assessment

The regular, frequent, and intimate contact that nurses have in their care of people affords them an opportunity to detect subtle cognitive changes early in the development of confusion (Gagnon et al. 2000). This should be augmented with a multidisciplinary approach in consultation with colleagues, and with the family. Family meetings are useful in identifying issues that might be of concern to the patient, and in allowing family members to have their concerns heard.

'Nurses have an opportunity to detect subtle cognitive changes early in the development of confusion.'

The Box on page 223 describes a case in which nurses noted early signs of confusion in a patient they knew. As a result, investigations and appropriate management were instituted, thus preventing a significant worsening of the person's condition.

Screening instruments

The development of the *DSM* criteria (see page 216), in providing diagnostic criteria for delirium, provoked the development of a plethora of assessment tools for the purposes of screening, rating, and diagnosing confusion. Most of these instruments have been developed with a view to geriatric and psychiatric nursing, but some have been validated for use in palliative care. The use of a screening instrument does not replace an astute clinical assessment, but it aids in assessing those persons who are suspected of being confused, and can lead to helpful specific evaluation. Nurses can administer most confusion-screening instruments.

One example of such a screening instrument is the 'Confusion Rating Scale' (Williams 1991). It is an observational screening, intended for use and documentation once on each shift, with the nurse caring for the person giving a score for each of four domains of patient behaviour, as follows:

▶ disorientation in time, place, or person;
▶ communication;
▶ inappropriate behaviour; and
▶ illusions or hallucinations.

A positive score in one or more of these four domains might be due to delirium, but might also be due to dementia, depression, or a psychotic illness. Further assessment is therefore necessary. The 'Confusion Assessment Method' (CAM) is a useful diagnostic tool that can be used in many situations, including palliative care (Inouye 1990).

During the course of a brief interaction with the person, the clinician assesses for the following features:

▶ acute onset and a fluctuating course;
▶ inattention;
▶ disorganised thinking; and/or
▶ altered consciousness.

A diagnosis of delirium is dependent on the presence of *both* of the first two features, and one of either the third or forth.

Search for a precipitating cause

Once a clinical diagnosis of delirium has been made, further clinical assessment and investigations relevant to the person's condition will confirm the likely cause.

A review of the current medications is important in any assessment of delirium, and those that might cause confusion should be reduced or ceased.

Noting early changes

Mrs GM, aged 52, was admitted for respite. She had been diagnosed with breast cancer and bony metastases. On admission, Mrs GM required some increased analgesia but was otherwise well. During her time as an inpatient, nurses got to know her well. Two days before she was due to be discharged home, it was noticed that Mrs GM was unable to concentrate fully when discussing discharge arrangements with the nurse. This was unusual and prompted further investigation before the patient was discharged to home care.

Further screening showed she was, indeed, clinically confused, and blood tests revealed hypercalcaemia. This was treated, and Mrs GM's confusion settled, although it did not entirely resolve. However, Mrs GM was able to return to her home in a stable state, and with her carers aware of the need to monitor this condition.

Rotation of opioids can provide a partial or full resolution of confusion in some people (Ashby, Martin & Jackson 1999).

Physical problems, especially those related to bowel and bladder function, should be reassessed. Many of these contributing problems can be managed relatively easily.

Special investigations following routine observations can pinpoint the cause. For example, a raised temperature might suggest that the patient has an infection. Suitable investigations might include a chest X-ray or a urine test. Other tests, such as blood tests might be help to identify the cause in particular cases. Hypercalcaemia should be considered as a cause in persons with squamous cell lung cancer, breast cancer, and multiple myeloma because these tumours often metastasise to bone—although it should be noted that hypercalcaemia can also occur without bony metastases. Renal failure is especially prone to cause problems in persons receiving opioids due to decreased metabolism of the drugs and their metabolites.

Management of confusion in palliative care
General
Sometimes confusion is not distressing to the person (Davis et al. 2001). Occasionally, patients describe having seen or spoken to someone who has died. This does not always distress people, and they often say they actually find comfort in the experience. They are able to describe in detail the conversation, and speak of it as being very real. In this situation, support and an opportunity to share the experience is the appropriate management.

'All management approaches must respect personal, cultural, spiritual, and family wishes.'

All management approaches must respect personal, cultural, spiritual, and family wishes. However, any underlying causes should be treated, if this is an appropriate option.

Environmental issues
Intervention with respect to environmental issues is aimed at support and re-orientation. Simple measures can be very effective. These include:

▶ clear and concise communication;
▶ continuity in carers whenever possible and practical;
▶ ensuring that the immediate area around the patient is safe and uncluttered, whether the person is at home or hospitalised;

❯ placing familiar items near the patient (such as a clock or favourite rug) can provide reassurance;
❯ avoiding harsh or sudden lights or noises (with a dim night light for re-orientation);
❯ music (for those persons who enjoy it);
❯ ensuring that patients have hearing aids and spectacles in place; these are simple measures, but surprisingly effective; and
❯ providing a low bed can prevent falls and injuries.

Family education

Family members can feel distressed, embarrassed, and overwhelmed by their loved one's behaviour. They often need support and guidance to help them to understand the situation. Family members should be provided with opportunities to discuss issues of concern to them.

Treatment of confusion

It is important to treat the delirium itself, as well as the underlying cause (if diagnosed, and if treatment appropriate). Delirium is often unpleasant for the person and, as Casarett and Inouye (2001) have observed: '. . . the patient's time is limited [so] it is reasonable to treat the delirium before, or in concert with, a diagnostic evaluation'.

Pharmacological treatment

The goal of pharmacological management of delirium is to provide relief of distressing symptoms without sedating the patient. Some of the commonly used drugs are:
❯ haloperidol;
❯ newer antipsychotics; and
❯ benzodiazepines.

Haloperidol

Haloperidol (Serenace; Haldol) is an antipsychotic drug with a rapid onset of action. It is considered the cornerstone of the pharmacological approach to confusion because it improves cognitive function in acute confusion. Symptom improvement is usually evident within hours, often before the underlying cause is treated. The recommended dose is 0.5–1.0 mg repeated half-hourly until a response is achieved (Casarett & Inouye 2001). Once an effective titrated dose over 24 hours has been established, the daily requirement is given in divided doses every 12 hours.

Newer antipsychotics
The newer antipsychotics are currently available in Australia as oral medications only. They include olanzapine (Zyprexa) and risperidone (Risperdal). There is some evidence that these are useful drugs in the management of delirium in palliative-care patients (Passik & Cooper 1999).

Benzodiazepines
Benzodiazepines have a more sedating effect than haloperidol. Useful benzodiazepines in the management of delirium include clonazepam (Rivotril) and midazolam (Hyponovel). Clonazepam is a long-acting agent that can be administered orally (as a tablet or as sublingual drops), or subcutaneously. Midazolam is a short-acting agent that is administered subcutaneously or intravenously.

Rehydration
If dehydration is thought to be the cause of confusion, rehydration is required. This can be achieved slowly subcutaneously. Further discussion on hydration in the terminal phases of palliative care can be found in Chapter 13 (page 187).

Management of terminal restlessness
Medications
The management of terminal restlessness is similar to that of confusion. The most significant difference in management is in the pharmacological approach.

The drugs of choice for terminal restlessness are the benzodiazepines because of their sedating, anxiolytic, and anticonvulsant effects (Burke 1997). They rarely cause side-effects. In particular, they do not cause increased central nervous system excitation, which can exacerbate any tendency to myoclonus. Benzodiazepines are particularly effective when alcohol withdrawal is contributing to the person's restlessness. The dose is titrated according to patient response, balancing control of symptoms against sedating effects—with the aim of keeping the person rousable. Unfortunately, this is often not possible and sedation of the patient is required (Hardy 2000). About 25% of people who exhibit terminal restlessness in the last days of their lives will require sedation (Ross & Alexander 2001).

Antipsychotic drugs such as haloperidol are usually not recommended because they provide inadequate sedation and can lower the seizure threshold.

Ethical issues in sedation

The main issue that arises in using sedation for confused patients—both those with terminal confusion and those with a potentially reversible delirium—is the question of treating people who are unable to consent to the treatment. Most treatments in palliative care are discussed with the person concerned, and sometimes the family. The person is an active partner in the treatment plans. In contrast, a confused patient is unable to understand his or her illness, and unable to discuss the treatment options. A confused person might be unwilling to accept any treatment, including analgesia, because of paranoia about being 'poisoned'. Most clinical staff accept that if a confused patient is extremely agitated and unwilling (or unable) to take oral medication, '. . . it is appropriate and justifiable to give a sedative by injection to relieve distress, restore dignity, and enable analgesia to be given if required' (Randall & Downie 1999).

In some cases it is not possible to cease the sedation, either because no cause or other appropriate treatment can be found for the restlessness, or because any lightening of the sedation causes the person to become severely agitated again, with behaviour that poses a risk to his or her care. Although these situations are uncommon, it might be necessary to continue strong sedation for some time, with ongoing discussions about terminal sedation occurring among members of the team, and with the family.

In most cases in which the level of necessary sedation is such that the patient is unaware of his or her situation, the person is said to be 'terminally confused', and is dying. As in all palliative-care situations, it is vital to explain the situation and likely outcomes to the family, and to discuss what treatment is planned and what the effects of this treatment are likely to be.

Conclusion

Acute confusion in palliative care is under-recognised, and is therefore not treated optimally. There is a need for the possibility of acute confusion to be monitored throughout the illness, with a view to early identification and appropriate management. It is important to recognise the impact of emotional distress in complicating confusion and terminal restlessness. It is also important to embrace all realms of patient care, including emotional, social, physical, spiritual, and cultural factors when assessing and managing confusion. This is an under-researched, but important, issue in clinical palliative care.

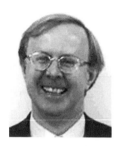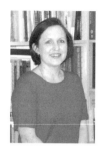

David Kissane

David Kissane is is a consultant psychiatrist and professor of palliative medicine at the University of Melbourne (Victoria, Australia). He is also director of the Centre for Palliative Care, which was formed in 1996 as a consortium of Melbourne care providers and institutions involved with palliative care. David's research interests include observational studies of adaptation to cancer, therapeutic interventions to enhance coping, and outcome studies of bereaved families. In the past five years, he has produced 46 refereed articles, chapters, monographs and non-print media publications. David is on three editorial boards, and reviews for ten journals and seven research funding bodies.

Patsy Yates

Associate Professor Patsy Yates is director of research for the Centre for Palliative Care Research and Education (Queensland, Australia), and is director of postgraduate programs in the School of Nursing, Queensland University of Technology. She has extensive experience in clinical practice, education, and research in cancer and palliative care and, for the past six years, has held an academic and clinical appointment with the Division of Oncology at Royal Brisbane Hospital (Queensland, Australia).

Chapter 16

Psychological and Existential Distress

David Kissane and Patsy Yates

Introduction

In palliative care, all members of the treatment team must be competent in the clinical response to distress. Given their intimate relationships with the dying and their carers, nurses are especially important in this regard. They need to be adept in the recognition, diagnosis, and management of distress, including skills in advocacy and referral when particular professional help is required. A framework (or taxonomy) of distress helps nurses to approach these issues with purpose and clarity.

> 'Nurses need to be adept in the recognition, diagnosis, and management of distress.'

Distress can be defined as an unpleasant emotional experience arising from psychological (affective, behavioural, cognitive), physical, social, or spiritual issues. This experience requires a coping response as the person adapts to the challenges of life. *Existential distress* is more specifically defined as that distress which arises from confrontation with the essence of existence—the issues of death, the meaning of life, aloneness, responsibility, freedom, choices, and a sense of personal worth (Yalom 1980).

There are many potential causes of transient distress in palliative care, including insensitive comments, long waits in clinical departments, and disease symptoms. Such potential causes of distress should be an important focus of attention in everyday nursing practice, because the disruption and worry they cause is often unnecessary. More prolonged mood disturbance also needs to be a major focus of nursing practice. Existential threat is more likely to cause persistent anxiety or depressive symptoms requiring intervention. Although it is not a traditional medical diagnostic category, existential suffering is a substantial cause of distress.

There are key stages in life when individuals are more likely to grapple with existential distress. Transitional periods in life—such as adolescence, mid-life, and terminal illness—can be times when life events (such as bereavement, relationship breakdown, natural disaster, unemployment, financial loss, and health problems) disrupt usual routines. Clinicians need to be especially aware of the existential component of distress at these times.

Whereas most physical symptoms can be fairly effectively treated with modern palliative care, existential distress poses special problems because it is a threat to personhood—the sense of who a person really is (Cassell 1982). Such distress is more than pain, anxiety, or depression.

Communication about death and dying is one of the most formidable nursing tasks. Nurses must balance honest discussion of prognosis with the promotion of hope. In achieving this balance, nurses can think in terms of the authentic 'living out' of the life that remains (Butow, Kazemi & Beeney 1996). The ideal of the possible cure of cancer can mean that doctors and nurses become perceived as omnipotent healers. When cancer progresses, people can feel abandoned. A comment such as 'there is nothing more I can do for you' can doom a person to abject dejection.

'A comment such as "there is nothing more I can do for you" can doom a person to abject dejection.'

Nurses have an especially important role in helping with such distress. Many of their everyday interactions with patients can foster hope, preserve dignity, and enable achievement of personal goals. This is the essence of good palliative-nursing practice, and an integral component of the overall multidisciplinary management plan. To provide effective support for the dying, nurses require a sound understanding of potential sources of existential distress in individual people, and competence in tailoring their responses to patients' needs.

Forms of existential distress

A typology of existential suffering is set out in Table 16.1 (page 232). For each existential issue, there is a mature response in which the individual can achieve resolution with equanimity. Such people not only appear composed but also, when asked, will reveal a sense of spiritual transcendence that aids acceptance of their circumstances. However, when distress supervenes, certain symptoms can emerge. From this state it is possible that further deterioration will lead to a clearcut psychiatric disorder. On other occasions, chronic distress follows and needs to be treated on its own merits.

In practice, there is overlap between these mental states and several can coexist in any given person. Thus a person with a controlling and rigid personality style might be greatly distressed by a colostomy, leading to a loss of dignity, fear of loss of control, and social withdrawal—all of which lead to greater aloneness and loss of the purpose that life once held. Adjustment and depressive disorders can then develop. Until attention is paid to the existential issues, any resolution of such a person's psychiatric state will be temporary and relapsing.

There have been few formal studies of existential distress in palliative care. One study of 162 terminally ill patients in a Japanese hospice found meaninglessness (present in 37%), hopelessness (37%), role loss (29%), dependency (39%), and concern about being a burden (34%) were common causes of distress (Morita et al. 2000).

Assessing psychospiritual distress

Sensitive nurses have an intuitive awareness of the 'troubled nature' of those in their care, but routine enquiry about existential concerns is the only method of avoiding neglect of such issues. If nurses are comfortable in discussing these matters, the person might return to the topic in his or her own time.

Creating time, space, and privacy are essential to facilitating discussion. People might feel that they do not have the words to describe how they feel, might not want to be a burden, might fear breaking down, might be ashamed of admitting coping problems, or might perceive that the nurse is too busy or uninterested. On the other hand, nurses might fear causing distress for patients, might feel out of their depth, or might feel that the existential or spiritual domain is not an appropriate part of care. Many nurses also feel they have little

Table 16.1 Clinical forms of existential distress

Existential challenge	Successful adaptation	Existential distress	Common symptoms	Related psychiatric disorders
Death	courageous awareness and acceptance	death anxiety	fear of process of dying or being dead; panic at physical symptoms; troubled by uncertainty of future; loss of spiritual or religious beliefs	anxiety and panic disorders (such as agoraphobia); generalised anxiety disorder; acute stress disorder; adjustment disorder with anxious mood
Meaning	spiritual peace and sense of a fulfilling life; courage to live it out fully	demoralisation	sense of pointlessness; loss of spiritual direction; loss of a role; helplessness; desire to die	'demoralisation syndrome' depressive disorders
Grief	sad but resigned to closure of life and need to say goodbye	complicated grief	intense tearfulness, sadness, anger; sense of unfairness; depressed mood	depressive disorders
Aloneness	accompanied and supported by family and friends	existential aloneness	isolated; sense of complete aloneness in life	dysfunctional family; absence of social support; relationship problems

(Continued)

Table 16.1 Clinical forms of existential distress continued

Existential challenge	Successful adaptation	Existential distress	Common symptoms	Related psychiatric disorders
Freedom	acceptance of frailty and reduced independence	loss of control	angst at loss of control; obsessional; trouble with decision-making; unrealistic choices; lack of treatment compliance; fear of dependency	phobic disorders; obsessive compulsive disorders; substance abuse
Dignity	dignified despite infirmity, disfigurement, or handicap	loss of worth	angered or distressed by illness; shame; body image concerns; fears being a burden to others	adjustment disorders

time to assess and address people's concerns comprehensively. It is not uncommon for nurses to use communication simply as a means of providing information, rather than a means of gaining an indepth understanding of patient and carer concerns. Because of these barriers, it is the responsibility of the nurse to take the initiative in signalling an interest in feelings as well as physical wellbeing.

Open-ended inquiry is the usual approach adopted to lead into a psychospiritual discussion. Simple questions can initiate discussion:

▶ 'How are you getting on?'
▶ 'How do you feel you are coping?' or
▶ 'Is there something worrying you that you would like to discuss?'

If the person's demeanour, facial expression, body language, or comments signify distress, the nurse can respond to the cue with a more direct inquiry:

- 'You seem distressed today. Do you want to tell me about it?'
- 'What are you specifically worrying about?' or
- 'What are your greatest fears at this time?'

Many people need more help to steer them towards the crux of their concerns. Their fears are often nebulous, vague, and non-specific. They are not sure what to ask because they lack insight into the course of illness and the potential range of treatments. A useful approach is to use the story of the death of a relative or friend to identify the fears that the person holds for his or her own journey:

- 'What horrified you about the death of X?'
- 'Did you talk to X about her experience?'
- 'Is it possible that X actually coped better than you thought?'

Once the nurse realises that the distress appears to be of an existential nature, the following systematic questions help to assess the person's coping and adaptation:

- 'Are there particular fears you have about the process of dying or what happens after your death?'
- 'Does your life continue to have purpose and meaning?'
- 'What hope do you hold for your future?'
- 'Does sadness come in waves and in specific circumstances, or is it constant and persistent?'
- 'Are you troubled by a sense of loss of control over your life?'
- 'Do you hold on to your sense of self worth, your dignity as a person?'
- 'Do you feel supported or terribly alone?'

The nurse should listen carefully to the responses and, if necessary, follow them up until the person's situation is well understood. Although the discussion that follows might raise issues of a personal nature, this type of questioning can help the nurse to gain a deeper understanding of the particular sources of a person's distress, and allow a more appropriate response to an individual's concerns. Inviting people to discuss existential concerns in this way provides an opportunity for them to share otherwise private and unrecognised sources of suffering. However, such questions are a guide only, and should not be used rigidly as a recipe. The method and timing of raising these issues depends on cues from the person or carer about their readiness to engage in such discussions.

Standardised screening instruments can also be used. Examples include the General Health Questionnaire, Brief Symptom Inventory, or Beck Depression Inventory. However, the validity of such screening tools in the palliative-care setting has not been established, and the use of standardised instruments with people who are very seriously ill might cause additional unnecessary distress and burden (Grealish 2000). Screening instruments certainly do not replace a comprehensive clinical assessment of each individual patient. Such instruments can only indicate if a patient has a particular psychiatric symptom suggestive of a diagnosis (Lloyd-Williams 2001). A clinical decision about how to treat and whether to refer is still required.

Promoting hope while supporting grief

Mourning is inevitable for people with advanced illness as they come to terms with the many losses that can result from their illness, its treatment, and its progression. In a trusting and safe environment, people will share their grief with relatives, friends, nurses, and doctors. These people must allow enough time to listen to the person's distress. Sharing grief facilitates healing. Recognition and acceptance of grieving can be very reassuring for many people who are caught up in a turmoil of emotions.

> 'Sharing grief facilitates healing.'

Grief waxes and wanes throughout the progression of an illness, and nurses should therefore ensure ongoing assessment, and respond sensitively to changing needs.

It is important for nurses to focus on hope, for hope is the lifeline for continued involvement with the life that remains. Frank truth-telling can destroy hope if clinicians do not acknowledge that they can be wrong in estimating prognosis (Christakis 1999). If a person has received more bad news, nurses can assist by reminding the person to keep some hope alive, by being present to answer questions, and by giving information, listening, and comforting. The nurse can check the person's understanding, and re-emphasise what can be done. The willingness of the nurse to be present and share these difficult times helps to establish trust and allows exploration of the hopes and desires that are important for the person as he or she progresses through the illness.

Helpful questions to ask at this point include:

▶ 'Does your grief help or hinder your ongoing life?'
▶ 'Imagine that you fare better than predicted. If you are still alive in one or two years' time, would you want to have grieved all that time?'
▶ 'Could your grief be premature? Perhaps it would be better postponed until your life is truly coming to a close?'

Discussion can then focus on the present, with its agenda. The nurse can invite the person to move from a state of generalised hope for the future to particular hopes to take up here and now. Achieving a balance between grief and hope can be a tightrope, but getting this balance right is critical to adaptive adjustment. Several writers have described helpful strategies for nurses in fostering hope in these difficult situations (Ersek 2001; Herth 1995; Penson 2000).

Helping death anxiety

The wish to continue living is a potent life force that is present in most people until the moment of death, and fear of death grows as death approaches. For those fortunate enough to live long and fulfilling lives, acceptance of dying can develop, and anxiety regarding death is inversely proportional to life satisfaction (Yalom 1980). But for other people, anxiety regarding death is present to varying degrees—either as a fear of the process of dying or as a fear being dead. Uncertainty over when this will occur adds to the distress.

This anxiety can present as:
▶ dread, agitation, or panic;
▶ maladaptive behaviours;
▶ poor coping (such as avoidance, poor compliance, and nightmares); or
▶ somatic symptoms.

These presentations can vary from mild to extreme, and might be diagnosed as adjustment disorder, panic disorder, or anxiety disorder (APA 1994). In these cases, relaxation and meditation can promote a sense of calm and control. Antianxiety medication with long-acting benzodiazepines or antidepressants can also be helpful for very distressed people. Nurses should be aware that severe anxiety might require referral for specialised management.

However, for the majority of people, inviting them to talk about their fear helps them to put unspoken thoughts into words. Sharing their fears helps people to feel understood and supported.

Many people ask questions about what it is like to die. The nurse needs to feel comfortable in describing the process of failing health, reduced appetite, gradual weight loss, greater need to sleep and rest, and gradual progression to drowsiness and coma. The nurse can give reassurance about effective pain control and the capacity of nurses to control symptoms and sustain a peaceful state.

Precise information about the range of modern palliative approaches to symptom control can do much to reassure frightened patients. Nurses can stress that progress has been made in recent years—in contrast to the memories that people might carry of 'bad deaths' that they have witnessed in the past.

Recognition and treatment of Demoralisation Syndrome

If a person reviews his or her life, and feels that there has been a lack of purpose or absence of fulfilment, this can cause despair associated with a feeling that life has been wasted. A demoralised person might be heard to say: 'I can't see the point any more; there's no reason to go on'. A demoralised person lacks meaning and purpose in life, and becomes trapped in a conviction that life is futile. Such a person might desire death, but not with the acceptance that life has been satisfying and fulfilling, as is commonly seen in elderly people who patiently await their deaths. Rather, a demoralised person can await death with impatience—because life is perceived as meaningless and might as well be ended. Suicidal thoughts can develop in a demoralised person who can see no other way out (Kissane, Clarke & Street 2001). However, such people might not be clinically depressed, and can be perceived by clinicians as having rationally chosen suicide as a merciful conclusion to their lives (Kissane 2001).

Such changes in morale can span a spectrum from *disheartenment* (mild loss of confidence) through *despondency* (starting to give up), and *despair* (losing hope), to *demoralisation* (having given up). Although the mild end of this spectrum is an understandable response to adversity and requires appropriate supportive responses from nurses that enhance a person's hope and sense of self-worth, the severe form is pathological because it is maladaptive, causes considerable personal distress, and has the potential to generate greater harm if there is further deterioration and the possibility of suicide. Given this degree of morbidity, demoralisation syndrome meets the usual requirements to be considered as an illness (Kissane, Clarke & Street 2001).

Demoralisation syndrome can be formally defined as a psychiatric state in which hopelessness, helplessness, meaninglessness, and existential distress form the core phenomena. The diagnostic criteria for demoralisation syndrome are:

> 'Changes in morale can span a spectrum from *disheartenment* through *despondency* and *despair*, to *demoralisation*.'

▶ symptoms of existential distress (meaninglessness, pointlessness, hopelessness);

▶ a sense of pessimism, 'stuckness', helplessness, and loss of motivation to cope differently;

▶ associated social isolation, alienation, or lack of support; and

▶ these phenomena persisting for more than two weeks.

Hopelessness and helplessness arise from the experience of feeling trapped or not knowing what to do, and often occur in the context of alienation and social isolation. The existential distress includes despair and angst, even extending to people losing a sense of who they are. Sometimes intense anxiety can lead to desperation to obtain relief, and an imminent risk of suicide. The thoughts of a demoralised person are dominated by pessimism, exaggeration, generalisation, and 'all-or-none' thinking in which the world is seen in 'black-and-white' terms. There can be negative self-labelling that lowers self-esteem. The person is still able to interact with the environment, but without enthusiasm—because he or she lacks motivation, and has no perception of a worthwhile future.

Demoralisation can be contrasted with depression. Demoralisation is characterised by a sense of incompetence through loss of meaning and purpose, whereas depression is characterised by a loss of pleasure or interest in life's activities. In addition, although demoralised people lack *anticipation* of pleasure, they can still enjoy pleasure *in the present*. In contrast, depressed people lose *both* anticipatory pleasure *and* pleasure in the present.

It has been known for some time that a wish to die is more highly correlated with a sense of hopelessness than with the severity of depression (Beck, Kovacs & Weisman 1975). This finding has been confirmed in several studies of the terminally ill (Chochinov, Wilson & Enns 1998; Owen et al. 1994; Breitbart, Rosenfeld & Passik 1996; Breitbart, Rosenfeld & Pessin 2000). Furthermore, desire for death fluctuates with changes in hopelessness during the terminal stages of an illness (Chochinov et al. 1999).

Untreated demoralisation commonly, but not always, develops into clinical depression, and a demoralised state should be noted when depression is being treated—in case demoralisation triggers subsequent relapse.

> 'A wish to die is more highly correlated with a sense of hopelessness than with the severity of depression.'

Demoralisation is associated with people who are elderly, disabled, disfigured, dependent, and socially isolated, especially if they are concerned about being a burden, fear a loss of dignity, or express desires for death or active suicidal thoughts. The relative lack of attention to demoralisation is understandable because it has been considered to be a form of 'subthreshold depression'. But it is now being recognised as a separate and clinically important mental state (Kissane Clarke & Street 2001).

Pharmacological therapy for comorbid anxiety and depressive states should not be overlooked.

Therapeutic approaches to management of demoralisation syndrome include:

▶ ensuring continuity of care and active symptom management with empathy and reassurance;

▶ the use of meaning-based therapy to counter boredom and to explore meaning and purpose in life; these therapies include goal-setting, task orientation, and role delineation;

▶ cognitive-behavioural therapy (reality-testing, problem-solving, and reframing of pessimism, sense of failure, or shame);

▶ interpersonal therapy (nurturing of relationships and adaptation to change);

▶ family therapy (support for carers and promotion of healthy family functioning);

▶ life review narrative therapy with attention to spiritual or religious issues; and

▶ pharmacological therapy for anxiety and depressive states.

These approaches are directed primarily at enhancing meaning and fostering hope. For example, generalised hope provides the climate to develop particular hopes and rescues a person at times when specific hope seems no longer realistic. Support of grief and uncertainty can also empower a return of hope and meaning. Relationships that counter alienation and isolation are fundamental to sustaining this support, and can highlight continuity of the person's role and identification of any tasks that still remain. This includes ongoing conversations with family members, affirming their worth, and expressing gratitude for times shared. The overall emphasis is on 'being' rather than 'doing'.

Nurses working with demoralised patients can contribute to such therapy in numerous ways. During everyday conversations, nurses can do much to enhance a person's sense of self worth by actively listening to the person's past and present life experiences, and by acknowledging the value of these experiences. Nurses can encourage family and friends to be present and involved in supportive social interactions. This informal support can be important in providing emotional support, practical help, and companionship.

> 'Approaches are directed primarily at enhancing meaning and fostering hope.'

Reorganising care schedules and daily routines can also be of benefit by allowing a dying person to maximise participation in activities that give joy and allow a continuation of normal functions. Nurses can provide comfort, maintain privacy, and help the person to feel good about his or her appearance and environment—all of which can enhance a person's willingness to engage in meaningful social interactions and activities.

Nurses can draw on a range of other services if available—including volunteers, diversional therapists, and hospice day centres. All of these services can provide additional opportunities for participation in activities that can enhance meaning and purpose in everyday life, and overcome boredom.

Actively managing anxiety and depression

Standard psychotherapy and pharmacological management for patients who experience anxiety and depression is sometimes required. Relaxation and meditation therapies are useful for anxiety disorders, as is judicious use of minor tranquillisers and hypnotics. Concern over physical dependence on benzo-diazepines is not an issue in terminal care, but selection of long-acting agents avoids the rebound wakefulness often seen with standard short-acting hypnotics. Antidepressants have proven efficacy as both anti-panic agents and in the treatment of depression.

The treatment of depression in palliative care thus includes supportive therapy that restores self-esteem, enhances relationships, mourns losses, and is task-oriented with goal-setting for the future.

This can be combined with antidepressant medication selected from the following:

▶ *selective serotonin reuptake inhibitors* (SSRIs) such as sertraline (Zoloft) 50–200 mg, paroxetine (Oxetine, Paxtine, Aropax) 10–40 mg, citalopram (Celapram, Cipramil) 10–40 mg, fluvoxamine (Luvox) 50–300 mg, and fluoxetine liquid 20 mg/5 mL (Lovan liquid) by nasogastric tube or percutaneous enterostomy gastrostomy (PEG) administration;

▶ *selective noradrenergic reuptake inhibitors* (SNRIs) which are useful for severe depression and as co-analgesics; these include as mirtazapine (Mirtazon, Avanza, Remeron) 15–60 mg, venlafaxine (Efexor) 37.5–375 mg (divided doses, or slow release);

▶ *tricyclics* such as dothiepin (Prothiaden, Dothep) 75–300 mg, nortriptyline liquid 2 mg/mL (Allegron) for nasogastric or PEG administration

▶ *reversible inhibitors monoamine oxidase type A* (RIMAs) such as moclobemide (Aurorix) 150–600 mg; and

▶ *tetracyclics* such as mianserin (Tolvon) 10–120 mg;
Psychostimulants can also be used. These include:

▶ methylphenidate (Ritalin) 5–20 mg; and

▶ dexamphetamine 5–20 mg.

Lithium and non-selective monoamine oxidase (MAO) inhibitors should generally be avoided, and require specialist supervision if their use is considered desirable.

The effective application of these therapeutic options is often dependent on nurses identifying people with special needs, and communicating this to other members of the treatment team. Studies have suggested that the detection and referral of such people might be an area of difficulty for nurses (Stromgren et al. 2001; NBCC 2000, personal communication). The low referral rate revealed in these studies can be partially explained by a lack of available specialist mental health personnel to whom patients can be referred, and the general unwillingness of these people to accept help. Nurses working in palliative care therefore require skills in detecting psychological disorders, and should advocate for additional specialised care if indicated.

> 'Nurses working in palliative care require skills in detecting psychological disorders.'

Helping the family and community

Effective palliative care requires the engagement of all family members in the circle of care through effective communication. Attention should be paid to the overall quality of family functioning—that is, how well the family pulls together, and whether family members mutually support one another, openly communicate, and resolve conflict. Attention to these matters will optimise the capacity of family members to support their dying relative. This approach will also help to prevent subsequent bereavement morbidity among family members. Meetings conducted in the home are greatly appreciated, but a neutral office setting is recommended when conflict is prominent in the family. A palliative-care domiciliary nurse is well placed to arrange family meetings and attend with a medical practitioner or social worker. A domiciliary nurse's intimate knowledge of the family can be of great assistance in targeting relevant issues and family concerns.

For the majority of people receiving palliative care, families form the primary network of support. Attention to family functioning is very important if isolation and alienation are to be avoided. A useful model of family intervention has been described by Kissane and Bloch (2002) to guide practitioners in the conduct of family meetings and the provision of continued support for the carers.

Will you help me to die?

Approximately one patient in ten desires death and asks for help with their dying (Chochinov et al. 1995). The nurse whom people have grown to trust might be the person who receives this request. This should be recognised as a 'cry for help' that requires sensitive support and active listening to identify fears. A key nursing role is to help the person identify the most appropriate clinician to assist with these concerns, and to reassure the patient that much assistance can be given.

Some people express concern about becoming a burden to their families. In addition, they might fear an undignified death. It is important to explore their expectations and attitudes with respect to these matters. They might have witnessed a death that they perceived as being undignified. In such circumstances, it is important to reassure people about the improved options that modern palliative care provides. Pain is controllable with modern analgesia and anaesthesia; indeed, existential challenges constitute a greater barrier to the relief of suffering. Nonetheless, suffering might not be able to be fully ameliorated. The nurse's task is to support and 'accompany' the dying person on his or her journey. For some people, a spiritual means of transcendence of suffering might prevail; for others, pharmacological relief with deep sleep might be needed. Continued care and support of family and staff is sustained until death.

An unspoken myth within our culture is the expectation of an heroic death in which the individual reaches a state of open acceptance that he or she is dying and can courageously share this reality with family or friends (Seale 1995). In practice, many people fear that they will not reach this unspoken goal. For them, a compromise is a managed death through which they hope to retain some sense of mastery over the manner of their dying, including the timing. This choice leaves them in control, but it is often at the expense of further potential life. Most family onlookers rate the quality of life of the ill person as being substantially worse than the patient does, and such perceptions can predispose family members to a similar fear of loss of dignity (Curtis & Furnisher 1989; Blazeby et al. 1995; Sneeuw et al. 1997). The nurse needs to offer reassurance and help people to appreciate the reality of the situation, promising to accompany the patient through any hard times that might lie ahead.

> 'The nurse's task is to support and "accompany" the dying person on his or her journey.'

Conclusion

The nurse becomes aware of distress in people through their gestures, bodily demeanour, innuendo, or quiet tears, and this is often revealed while physical care is being attended to. The nurse is well placed within the treatment team to listen to the person's issues and concerns, and to advocate for his or her needs. However, the nurse is not trained professionally to treat and resolve all sources of distress. Often the nurse's most important role is to raise concern about this distress within the multidisciplinary team, so that others who *are* appropriately trained can respond. Nurses must be confident in their advocacy, and must be persistent until other health professionals have duly attended to their patients' needs.

The nurse's sensitive and compassionate care of the terminally ill is the bedrock of clinical care because it continues when cure is no longer possible, and is sustained until death finally intervenes. Even then, the support of the nurse remains vital for the bereaved who, as carers, have usually formed special relationships with the nursing team and will continue to look for this support. The nurse has a pivotal role in assisting with emotional distress through the care delivered to patients and their relatives—a privileged role as comforter in what, for some, are dire times.

'Nurses must be confident in their advocacy, and must be persistent until other health professionals have duly attended to their patients' needs.'

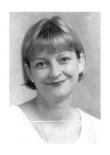

Kate White

Dr Kate White has an extensive background in palliative care in the areas of clinical practice, education, and research. She is currently associate professor of Cancer and Palliative Care at Edith Cowan University (Perth, Western Australia). Kate's research areas have focused on sexuality, women's cancers, rural health care, and communication and psychosocial aspect of care. Her PhD focused on patient's perceptions of quality of life during palliative care. Kate represents palliative-care and cancer nurses on a number of national and state bodies.

Chapter 17

Sexuality and Body Image

Kate White

Introduction

The focus of this chapter is sexuality and body image in people receiving palliative care. The message often given to these people by the health-care team, directly or indirectly, is that sexuality; body image, and sexual function are not priority issues at this time of their lives. The reality for many individuals is very different. The purpose of this chapter is twofold. First, the chapter aims to highlight why sexuality and body image need to be considered in the palliative-care context. Secondly, the chapter outlines strategies to assist nurses to discuss and respond to sexuality issues that can arise in the palliative-care setting.

Although there is no consensus on the definition of sexuality, it is widely recognised that sexuality is an integral component of who each person is, and is central to each individual's uniqueness (Masters & Johnson 1980). Sexuality is fundamental to the way people share intimacy, experience physical closeness, view themselves as sexual beings, and are perceived by others (Dennison 2001). Sexuality and body image are closely linked with roles and relationships within families, at work, and in society (Rice 2000; Dennison 2001). Sexuality includes, but should never be limited to, sexual intercourse and sexual function. Body image is an important aspect of sexuality.

Sexuality and body image in palliative care

Cancer and other life-threatening disorders, and treatment for these conditions, have profound physical and emotional effects on all aspects of people's lives, including sexuality and body image (see Table 17.1, below).

It is unknown how many palliative-care patients experience problems or concerns regarding sexuality and altered body image. The questions are rarely asked. In a survey of symptom burden in 348 hospice patients, although only 16% of patients reported concerns regarding body image or sexual function,

Table 17.1 Sexuality and body image issues in life-threatening illness

Issue	Reason
Infertility	medications
	surgery
	hormonal treatment
	radiotherapy
	chemotherapy
Altered body image	surgical removal of tissue or organs
	weight loss or gain
	loss of muscle function and tone
	alopecia
Impotence	surgery
	medications
	radiotherapy
	vascular or neurological factors
Premature menopause	surgery
	radiation therapy
	chemotherapy
	hormonal therapy
Loss of libido	medications
	psychological distress
	physical limitations
	altered body image
Loss of sexual function (physical genital impairment)	pelvic radiotherapy
	surgery
	neurological deficits

Author's presentation

these questions had not been not asked of more than 60% of the patients (Kutner, Kasner & Nowels 2001). However, discussions with palliative-care nurses indicate that sexuality and body image issues frequently arise in caring for their patients.

The lack of assessment of sexuality is an issue for all palliative-care staff, given that the importance of sexuality as an integral component of an individual's quality of life does not decrease in the palliative-care phase (Fallowfield 1992; Shell & Smith 1994). There is now an extensive body of literature that describes the effect of cancer on sexuality and body image. Those at greater risk of such problems are those with a high investment in body image before their

> 'Nurses indicate that sexuality and body image issues frequently arise in caring for their patients.'

diagnosis, those in unsupportive relationships, those with pre-existing relationship problems, those who were single at the time of diagnosis, and those with a history of psychological illness (Kissane, White & Cooper 2002).

As shown in Table 17.2 (page 248), there are several physical and emotional factors in the palliative-care context that can affect an individual's sexuality and body image. This is a not a definitive list because any problem that has potential to diminish sexual functioning, feelings of sexual attractiveness, or relationships can have a negative effect on an individual's sexuality (Rice 2000).

In discussing sexuality issues, there remains a tendency to focus on sexual function, and on associated conditions such as dyspareunia, impotence, premature menopause, and infertility. However, for the majority of palliative-care patients, fatigue is the most common physical problem (Neuenschwander & Bruera 1998). Fatigue affects sexuality in a number of ways, including inability to maintain a role, decrease or loss of sexual desire, limited energy to focus on relationships, and decreased ability to maintain personal grooming or hygiene. It can be extremely challenging to 'feel sexual' when a person is unable to shave, blow dry hair, clean teeth, or shower. Similarly, any unrelieved symptom has the potential to affect sexuality. Unrelieved suffering can be overwhelming, and can block out all other aspects of an individual's life. Pain, nausea and vomiting, constipation, and dyspnoea are all commonly experienced by palliative-care patients.

Each of these symptoms has potential to affect an individual's sexuality. Prompt assessment and intervention are essential in limiting the effect of these symptoms on all aspects of quality of life. Awareness of the potential adverse effects of medications on sexuality is crucial. A range of medications commonly

Table 17.2 Sexuality and body image factors in palliative care

Symptom or treatment	Effect on sexuality
Fatigue	loss of libido; decreased physical ability; decreased ability to maintain personal grooming
Depression, anxiety, grief	loss of libido; possible effect on relationship (including ability to communicate concerns; disinterest in sexuality and appearance)
Pain	physical limitations due to pain and discomfort; decreased desire
Altered body image	loss of self-esteem; altered perception of attractiveness
Loss of role	loss of self-esteem and effect on self-perception
Unrelieved symptoms	increased suffering; fatigue; loss of desire and libido
Symptoms that cause loss of dignity (for example, incontinence)	negative effect on body image and sexuality; embarrassment
Medications (for example, opioids, antidepressants)	loss of libido; altered body image
Malodour	altered body image; effect on relationships
Loss of independence	perception of self, sexuality, and body image
Halitosis, dry mouth	embarrassment
Dyspnoea	loss of energy
Neurolytic procedures	coeliac plexus block; dry ejaculation

Author's presentation

used in palliative care (such as steroids, opioids, and antidepressants) can affect libido, potency, and body image. Mouth care is an important aspect of palliative care. It is equally important in sexuality if people experience difficulties in communicating or kissing because of oral problems.

Alteration in body image can have a profound effect on an individual's self-worth and sexuality (Rice 2000). Disfiguring surgery, a stoma, weight loss or gain, alopecia, insertion of tubes for feeding or hydration, and changes in clothing are some of the alterations in appearance experienced by people receiving palliative care. Concerns regarding alteration in body image can affect relationships, and can lead to communication and sexuality problems if not addressed. Psychological distress, such as depression, anxiety, or grief alters an individual's sense of self, ability to participate in relationships, and ability to engage in life generally (Rice 2000). Loss of sexual desire or a decrease in sexual pleasure is a common symptom of depression (Massie & Popkin 1998).

Loss of dignity can have a profound impact on any individual. There are many potential causes of loss of dignity in palliative care. Incontinence is frequently feared, and can be a source of significant distress if it occurs. Another concern for some people is being dependent on another for assistance with personal hygiene or toileting, or simply being seen in their nightwear or without a wig. These are everyday activities for palliative-care nurses, but they require sensitivity to ensure that the individual's dignity is maintained and that his or her sexuality is respected.

Silence about sexuality

Despite the volume of literature regarding sexuality, it remains a neglected area in palliative-care nursing (Jenkins 1988; Schover 1991; Fallowfield 1992; Shell & Smith 1994, Rice 2000). This is of particular concern, given that people identify nurses as the preferred health professional with whom to discuss sexuality (Waterhouse & Metcalfe 1991), and given that simple interventions such as supportive listening and provision of information can make a difference (Schover 1999; Dennison 2001). It is also of concern that fewer then 10% of cancer patients raise sexuality issues unless specifically asked. That nurses find this to be a difficult area to explore with people is not surprising, given the fact that few nurses receive education in this area. Several factors have been identified as major barriers for nurses in addressing sexuality issues. These include lack of knowledge and skills (Chamberlain Wilmoth 1994), fear of causing distress (Rice 2000), misconceptions regarding sexuality, personal biases and prejudices (Waterhouse & Metcalfe 1991), or structural issues such as a lack of privacy (Schwartz & Plawecki 2002).

Palliative-care nurses need to be knowledgeable about the effect on sexuality of life-threatening diseases and their treatments if they are to respond to this important aspect of quality of life. This knowledge allows nurses to anticipate problems, assess

'People identify nurses as the preferred health professional with whom to discuss sexuality.'

each person's response, and plan care accordingly. Communication skills are crucial to the sensitive exploration of issues related to sexuality (Schover 1999). There is evidence to suggest that education in communication skills for palliative-care nurses requires frequent review and update (Wilkinson 1999). Knowledge and effective communication skills will assist nurses to overcome any lack of confidence they might have in exploring these sensitive topics.

The values and beliefs held by nurses can have either positive or negative effects in this respect. Nurses need to be aware of their own values and beliefs regarding sexuality. They should not dismiss these values and beliefs, but they should ensure they do not lead to assumptions being made regarding their patients. In making judgments on appropriate sexual behaviour, nurses need to be aware of how their own values and beliefs influence their judgments (Wright 1996). Similarly, care should be taken not to make assumptions about what might be important to the person in their care (Rice 2000). Common misconceptions include:

▶ age—that is, assuming that sexuality is no longer important to individuals of mature years;
▶ heterosexuality—ignoring the possibility of homosexual relationships;
▶ being single—assuming that sexuality is not an issue for those not in a relationship; and
▶ palliative-care status—assuming that sexuality is not important to palliative patients by assuming that advanced disease precludes interest in sexuality and sexual function.

Approaches and strategies
General approaches
Several strategies can be implemented to support sexuality in a person receiving palliative care. These include:

▶ recognition of the importance of sexuality;
▶ listening to patients' concerns;
▶ assessment;
▶ creating a space for sexuality to be expressed and maintained;
▶ respecting and supporting self-image;
▶ instigating interventions that support the expression of sexuality; and
▶ maintaining a person's dignity.

The cornerstone of interventions for supporting sexuality has been the P.LI.SS.IT model (Annon 1976). This model focuses on four key interventions, with the name of the model being an acronym formed from the first one or two

P.LI.SS.IT model for interventions regarding sexuality

The cornerstone of interventions for supporting sexuality has been the P.LI.SS.IT model This model focuses on four key interventions, with the name of the model being an acronym formed from the first one or two letters of these interventions:

- permission (P)—legitimising the inclusion of sexuality into care by including it in the initial history in conjunction with other systems;
- limited information (LI)—formal and informal sharing of the sexual side-effects of treatment in conjunction with education of other treatment side-effects
- specific suggestions (SS)—discussion of specific techniques that can be used to minimise sexual alterations caused by treatment; and
- intensive therapy (IT)—treatment by a specialist for sexual dysfunction and relationship issues that have resulted from cancer therapy.

Adapted from Annon (1976)

letters of these interventions (see Box, above). Despite being widely discussed in the nursing literature, it has not been widely adopted in clinical practice. However, it is a potential model to guide practice.

Recognising the significance of sexuality and legitimising the person's concerns is of paramount importance in supporting that person's sexuality. This requires supporting the person's expression of his or her concerns in an open and non-judgmental manner. Many nurses fear that asking about sexuality might cause distress to people, or fear that they do not know how to respond to the people's concerns (Clifford 1998). However, as with any area of palliative care, most patients require someone who will listen and validate their concerns. Listening skills are essential. It is important that concerns raised by people are not dismissed or 'normalised'. Comments such as 'most people experience these concerns' might seem to be supportive. However, such comments frequently end the conversation, and can be perceived by the person as being dismissive of his or her concerns. Responding in an open and exploring manner is supportive, and allows nurses to obtain a more detailed assessment of the issues.

Assessment

Assessment is a key component of the nurse's role, given that the majority of palliative-care patients will not disclose sexuality concerns. This assessment needs to be undertaken when privacy can be ensured.

The assessment can occur at different levels. For most people a less complex and detailed assessment is all that is initially required (see Box, page 252).

Level One Sexuality Assessment

- How has [health problem] affected your role as wife/husband/partner/parent?
- How has [health problem] affected how you feel about yourself as a woman/man?
- What aspects of your sexuality have been affected by [health problem]?
- How has [health problem] affected your ability to function sexually?
- How significant has this impact been?

Adapted from Woods (1984) and Wilmoth (1994)

These simple questions give permission for people to raise their concerns, and they show that the nurse is willing to discuss these concerns. For more detailed history-taking and assessment there are several assessment tools that can be used to guide this process (Bruner & Boyd 1999). Sexuality assessment should also include an assessment of the information needs of the patient and his or her partner.

Tailored information and referral

Tailored information can play a major role in addressing concerns about sexuality (Dennison 2001). It should never be assumed that people have been informed or will recall information on the side-effects of treatments related to sexuality and sexual function. Assessment needs to include the person's understanding of his or her disease and treatments, and how these can affect sexuality. Patients should receive information that is tailored to their needs, using visual aids to assist understanding, and ensuring that any misconceptions are corrected (Dennison 2001).

The concerns raised by some people will be beyond the remit of the palliative-care nurse. These people require referral to professionals with appropriate expertise. In assessing concerns regarding sexuality and sexual function it is important to be aware that some issues might be of long standing and not related to the diagnosis of a life-threatening illness. Long-standing relationship problems or sexual dysfunction require specialist expertise. It is important that nurses establish a network of referral for specialised services (Rice 2000). The person might require the services of family planning organisations, women's health nurses, general practitioners who specialise in women's health, relationship counsellors, or sexual therapists. Cancer information services can also be a valuable source of information. It is essential for the nurse to know about the services that are available, how to access them, and when to refer. The suggestion of a referral can be challenging for the person, and permission must be obtained before making the referral. For the majority of people, acknowledgment of the problem and recognition that something can be done helps to overcome their concerns regarding referral. Care should be taken not to stigmatise the person in this process.

Creating a space for sexuality

Creating a space for sexuality can be challenging in institutional settings, but it is achievable. Access to double beds for couples to maintain physical contact is often mentioned as one approach. But there are several other ways in which nurses can create an environment that is supportive of an individual's sexuality, both in the home and in the clinical setting.

Open dialogue among the nurse, the person, and his or her partner is crucial. The most important thing that can be done is to recognise each individual as a sexual being. Respecting and fostering self-image is an important strategy to support the individual's sexuality. This includes attention to personal grooming, assisting people to obtain prostheses that can reinstate body form, encouraging people to maintain normal activities if possible, supporting them to maintain important roles (for example, aspects of the person's mothering role), and wearing normal clothing if this is possible.

'The most important thing that can be done is to recognise each individual as a sexual being.'

Simple events can improve body image—such as getting dressed in day clothes, ensuring that men have a daily facial shave, and purchasing clothes that fit after recent weight loss or gain. The story of Bernadette (Box, page 254) demonstrates how a sensitive nurse can make a significant difference to a person's sense of wellbeing.

Involving partners

Specific strategies need to be tailored to the individual. Partners can be involved in providing personal care, or couples can simply be provided with private time without interruptions for them to communicate and be intimate. Using showering or bathing as an opportunity for physical closeness and intimacy is one example. This requires that privacy is ensured, and additional strategies can include the use of music, soft lighting, or aromatherapy to 'de-institutionalise' this experience.

However, for some people, having partners involved in their physical care decreases their perception of sexuality and desirability, and they can find that

Bernadette

Bernadette was a 48-year-old woman with metastatic breast cancer. She had never allowed anyone; including her husband and children, to see her without her wig and her make-up. When admitted with spinal cord compression, a major concern for Bernadette was that staff, fellow patients, or family would see her ungroomed and without her wig.

The palliative-care nurse arranged for a hand mirror so that Bernadette could apply her make-up each morning, ensured that her side locker was accessible, arranged for Bernadette to be showered before visiting hours, and arranged for night staff to pull the curtains closed so that Bernadette could apply a scarf to sleep in without fellow patients seeing her without her wig.

the shift from 'lover' to 'caretaker' compounds the loss of sexuality (Schover 1997). The story of Joanne and Paul (Box, page 255) is an example of how this can be a problem.

Teaching and encouraging partners to use techniques such as soft-stroke massage encourages the maintenance of physical touch, as well as providing opportunities for communication and closeness. Maintaining social activities, if possible, can also have a positive effect on an individual's sexuality. Eating out, going to the hairdresser, and socialising with friends can all assist to maintain a sense of sexuality. These activities need to be tailored to each individual's current health status.

Providing intimate care

How nurses provide intimate care has always been a challenge, particularly because nurses receive limited preparation for this aspect of their role (Lawler 1991). Respect for an individual's privacy and maintenance of dignity are essential components of providing intimate care and respecting an individual's sexuality. Regrettably, most visitors to adult hospitals have seen a patient walking down a corridor with the back of a hospital gown flapping, exposing the person's buttocks. Regardless of how busy a nurse might be, and regardless of whether the person is unaware, care should always be taken to respect an individual's personal appearance.

'Support for partners is also important in addressing issues of sexuality.'

Support for partners is also important in addressing issues of sexuality. Many partners can experience significant difficulties. The words of the partner of

Joanne and Paul

Joanne was being cared for by her husband at home. The community palliative-care nurse noted increasing tension between Joanne and her husband, Paul. While Paul was out, the nurse explored this with Joanne.

Joanne said that Paul wanted to provide all aspects of her physical care, including showering and taking her to the toilet. For Joanne, this was not only undignified, but also reiterated, on a daily basis, how their relationship had changed. She noted that: 'He used to undress me in a sexual way; now it is like I am a child. I hate every minute of it.'

The nurse explored with Paul and Joanne how they had previously expressed their physical closeness and intimacy. She arranged for community nurses to undertake the daily showers. In addition, Paul arranged intimate dinners each week, learnt how to massage Joanne, and explored approaches to maintaining their sexual relationship.

Negotiating a complex issue

'I mean sex is always a problem in relationships. Let's face it. There's always a problem with who wants more sex and who wants less sex, and so on. And about who's going initiate it and who's not going to initiate it, and so on. And what you feel is you've got to let the woman initiate because obviously you're not going to impose your [pause] desires, you know, because obviously you don't die from not having it. But that of course puts strains on the relationship as well. Because you're not initiating it, she thinks: "He doesn't love me any more".'

a young woman with cancer, as recorded in the Box above, demonstrate how negotiating the complex issues of a sexual relationship can be fraught with misunderstandings if communication is not maintained.

Partners might seek advice on how to be supportive regarding sexuality. Central to this is open communication and, if possible, ensuring that both partners join in the discussion with the nurse. Practical suggestions tailored to the person's current situation is important, with open and honest communication being pivotal to the success of any intervention.

Cultural issues

Cultural sensitivity is crucial to all areas of palliative-care practice, including sexuality. In some cultures it is inappropriate for staff members to raise or discuss issues related to sexuality with patients of the opposite sex. Palliative-care nurses need to be informed about different cultural groups and beliefs to ensure that culturally sensitive care is provided.

Conclusion

Sexuality is an integral component of every individual. Consistent with the philosophical approach of holistic care, attention must be given to addressing the sexuality concerns of palliative-care patients. Support can be provided by nurses through recognition that sexuality is an integral component of quality of life, by assessing sexuality concerns, and by responding appropriately in a non-judgmental manner. Institutional palliative-care services need to develop policies that are supportive of patient sexuality. Individual nurses and service providers have a responsibility to ensure that the health-care team is knowledgeable and skilled in assessing sexuality concerns in those in their care.

> 'Support can be provided by nurses through assessing sexuality concerns, and by responding appropriately in a non-judgmental manner.'

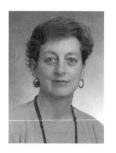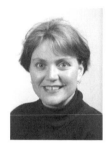

Pauline McCabe

Dr Pauline McCabe has worked as a nurse, midwife, naturopath, and acupuncturist. In higher education she has focused on the integration of nursing and natural therapies in her teaching, writing, consultation, and research. She has had a leading role in developing policy for the nursing profession regarding the integration of complementary therapies into practice, and edited Ausmed's publication *Complementary Therapies in Nursing and Midwifery*. She is currently senior lecturer in naturopathy at the School of Nursing and Midwifery, La Trobe University, Melbourne (Victoria, Australia).

Amanda Kenny

Amanda Kenny is a registered nurse and midwife with extensive experience in rural health care where she gained valuable insight into the issues affecting the health status of people requiring palliative care. Amanda is currently a lecturer in nursing at La Trobe University, Bendigo (Victoria, Australia) where she teaches both palliative care and complementary therapies. She is interested in the evidenced-based use of complementary therapies for nursing practice. Her current research focuses on service delivery in Victoria's rural hospitals.

Chapter 18

Complementary Therapies

Pauline McCabe and Amanda Kenny

Introduction

The use of complementary therapies in palliative care has a very long history. Many 'natural therapies' have traditionally been used in nursing and have been understood as normal nursing care. These have included touch, massage, listening, prayer, the use of scents (now called 'aromatherapy'), energy therapies (therapeutic touch, reiki), diet, music, relaxation techniques, foot massage (reflexology), the therapeutic use of water (hydrotherapy), meditation, visualisation, and the provision of a healing or sacred environment. In a sense, the inclusion of what are now called 'complementary therapies' is really no more than a development of traditional nursing practices. Many of the early nursing arts were foregone as 'high-tech' nursing became the norm. However, in palliative care, natural and complementary therapies add to the nursing arts and can provide nurses with a much wider range of interventions in the provision of patient comfort.

There is a worldwide swing to natural therapies as people attempt to create their own forms of health care by integrating medical and natural therapies according to individual needs. In Australia, approximately 60% of people now use some form of natural therapy (Scherer Australia 1998). This is reflected in the increasing use of natural therapies by cancer patients to complement medical treatment. Consequently, many dying patients will be comfortable with the integration of these therapies into nursing care. Indeed, the area of palliative care is frequently cited as one of the main clinical areas in which complementary therapies are used (Rankin-Box 1997). In the United Kingdom it has been suggested that 70% of palliative-care hospices utilise massage and aromatherapy as therapeutic modalities instigated by nurses (Vickers 1996b).

Current research supports the contention that the use of these therapies by palliative-care patients is increasing, with studies having been conducted on the use of acupuncture, massage, reflexology, acupressure, shiatsu, aromatherapy, herbs, and reiki. The use of complementary therapies can be understood as an empowerment strategy that can be used by palliative-care patients and their families to regain a sense of control over their illness and its management (Turton & Cook 2000), and it has been argued that one of the major benefits of complementary therapies in palliative care is that they encourage self-reliance (Shenton 1996). The notion of palliative-care patients embracing complementary therapies in their quest to find a more caring delivery of service is a constant theme in the literature (Shenton 1996).

Evidence-based practice

One of the greatest challenges for nurses who choose to incorporate complementary therapies into clinical practice is the lack of substantive research that validates these therapies. However, developing research into complementary therapies is not without its problems. It is sometimes difficult to provide rigorous, validated evidence as to why some things seem to work. Many nurses have had anecdotal success with various complementary measures, but are uncertain whether it has been the therapy or 'being with' the person that has provided the benefit.

'Many nurses . . . are uncertain whether it has been the therapy or "being with" the person that has provided the benefit.'

Although there is difficulty in applying some research techniques to complementary therapies, this is not a reason to abandon their use (Vickers 2000). Although there is a need for nurses to have a sound evidence base to justify the use of complementary therapies, this must be balanced (Rankin-Box 1997). Demands for complex research trials have little relevance for most clinically based palliative-care nurses who are struggling to provide quality care within an increasingly demanding and economically constrained health-care system. Research must be directed at highlighting the practical application of these therapies and their value as a complement to conventional medicine, particularly in the palliation of symptoms.

Complementary therapies and symptom control
Overview
Nursing is the cornerstone of effective palliative care, and the palliation of physical symptoms is one of the nurse's primary roles (Abrahm 1998). More than 60% of palliative-care patients have a primary diagnosis of cancer, and many of these are suffering from pain, dyspnoea, narcotic-induced constipation, nausea and vomiting, and sleep problems. Other illnesses encountered in palliative care are end-stage cardiac disease, HIV/AIDS, and end-stage respiratory disease. All of these conditions have many severe physical symptoms.

The case of Meg (Box, page 262) illustrates how various complementary therapies can be used to provide a sense of control and independence in the presence of severe symptoms.

Pain
Of all the physical symptoms that can be experienced by people receiving palliative care, pain is most associated with fear and trepidation. For families, pain relief and pain management are their greatest concerns. Although pharmacological analgesia is central to the management of pain, complementary strategies can enhance pain relief and provide significant patient comfort. Patients are increasingly considering complementary approaches to pain management (Gecsedi & Decker 2001).

'Patients are increasingly considering complementary approaches to pain management.'

Acupuncture
There is good evidence to suggest that acupuncture can be of benefit in pain control. Various studies have found statistically significant increases in pain threshold when acupuncture is used for pain relief (Vickers 1996a). Another

study showed that acupuncture can produce a significant decrease in pain scores and morphine requirements (Hidderley & Weinel 1997).

Reflexology

The use of foot reflexology on patients with breast and lung cancer can result in significantly decreased pain and anxiety (Stephenson et al. 2000).

Meg

Meg, a 38-year-old sole parent of three daughters, had been diagnosed with breast cancer and had undergone mastectomy. There was axillary lymph node involvement. Preoperatively and postoperatively her surgeon prescribed arnica, a common homoeopathic remedy that is thought to minimise shock, bruising, and bleeding and assist in the healing of traumatised tissues.

Meg's treatment included radiotherapy, and chemotherapy. She had read of a study that reported the use of niaouli and tea-tree oils applied as a thin film before radiation to prevent burning and scarring. Meg obtained her surgeon's agreement for her to use these oils before and after radiotherapy. Various herbs were also part of her health regimen.

Three months after her surgery Meg experienced lower back pain and difficulty with movement. A CT scan showed bony metastases in her lumbar region and she was referred to a palliative-care nurse.

Meg's condition rapidly deteriorated. She was determined to avoid high doses of opiates because she wanted to 'stay with it' for her children. She was taught simple relaxation techniques, including imagery. Meg suffered severe bouts of nausea and believed that she gained relief from pressure on her 'pericardium 6 point'. She sipped peppermint tea infused with ginger for nausea.

Meg's eldest daughter, Kate, was very keen to be involved in her mother's care. Kate was taught simple massage techniques and the basic principles of reflexology. Meg talked about cherished moments with her daughters as they enthusiastically provided foot massages.

Meg continued to burn essential oils and used various oils in aromatherapy. Bergamot was used for its uplifting qualities, peppermint oil for nausea, sandalwood for relaxation, and lavender to help her sleep. A towel soaked in warm water with lavender oil and applied to her abdomen seemed to reduce the nausea. The therapies complemented her medical treatment and she died peacefully surrounded by her family and friends.

For Meg, complementary therapies assisted in gaining some control over her illness. She talked about the fact that she could choose whatever therapies that she wanted and that this gave her some sense of independence. She stated that when everything else was out of her control she could still choose something that made her feel better.

Relaxation techniques

The scope of non-pharmacological strategies to manage pain has broadened considerably over the past decade or so. The most popular non-pharmacological strategies are breathing, imagery, music, and meditation (Kwekkeboom 2001).

Patients with advanced cancer using relaxation techniques have reported reductions in pain and have been found to have a significant reduction in non-opiate analgesics, indicating better control and less need for breakthrough pain relief (Sloman et al. 1994).

Nurses should be encouraged to explore relaxation techniques that are effective in managing pain (Kanji 2000).

'Patients with advanced cancer using relaxation techniques have reported reductions in pain.'

Music therapy

There have been numerous studies supporting the use of music therapy in the alleviation of pain in palliative care (for example, O'Callaghan 1996).

One of the biggest challenges for nurses in palliative care is the amelioration of pain from bone metastases. Bone is a common metastatic site for cancers of the breast, prostate, and lung. Approaches to the management of this difficult problem should be multifaceted and can include such things as relaxation therapy, guided imagery, music, meditation, and therapeutic touch (Maxwell, Givant & Kowalski 2001).

Nausea

Acupuncture and acupressure

Acupuncture is a potentially beneficial therapy for palliative-care patients experiencing nausea and vomiting (Vickers 1996a).

Acupressure is a technique that involves manipulating the same acupoints as acupuncture (Harris 1997). It can easily be incorporated into nursing practice, and can be taught to patients and their carers. Acupressure has been shown to decrease nausea among women undergoing chemotherapy for breast cancer (Dibble et al. 2000). In particular, acupressure on acupoint pericardium 6 (PC6)—located on the anterior surface of the forearm proximal to the wrist—can reduce nausea and vomiting in patients undergoing chemotherapy (Price, Lewith & Williams 1991) and has been used to treat nausea and vomiting in children with aggressive cancers (Keller 1995). It has also been suggested that acupressure wristbands worn by palliative-care patients might decrease the incidence of nausea and vomiting (Brown et al. 1992).

Other therapies involving pressure include the role of shiatsu in palliative care. It has been suggested that this might be of value in pain management, control of nausea, and relief of anxiety (Stevenson 1995; Brady et al. 2001).

Other therapies in nausea

Self-hypnosis, music therapy with guided imagery, and relaxation exercises have been shown to decrease the severity of paediatric nausea and vomiting (Keller 1995). Clinical relaxation programs that include massage, guided imagery, and progressive muscle relaxation appear to shorten the emetic period following chemotherapy (Fessele 1996).

It has also been suggested that aromatherapy can be beneficial. There are indications that the use of peppermint oil in electric burners can reduce the incidence of nausea in cancer patients receiving high-dose chemotherapy (Hudson 1998).

Anxiety

Massage can contribute to feelings of relaxation, calmness and wellbeing, but few studies have been conducted in palliative care (Vickers 1996b). However, aromatherapy massage is increasingly being used in palliative care to induce relaxation—offering support and improved quality of life to people with limited treatment options and a poor prognosis (Hadfield 2001).

Aromatherapy massage with 1% roman chamomile essential oil in palliative-care patients has produced immediate positive improvement in anxiety, with a persistent effect on physical symptoms and a consistent fall in anxiety scores over time (Wilkinson 1995).

Quality of life and empowerment

Shiatsu, reflexology, and TENS

Shiatsu can be of benefit in promoting quality of life in persons receiving palliative care, with significant improvements in energy levels, relaxation, confidence, symptom control, clarity of thought, and mobility (Cheesman, Christian & Cresswell 2001).

People in the palliative stage of cancer have reported that their quality of life improved as a result of treatment with reflexology (Hodgson 2000), and it has been suggested that transcutaneous electrical nerve stimulation (TENS) can improve the quality of life and relieve fatigue in palliative-care patients (Gadsby et al. 1997).

Art therapy

Creative arts such as music can reduce anxiety and depression when used as part of a philosophy of healing the whole person (Hirsch & Meckes 2000; Biley 2000).

Art therapy can assist dying people to face pain and depression, lead a more meaningful life, and be creative in the 'art of living' (Deane, Carman & Fitch 2000). Terminally ill people with advanced cancer who were given an opportunity to participate in the making of a sculpture found it to be an empowering experience in which they went 'beyond' their illness and invested energy in something worthwhile (Shaw & Wilkinson 1996).

Complementary therapies in HIV/AIDS

Imagery, massage, and relaxation have been reported by HIV/AIDS patients as contributing to increased coping and feelings of being in control, with 98% reporting that they 'felt better' (Sparber & Lin 2000).

Supporting carers

Research has indicated that carers of palliative-care patients often face declining strength and poor health status (Kristjanson et al. 1996; Weitzner, Moody & McMillan 1997). The majority of palliative care patients are more than 65 years of age, and many caregivers are also of this age. All in all, caregivers are also in need of support and care.

MacDonald (1998) studied the effects of an outreach project that used massage as a respite intervention for primary caregivers. Recipients of this program reported reduction in physical and emotional stress, physical pain, and

'Caregivers are also in need of support and care.'

sleep difficulties. For many recipients, massage become part of the bereavement process as their loved ones died before the sessions were completed. Massage assisted carers with readjusting to life following bereavement, and provided emotional support.

Holistic nursing and complementary therapies

The concept of holistic nursing has received some criticism in recent years. This is partly due to the increased workloads of nurses, and partly due to a work environment that values technology, the medical model, task achievement, and professional detachment (Mackey 1998).

Complementary therapies can be part of the interventions used in holistic care, but they are not the same thing as holistic care (Taylor 2001). It is possible to use a complementary therapy in a detached and mechanistic way.

A holistic understanding of healing in palliative care holds that healing is possible at some level of being until the moment of death (Dossey et al. 1995). When a trusting relationship is developed, a nurse can be chosen to take a dying person's confession, or can facilitate a meeting in which a person makes peace with someone before dying. Spiritual and emotional healing of this nature can be supported by complementary therapies such as massage, listening, and music. Gentle touch and a healing environment can convey the kind of compassion and empathy needed to develop a therapeutic relationship. When the nurse is open to the patient and works with a healing intent, even the simplest tasks become sacred.

Needs cannot be generalised in dying people. Each person has unique requirements at certain times to maintain comfort. The senses are pathways to the inner mind and body, and complementary therapies provide options for soothing troubled senses. Music, aromas, touch, tastes, warmth, water, colour, and soft clothing are examples of environmental influences that can be manipulated to suit the individual. A nurse with healing intent can employ these tools to create the special environment appropriate to the patient.

Professional issues

To clarify the status of complementary therapies within nursing, guidelines have been developed by several professional bodies (RCNA 2000; ANF 1998; NBV 1999). These guidelines do not prescribe which therapies can be practised by nurses (who are free to qualify in whatever therapies they choose), but they do offer guidance on the role of complementary therapies with respect to professional and legal issues, education, practice standards, collaboration and referral, and development of workplace policy.

Standards of practice

Whatever therapies they are practising, nurses must hold to the professional standards applying to nursing practice. In Australia, the major standards include the Victorian *Nurses Act 1993*, the Australian Nursing Council Inc. (ANCI) Competency Standards, and the ANCI Code of Professional Conduct and Code of Ethics. The professional standards developed by natural therapy associations also apply if a nurse is using a relevant therapy (NBV 1999). In other jurisdictions, different standards and codes of ethics apply.

Education

A commitment to education is required to practise complementary therapies effectively and safely. Because of the growing interest in these therapies, an increasing number of universities is offering complementary therapy subjects in nursing curricula, but some are introductory only and do not equip the student to practise a therapy.

It is difficult for professional nursing bodies to accredit private courses because of the large number and changing nature of available courses. Nurses are therefore responsible for choosing a course that is of a standard appropriate to nursing practice. The course should be recognised by a relevant professional association. Continuing education in the therapy is essential, and the nurse should have access to experts in the field for consultation if necessary.

Legal and ethical aspects

As with any procedure, it is necessary to receive informed consent from the patient before using any complementary therapy. If the person is unable to do so, consent can often be obtained from a relative or guardian. If this is not possible the nurse may, as a competent professional, use a complementary therapy if it is considered to be in the person's best interest. The use of such therapy as a nursing intervention should be documented in the patient's notes— including the nursing goal, the therapy used, and the outcome.

Professional guidelines recommend that professional indemnity insurance be obtained. The Australian Nursing Federation (ANF) insures all its members for practice of any complementary therapy, except chiropractic and osteopathy. The nurse must have completed a course of a standard recognised by the relevant profession. Nurses who are not ANF members are advised to seek their own insurance.

The same duty of care that applies to any health care work applies to use of complementary therapies. If any breach of duty of care occurs, patients have redress through the common law, state health complaints commissions, and professional regulatory bodies (Lancaster 2001).

In making these prudent observations regarding informed consent, indemnity insurance, and duty of care, there is no suggestion that complementary therapies are any more dangerous than conventional medical and nursing care. Used appropriately, by trained staff, these therapies are very safe.

'There is no suggestion that complementary therapies are any more dangerous than conventional medical and nursing care.'

However prudence in matters relating to informed consent, professional insurance, and duty of care is advisable in the use of complementary therapies, as it is in all aspects of professional nursing care.

Developing workplace policy and dealing with change

For nurses contemplating the development of a policy covering use of complementary therapies in their workplaces, there are several strategies that can assist (McCabe 2001):

- organise a committee of like-minded colleagues;
- obtain the professional guidelines described above;
- read widely on the experiences of other nurses using complementary therapies in nursing practice;
- gather all available research and literature;
- learn to argue the case for complementary therapies; be clear that they will be used for nursing care and not medical work—that is, not for the treatment of disease but for the comfort and wellbeing of the patient;
- contact nurses in the area who have successfully integrated complementary therapies into practice and invite them to a meeting;
- decide which therapies can be offered initially; this will depend on the needs of patients, qualifications of nursing staff, and availability of suitably qualified practitioners;
- ascertain the level of support and dissent in the organisation;
- invite dissenting colleagues to a meeting and discuss their concerns openly; dissent often evaporates when people feel that their concerns are taken seriously and if accurate information is shared;
- advocate for nurses; recognise that nurses are professional health-care providers who can make decisions about appropriate and safe nursing care, and that this might include use of complementary therapies;
- advocate for patients; a wide range of nursing interventions needs to be available to best meet the requirements of terminally ill people;
- include in the policy a recommendation for evaluation of complementary therapy practices and regular review of the policy to ensure that the policy remains up to date with current practice.

Conclusion

Many 'natural' and 'complementary' therapies have long been part of traditional nursing nursing care. In a sense, the inclusion of what are now called 'complementary therapies' is really no more than a modern development of traditional nursing practices that were almost foregone as 'high-tech' nursing became the norm. In palliative care, natural and complementary therapies add to the nursing arts. Used skilfully and judiciously, these therapies can provide nurses with a much wider range of interventions in enabling the achievement of the ultimate aim of palliative care—patient comfort.

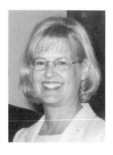 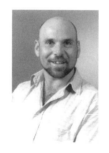 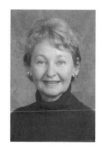

Linda Kristjanson

Linda Kristjanson is the professor of palliative care at Edith Cowan University (Perth, Western Australia). Linda holds a joint appointment at Sir Charles Gairdner Hospital where she serves as director of the Cancer Nursing Research Network. She is also the director of hospice research for Silver Chain Hospice Service in Western Australia. Linda obtained her undergraduate and master's degrees from the University of Manitoba (Canada) and her PhD from the University of Arizona (USA). She has received research funding from local and national organisations in Canada and Australia focusing on the palliative-care needs of patients and their families.

Peter Hudson

Peter Hudson is a senior lecturer in palliative care at the School of Postgraduate Nursing and the Centre for Palliative Care at the University of Melbourne (Victoria, Australia). Peter's PhD work focused on developing and evaluating a supportive intervention for families caring for dying relatives. He began working in palliative care as a district nurse in London (UK) in the early 1990s, and was employed for several years with a large Melbourne metropolitan community-based palliative-care service as a clinical coordinator. Peter has held several teaching appointments incorporating undergraduate, postgraduate, and distance education. He is an executive committee member of the Board of Directors for Palliative Care Victoria (Australia).

Lynn Oldham

Lynn Oldham is a research associate with the Cancer, Palliative Care, and Family Health Research Group at Edith Cowan University (Perth, Western Australia). Lynn's PhD work has involved the development and testing of a pain-management program for family caregivers of advanced cancer patients. Lynn has been working in palliative care for many years in both community and inpatient settings. She was the inaugural clinical nurse specialist at the Cancer Foundation Cottage Hospice (Western Australia), and is an executive committee member of Palliative Care WA.

Chapter 19

Working with Families

Linda Kristjanson, Peter Hudson, Lynn Oldham

Families of people receiving palliative care are profoundly affected by the challenges of the illness. They are called upon to cope with daily caregiving, alterations to their roles, and changing responsibilities within the family. Family members also confront shifts in the meaning of life and relationships as they come to recognise the terminal stage of the person's illness. These demands require changes in arrangements for physical care and practical difficulties with daily living while families are attempting to handle their own emotional distress about the person's care and concerns about the future (Bergen 1991; Ferrell 1998).

> 'Families of people are called upon to cope with daily caregiving, alterations to their roles, and changing responsibilities within the family.'

According to the World Health Organization (1990) the family is the unit of palliative care. Health professionals who endorse this approach and endeavour to provide family-centred care can, however, feel that they are not equipped to provide support for the family. Attention to the subject of family palliative care is a relatively recent development, and many health professionals have received little formal preparation for this type of care.

Although this chapter focuses on work with care of families in the palliative phase of a person's illness, family care must begin at the time of diagnosis and treatment (Hilton 1996; Weitzner, McMillan & Jacobsen 1999). Families who do not receive adequate information and support in the early phases of the person's treatment have more needs and less confidence in the health-care system, and cope less well than families who have been supported throughout the illness (Stetz & Hanson 1992; Thorne & Robinson 1988).

Provision of family palliative care requires attention to three key matters:
- the definition of the family requiring care;
- the most common needs of family members; and
- the most appropriate and useful interventions.

Each of these is discussed below.

Definition of the family requiring care

Families are comprised of individuals who might or might not be related through blood or legal ties. A family might be a married couple, or might be made up of a large network or relatives, close friends, and neighbours. Each family has its own unique biography that is shaped by the backgrounds, links, choices, and values of the people who comprise it. These people 'knit together' to define themselves as a family unit. Individuals within families have various needs, commitments, personal histories, resources, and goals. It is therefore difficult to agree upon a single definition of 'the family' (Kristjanson & White 2002).

In clinical practice, the most useful approach to defining and working with the family is to allow the person and his or her family members to define 'the family' themselves (PCA 2000). A lack of recognition of the unique nature of each family can lead to assumptions being about who makes up the family, and the needs of some family members being overlooked. Errors in acknowledging the family are more likely to occur if the family does not fit a 'conventional' definition of family

> 'Errors in acknowledging the family are more likely to occur if the family does not fit a 'conventional' definition of family.'

(such as a couple with two children). For example, partners in homosexual relationships can be neglected, as can stepchildren, family members who live geographically apart, and those without obvious formal ties to the patient.

'I was willing to do what needed to be done . . . '

'We had been divorced for years. Not a lot of tension . . . but a kind of distance that worked OK until he became ill. Then he needed someone and I guess I figured I would step in as much as I could. I wouldn't be able to live there, but would come in and check on him every day.

It was difficult because the doctors didn't quite recognise me, [as if] I wasn't Tom's wife any more. But we had been together 15 years and now I was willing to do what needed to be done . . . but I didn't have much chance to get information and learn about what was needed because there were questions about how much I was entitled to know.

You do what you have to do . . . but it would have been good to have felt that my role was valued . . . that it was seen.'

Authors' personal sources

The need for flexibility and understanding in defining the nature of 'family' is reflected in the experience of a former wife, as related in the Box above.

Nurses must remain accommodating and inclusive in their approach to identifying family members who require care and support. Examples of questions that might be asked to explore this are shown in the Box on page 274. Depending upon the situation, questions like these might also be used with family members themselves to expand the definition of family and ensure that people are not forgotten.

Needs of family members

Family members whose own needs are not met are less able to maintain their carer roles and are more likely to experience mental and physical health problems themselves (Blanchard, Albrecht & Ruckdeschel 1997; Ramirez, Addington Hall & Richards 1998).

Four types of family care needs are especially important:
- reassurance regarding patient comfort;
- family information needs;
- family practical care needs; and
- family emotional support.

Each of these is discussed below.

Reassurance regarding patient comfort

The greatest concern for families is to know that the patient is comfortable and not suffering (Bucher, Trostle & Moore 1999; Ferrell et al. 1991). This is

Defining the family as the unit of care

The following questions are examples of a general approach (to the person, or family members) that facilitates a wider understanding of the definition of family and ensures that people are not forgotten.

- When someone has a serious illness it can affect not only the patient, but also the whole family. It is important to us that we provide support to everyone in the family who might be affected. Can you tell me a little about the members of your family?
- Family does not always mean only blood relatives or legal relatives. Family can include people who don't live with you and others with whom you are close. It might be someone who is such a good friend that he or she feels like 'family'. Are there any people involved with you whom we should include or reach out to?
- Who in your family is likely to most affected by your illness? Who seems to be coping the best? Who needs the most information? Who needs the most support and practical assistance?
- What is the best way to share information about your illness and your care plan with you and your family?
- Are there family members or individuals whom you would prefer were not included in discussions about your care?

fundamental to the family's ability to cope—whether family members are providing care at home or whether they are observing the person's distress in the hospital or hospice setting.

The patient's pain has an intense effect on the family who can interpret it as a sign of progressive illness and impending death. However, families can contribute to poor pain relief because they are concerned about the use of opioids and the possibility of respiratory depression and addiction (Bucher, Trostle & Moore 1999; Glajchen et al. 1995). These anxieties about medication can lead to patients being under-medicated (Yeager et al. 1995). The experience of one family member who was worried about opiate medication expresses these fears (see Box, page 275).

Family members can also experience apprehension when the patient is experiencing other distressing symptoms—such as dyspnoea, fatigue, nausea, or anxiety. Family members who cannot comfort the patient effectively report feelings of helplessness and desperation when they witness unrelieved symptoms (Ferrell et al. 1991). This sort of family distress has been termed, 'vicarious suffering' (Kristjanson & Avery 1994). See the Box on page 275.

When the family witnesses a peaceful and comfortable death they report more satisfaction with care, and can reflect on the end stages of the patient's life

---

'I worry that he suffered . . . '

'He would wake in the night and be moaning and yet it hadn't been that long since his last medicine and I wasn't sure what to do . . .

He would tell me to go and get my rest, but I couldn't because I knew he was in such pain, but I was afraid of the drugs and the effects on him—especially at night. And your judgment isn't too good when you are tired.

I worry that he suffered on account of me not knowing what to do.'

Authors' personal sources

'I remember how awful it was . . . '

'I remember how awful it was watching her trying to get her breath. We didn't know what to do. She was sitting up and rocking and struggling for breath, and we tried all we could to comfort her and try and keep her calm, but we couldn't seem to make a difference. Even the oxygen wasn't enough.

And then the nurse came in and looked at her and said, we can give her something to ease her distress. And the medicine they gave her did the trick. She started to breathe more slowly and normally again. She could lie back and rest and we all felt her relief.'

Authors' personal sources

---

without undue distress. However, family members who witness a painful or distressing death are more likely to experience guilt and regret in the bereavement period because they chastise themselves for not being better advocates for the person (Kristjanson et al. 1996). It is therefore necessary to be attentive to patient comfort and to provide support for family members who observe distressing symptoms.

Family information needs

Family members need to receive information about illness and about how to care for the person. This sort of information is empowering. Families require information about how best to provide comfort, how to talk with other family members about the patient's illness, how to manage treatment and medication side-effects, how to anticipate changes in the patient's condition, and how to communicate with the patient and within the family (Ferrell et al. 1995; Scott, Whyler & Grant 2001). The information should be simple to understand, and specific to their needs at the time. Practical advice and focused information

---

'I kept panicking and thinking about it'

'I was a bit surprised at the autonomy that was given to the carer by the nursing staff—to be responsible for the dosage of morphine and that sort of thing. I kept panicking and thinking about it and ringing up at night and asking: "Am I doing the right thing?".'

Adapted from Hudson, Aranda & McMurray (2002)

---

provided by nurses is particularly useful in managing the day-to-day challenges of providing palliative care at home.

Carers can be surprised at how much autonomy and responsibility they are given, and often need information and reassurance regarding their role. The comment in the Box above, made by a woman who was supporting her dying husband, exemplifies the importance of guidance for family caregivers:

Family practical care needs

Families feel the burden of providing ongoing care, and need practical assistance. Various individual burdens can add up to a significant strain on family resources, and signs of caregiver fatigue can be missed or underestimated by health-care providers who observe family members briefly and intermittently. This lack of support occurs, in part, because family caregivers are viewed as resources rather than as potential recipients of care themselves (Leis et al. 1997).

Families in rural areas and families with elderly caregivers are especially at risk. A lack of available resources for families in rural areas can produce marked strains (Buehler & Lee 1992). In instances when the family caregiver is elderly and has health problems of his or her own, the demands of caregiving can be extremely taxing (Cobbs 1998; Given & Given 1998).

'Family caregivers are viewed as resources rather than as potential recipients of care themselves.'

The involvement of family members as carers must therefore take into account the finite resources of these people—which they might be stretching beyond their usual limits because of a sense of duty to care for the patient. This can produce caregiver fatigue, isolation, and 'burnout' (Jensen & Given 1991; Yang & Kirschling 1992). The comments of family members in the Box on page 277 exemplify how exhausting caregiving can be.

'I've never felt so trapped in my life'

'In my case I wasn't aware of how exhausting it is. I had to be available 24 hours a day . . . In three weeks I've had two-and-a-half hours out of this flat, I've never felt so trapped in my life.'

Adapted from Hudson (nd)

The role of family carer can also impose financial burdens. With a shift in care towards home-based community care, dying people are being cared for more often at home. Caregivers often have to take time off work to care for terminally ill people at home. The cost of family labour and family out-of-pocket expenditures can be significant, and might be an additional source of family stress (Kristjanson & White 2002).

Family emotional support

The ability of families to provide support to the patient and to manage home care depend to a large extent on the amount and quality of support they receive. The need for emotional support is paramount, as reflected in the comments of a family member in the Box below.

'The greatest stressful period of your life'

'Well, suddenly you're thrust into the greatest stressful period of your life. Your life's just turned over . . . You can't get your mind around it.'

Adapted from Hudson, Aranda & McMurray (2002)

Attention needs to be paid to the emotional needs of family members to ensure that their caring efforts are sustainable. These needs include support in coping with loss, uncertainty about the illness, impending death, communication within the family, and their own psychological distress (Kissane et al. 1994). The comments of one young father and husband reflect this need for emotional support (Box, page 278).

One of the most difficult experiences for family members to cope with is deterioration in the patient's mental status. Confusion, agitation, or personality changes can trigger feelings of loss in family members, and can create anxiety about the patient's safety. The family might feel that the person whom they knew has been lost, and can experience feelings of grief, anger, and despair. This can be particularly difficult to cope with amid the ongoing demands of physical care.

'This stuff is always in the back of my mind'

'I worry about what to say to the children. I don't know how much they really understand and I don't want to upset them, but I don't know the words to use.

I am not sure how I am going to cope on my own with them . . . I mean, raising teenagers isn't easy at the best of times, and without a mother this will be a real challenge.

I don't want to worry my wife about these things because she has enough to cope with. Not that I am normally a worrying type, but this stuff is always in the back of my mind, churning over and over.'

Authors' personal sources

Helping family members to communicate among themselves is a particular challenge. Families who communicated effectively before the illness cope more effectively during the illness than those with histories of poor communication (Higginson, Wade & McCarthy 1992). Nurses should be alert to difficulties and should help family members to talk through how they are going to share information and discuss concerns. They might need to be assisted in ways of avoiding conflict and communication mistakes.

Family members who have previously experienced a traumatic illness or death of a relative might be at risk of a more complicated bereavement reaction on a later occasion (Kristjanson & Sloan 1991; Kristjanson et al. 1996). Caring for these people during the palliative phase of illness requires a preventive approach to help them cope with the new crisis and maintain their own health (Kellehear 1999). Family members who have experienced a difficult death in a relative, or witnessed their unrelieved suffering are in particular need of help to cope with the memories and regrets associated with these experiences.

Appropriate and useful interventions

Nurses are well placed to take a role in planning, implementing, and evaluating strategies to support families. Interventions most helpful to families can be grouped into four categories:

▶ patient comfort;
▶ family information;
▶ family emotional support; and
▶ family practical assistance.

These are summarised in Table 19.1 (page 279).

Table 19.1 Family care interventions in palliative care

Family care need	Care interventions
Patient comfort	education about pain assessment & management (types of pain; use of pain medications; information about comfort therapies; information about disease progression);
	assess patient's comfort and develop comfort management plan with family;
	use of teaching tools (comfort diary, demonstration, videos);
	serve as back-up comfort consultation (inpatient or home care);
	help families know when to call health professionals for assistance
Family information	provision of generous amounts of information in simple language, supported by written resources;
	information about patient's disease, treatments, and changes in patient's condition;
	24-hour-a-day access to information;
	use of family conference for sharing information with all members;
	information about options for caregiving;
	signs and symptoms of impending death.
Family emotional support	helping families to identify ways of coping (for example, taking one day at a time, use of social support, seeking information to dispel uncertainty, knowing how to compartmentalise concerns);
	help families to identify positive aspects of care-giving role;
	help families to identify ways of caring for themselves, avoiding caregiver fatigue
	acknowledge importance of family members' emotional needs;
	facilitate referral to other health professionals and resources

(Continued)

Table 19.1 Family care interventions in palliative care (*Continued*)

Family practical assistance	help families to identify practical needs for assistance; identify needs for respite at early stage; provide practical assistance with patient care needs (for example, bathing, monitoring); provide information regarding resources available (for example, financial help, transport assistance)

Authors' presentation

Patient comfort

The most useful ways to assist families in providing patient comfort care at home are: (i) to educate them about basic pain-management principles and skills; (ii) to act as an advocate for the patient and family in ensuring that the patient's comfort needs are met; and (iii) to serve as a consultant to the family.

Basic pain-management principles include pain assessment and management, knowledge of pain types, current knowledge of all pain medications used in palliative care, knowledge of comfort therapies, and knowledge of disease progression.

Nurses can advocate for comfort management by establishing the pain-management needs of the patient and by developing a management plan with the patient, family, and the health-care team. Pain-management education should be ongoing, as should be evaluation of patient comfort and family needs in assisting with pain management. Educational strategies that are helpful to families include short, sequenced teaching sessions accompanied by written information, use of a daily comfort diary to rate and assess pain, and videotapes to demonstrate ways of moving people in and out of bed and into a chair.

Family information

Family members require information about how to provide comfort care, how to communicate within the family, how to conserve their own energies, and when to call for assistance. Home-care nurses are valuable sources of such information, and families appreciate 24-hour-a-day access to information (Kristjanson 1989). In rural communities, this is particularly important because the nurse is often the most accessible person to provide information. Family conferences are especially helpful in providing information and an opportunity to clarify questions (Kristjanson 1989).

Families should be made aware of the typical demands associated with supporting a dying relative so they can prepare themselves. Family members should be informed that they have a choice with regard to the amount and type of care they offer their relative. They should be advised about the resources and services available, and how to access them.

Provision of practical information that will help families to anticipate the next steps of the person's illness is especially helpful. This allows family members to know what to expect and decreases the chance that they will be caught in a moment of crisis, unprepared for a deterioration in the person's condition. Families value information about the signs and symptoms of impending death because it helps them to prepare psychologically for the person's death, and gives them time to call family members who might wish to visit (Grbich, Parker & Maddocks 2000; Hull 1992; Vachon 1998).

Family emotional support

Helping families cope emotionally involves the identification of ways in which they can manage the care situation and the uncertainties that they face. 'Taking one day at a time' is a useful strategy for managing uncertainty (Hull 1992). Other useful coping strategies include acceptance, rationalisation, and social support (Hull 1992; Leis et al. 1997). These approaches can help families to cope, to reach out for assistance, and to compartmentalise stresses into more manageable pieces. This can make the

> 'Taking one day at a time is a useful strategy for managing uncertainty.'

experience of caring for a dying family member less overwhelming, as the comments in the Box below illustrate.

It is helpful to advise families that many family carers have had positive experiences in supporting a dying relative. Too much emphasis on the negative aspects of the experience can inadvertently cause caregivers to expect a burden (Gaugler, Kane & Langlois 2000). It should therefore be pointed out that many carers experience elements of caregiving as satisfying (Nolan 2001; Scott 2001).

'I couldn't have survived without support'

'You may be stabbing in the dark, when you are doing it yourself, but it is great to know you can pick up the phone and get support.'

'I couldn't have survived without support, and that very support gave me confidence.'

Adapted from Hudson, Aranda & McMurray (2002)

Families should be advised of the importance of accepting their own emotional needs as being legitimate and valid. However, it should be noted that some family members might not want support because they believe that health-care resources and the time of nurses are limited. Family members should be advised that nurses view the family's needs as being important. Such an approach will encourage family members to mention their emotional issues and seek support.

Although nurses assume much responsibility for supporting families, they can also assist family members by introducing relevant members of the interdisciplinary team—such as pastoral-care workers, psychologists, social workers, and volunteers.

Family practical assistance

Most palliative-care patients want to die at home (Smeenk et al. 1998). For many families, practical assistance is essential if they are to maintain home-based care.

Respite services can be invaluable to families in sustaining their caregiving energies. Respite might take the form of admission of patients to hospital or hospice if they have intractable symptoms or if the family needs time to rest. Admission to hospital or hospice might also be arranged if the person is about to die and does not wish to die at home.

In-home respite might also be appropriate. This can take the form of assistance from a volunteer or friend to allow the primary family caregiver some 'time out'. A nurse or care aide can also provide assistance for several hours or overnight to allow the family to obtain some rest.

Many families require practical assistance with hygiene care of the patient. It should not be assumed that family members, regardless of how devoted they are, want to be responsible for this care or know how to do it. They might need practical help with how to move and toilet the patient, how to provide basic hygiene (such as mouth care), and how to attend to skin care. Sensitive discussion about the willingness of family members to take on these roles is important.

Families might also need help to organise transport to and from appointments. They might require financial assistance and advice on how to access resources. A referral to a social worker might be especially helpful. The palliative-care nurse can also advise and assist families in accessing other members of the multidisciplinary team.

Conclusion

Nurses should not be prescriptive about how they support families, and it is of utmost importance that interventions be commensurate with the family's needs. The family-care approaches presented in this chapter should be viewed as guides to help palliative-care nurses to assess and assist families.

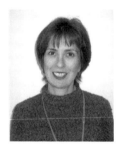 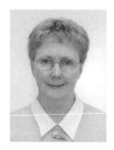

Donna Milne

Donna Milne is a registered nurse who has spent many years specialising in cancer nursing. The focus of Donna's master's degree was the needs and experiences of family caregivers of people with advanced cancer. Since completing this research, Donna has worked as a research fellow at the Centre for Palliative Care and the Victorian Centre for Nursing Practice Research at the University of Melbourne (Victoria, Australia). She is now working as a research fellow at the Peter MacCallum Cancer Institute, Melbourne. Donna has been involved in research projects on family caregivers, breast-care nurses, symptom management, bereavement risk assessment, and the implementation of evidence-based practice. Donna's role also involves teaching in communication skills, critical appraisal, and the development and utilisation of nursing research in the practice setting. Donna is involved with professional cancer nursing groups at a state and national level.

Regina Millard

Regina Millard is a member of the Sisters of Charity, Australia. She graduated from St Vincent's Hospital, Sydney (New South Wales, Australia) in 1971 and worked for 20 years as a registered nurse focusing on nurse education. After spending 12 months at the Institute of Religious Formation in St Louis (Missouri, USA), Regina's first position in palliative care was with the pastoral care team at Sacred Heart Hospice, Darlinghurst (New South Wales, Australia). She then began community-based palliative care in 1994 as a pastoral carer on the multidisciplinary team of Caritas Christi and the Order of Malta Hospice home-care service in Kew (Victoria, Australia). In 1998, this service became one of four partners in Eastern Palliative Care, the largest single provider of community-based palliative care in Victoria. Regina's special interests are in pre-bereavement and post-bereavement care of adults and children in family settings and groups.

Chapter 20

Bereavement

Donna Milne and Regina Millard

Despite recent advances in health care and health technology in the saving of life, care of the dying and their families remains an important health-care issue. The attention paid to grieving family members has been a particular focus of care in recent years.

The experience of bereavement has potential negative effects on the mental and physical health of people. Despite these negative effects, most people recover from their loss, and the psychological distress lessens over time, although the length of time that this takes varies from person to person. The challenge for nurses and other health professionals is to identify those who are not likely to adapt to their loss and who are therefore at greater risk of adverse bereavement outcomes.

Assessment of the risk of adverse bereavement outcomes is difficult. The first part of this chapter provides guidelines, based on the best available evidence, to assist in the identification of people at risk of adverse bereavement outcomes. The second part discusses the place of the health professional's own

> 'The challenge for nurses is to identify those who are not likely to adapt to their loss.'

bereavement history, notes the importance of grief education and understanding the person and family, and provides examples of different types of general bereavement support.

Assessment

Underlying assumptions

The guidelines presented in this chapter for bereavement risk assessment in family members are based on three important assumptions:

▶ that the risk of adverse bereavement outcomes can be identified;

▶ that grief is a normal reaction to bereavement that is usually managed effectively by the bereaved; and

▶ that if a risk of adverse outcomes is identified, people should be offered more intensive support and access to bereavement counselling services.

A full appreciation of these guidelines requires an understanding of: (i) the timing and people involved in risk assessment; (ii) the concept of 'complicated bereavement'; and (iii) the importance of targeting bereavement interventions. Each of these is discussed below.

Timing and people involved

It is reasonable for bereavement risk assessment to begin when death is expected in the near future (approximately three months), although there is no evidence to support a particular predeath timeframe.

Bereavement risk assessment is commonly focused on those closest to the dying person. Indeed, it is often confined to the primary carer because access to this person is facilitated by his or her role in the dying person's care. However, the assessment should encompass all people in the dying person's immediate family, as well as others with a significant relationship to the person. 'Family' is defined here as those people making up the closest social network for the patient, and is therefore not restricted to those related by birth or marriage.

The concept of 'complicated bereavement'

Complicated bereavement is a maladaptive response to loss marked by intense and prolonged mourning, depressive and anxiety disorders, and poor physical health. The risk of complicated bereavement depends on the extent to which a person is *susceptible* to adverse outcomes, but the identification of risk does not imply a *cause-and-effect* relationship—that is, that a high-risk person will necessarily experience complicated bereavement. Rather, the identification of risk indicates that this person might have difficulty dealing with his or her loss.

A person identified as being at high risk might cope well, whereas a person judged as being at low risk might, in fact, experience adverse outcomes. The assessment of risk of complicated bereavement outcomes is a process of balancing probabilities based on best evidence, clinical judgment, and input from the patient and family. This information can be used to provide preventative support or, if required, targeted bereavement resources.

Targeting bereavement interventions

Walshe (1997) has identified four reasons for targeting bereavement interventions at people who are at increased risk of complicated bereavement outcomes.

⏵ Most bereaved people are able to mobilise the coping strategies and inner strength needed to deal with their situation. Targeting bereavement interventions allows health professionals to maximise a bereaved person's coping abilities and to respect his or her resilience.
⏵ There is evidence that focused bereavement interventions do reduce risk and improve bereavement outcomes, whereas indiscriminate services can lack overall beneficial effects (Parkes 1980).
⏵ Resources for bereavement services are limited, making targeting of support necessary.
⏵ Provision of bereavement services that rely on self-referral assumes (perhaps wrongly) that those who need help are able to recognise and then act on this need.

The guidelines

The following guidelines for the assessment of complicated bereavement risk were developed within a palliative-care context, but are applicable to other settings in which people die, such as aged care (Aranda & Milne 2000). The guidelines can be used by all health professionals involved in the care of the dying, including nurses, doctors, pastoral-care workers, social workers, bereavement counsellors, and psychologists. Although some components of bereavement care, including predeath risk assessment, are the domain of all team members, specific team members are responsible for particular aspects of the assessment at different times.

A major limitation of the literature on complicated bereavement risk assessment (and bereavement in general) is the lack of attention paid to cultural factors. The majority of available research is undertaken in Western countries and involves Caucasian participants. Despite this, grieving is a universal response to the loss of someone close, and most cultures contain beliefs concerning the continuation of the person in some way beyond death (Rosenblatt 1993). This chapter cannot attempt to describe all the cultural variations surrounding death and bereavement, but it is important to understand that grief encompasses a wide range of responses, all of which can be legitimate within various cultural contexts. If an apparently unusual grief response is observed, assumptions about the meaning of the response should not be made until appropriate information is obtained. An important resource in this area is Parkes, Laungani and Young (1997).

> 'Grief encompasses a wide range of responses, all of which can be legitimate within various cultural contexts.'

These guidelines should therefore be used in conjunction with an awareness of 'cultural safety'—the acknowledgment of, and respect for, cultural differences. The application of the guidelines requires implementation of strategies in a manner that promotes and nurtures the cultural identity of the person and family (Ramsden 1998; Prior 1999).

A summary of the guidelines is presented in the Box on page 289, and the guidelines are discussed in the text below.

Guideline 1: Family members should be involved in assessment of risk of complicated bereavement outcomes.

Guideline 1 deals with the question of who should be assessed. Those most closely connected with the dying person are most likely to experience grief as a result of bereavement, with the intensity of the grief usually being proportional to the closeness of the attachment. A close relationship does not presuppose that the relationship is supportive or amicable. Indeed, close relationships might be ambivalent or even conflictual (Parkes 1975; Zisook, Shuchter & Lyons 1987; Gamino, Sewell & Easterling 1998).

In most family situations, the primary carer of the dying person is the person's spouse or child, and this person is most likely to be assessed for bereavement risk. Other members of the family are less often assessed. This narrow approach to assessment results from a combination of historical conventions, resource limitations, and restricted access to family members. It is important to move beyond assessment of the primary carer or primary relationship (Rando 1993).

The approach taken in these guidelines emphasises open communication and involvement of family members in risk assessment. Family members can be good predictors of their own response to loss. When working with families it can be useful to ask the following questions:

▶ Have you lost a close friend or relative to death at some point in your life?

Guidelines for assessment of bereavement risk

Guideline 1

Family members should be involved in assessment of risk of complicated bereavement outcomes.

Guideline 2

Complicated bereavement risk assessment forms part of the health care team's duty of care and is a process requiring input from a range of professionals involved in the care of the patient and family.

Guideline 3

Complicated bereavement risk assessment should commence at the point of referral to palliative care and continue through care provision, patient death, and early bereavement.

Guideline 4

Complicated bereavement risk assessment requires structured documentation, review in team meetings, and the use of family assessment.

Guideline 5

Complicated bereavement risk assessment involves four key categories of information—(i) the illness, terminal care, and the nature of the death; (ii) characteristics of the bereaved; (iii) interpersonal relationships (including family functioning); and (iv) characteristics of the deceased.

⏵ Do you still have difficulties with the loss?

An affirmative response to one or both of these questions might indicate unresolved grief and consequent higher risk of complicated bereavement outcomes (Zisook & Lyons 1989). Another useful question is:

⏵ How have you coped with previous losses?

Guideline 2: Complicated bereavement risk assessment forms part of the health team's duty of care and is a process requiring input from a range of professionals involved in the care of the patient and family.

Guideline 2 deals with the question of the team's involvement in an assessment. It is useful to have one person coordinate and take responsibility for recording the bereavement risk assessment. However, multidisciplinary input is important because it helps to ensure that a wide range of insights is gained in the assessment. Each discipline brings a different perspective on the person's life history and experience, and each contributes to the completeness of the assessment.

Other professionals who have had long-standing relationships with the family (for example, general practitioners and members of the clergy) can also be key informants on how individual family members are dealing with loss during early bereavement. If relevant, psychiatrists, psychologists, and counsellors might also be able to provide important information about coping abilities.

Guideline 3: Complicated bereavement risk assessment should commence at the point of referral to palliative care and continue through care provision, patient death, and early bereavement.

Guideline 3 addresses the question of the timing of an assessment. The information required to assess risk of complicated bereavement needs to be gathered from approximately three months before the death, and should extend into early bereavement.

Circumstances for the patient and the family change over the course of the illness, and information should be accumulated accordingly. There is little evidence to support the three-month predeath timeframe, but this period has been suggested on the basis of clinical experience and expert opinion. It is better to prevent complications, rather than instigate interventions after complications have already developed (Parkes 1993; Cleiren 1993).

Health professionals should think of bereavement as a continuum, with death being only one stage. One indication of how a person is likely to deal with grief after the death is how he or she deals with grief before the death (Bourke 1984). A person showing signs of complicated grief before the death is more likely to experience complicated bereavement outcomes following the death.

'Health professionals should think of bereavement as a continuum, with death being only one stage.'

To assist decisions about appropriate support, a summary of risk factors should be presented to the team as soon as relevant information has been gathered, and again at the time of death. In some instances specific support and grief education can commence before the death.

Guideline 4: Complicated bereavement risk assessment requires structured documentation, review in team meetings, and the use of family assessment.

Guideline 4 addresses the question of the documentation of an assessment. Documentation of the bereavement risk assessment is important, and review of all relevant information—from admission, to death, to early bereavement—is required. Structured documentation can consist of a checklist, a risk-assessment form, or some other form of structured family assessment.

Several complicated bereavement risk-assessment forms are mentioned in the literature, with most of these being measures of grief intensity. However, there is debate about the advantages and disadvantages of deciding on degree of risk based on a measure of grief intensity—given that people vary in their display of overt distress. Allocating potential risk a numeric score is therefore problematic, and outcomes do not necessarily correspond to the scores allocated. Any such score should be seen as one of a number of considerations that contribute to an understanding of the situation. Because of these difficulties, this guideline suggests the use of a checklist of factors that influence bereavement outcomes (see Appendix 20.1, page 300), together with clinical judgment and the family member's perceptions of risk.

Families who do not function well together as a unit are at increased risk of complicated bereavement outcomes (Kissane et al. 1998). One way to assess family functioning is to use the Family Relationships Index (Moos & Moos 1981). This is a simple and effective 12-item screening tool that assists in the identification of dysfunctional families. The tool screens for cohesiveness, expressiveness, and conflict within the family. Predeath work can then be undertaken with families who appear not to function well together with a view to increasing the likelihood of positive bereavement outcomes.

In assessing families, genograms can be particularly helpful if undertaken by someone with appropriate knowledge and skills (see page 297).

Guideline 5: Complicated bereavement risk assessment involves four key categories of information.
Guideline 5 addresses the four categories to be considered in an assessment:
▶ the illness, terminal care, and the nature of the death;
▶ characteristics of the bereaved;
▶ interpersonal relationships (including family functioning); and
▶ characteristics of the deceased.
   Each of these is discussed below.

Characteristics of the illness, terminal care, and nature of the death
The outcomes for the bereaved can be influenced by the duration of the illness and experiences surrounding the period of terminal care and death. There is greater risk of complicated bereavement if:
▶ the death is sudden or unexpected, particularly if the bereaved did not have an opportunity to discuss death with the deceased;

▶ the death occurred under traumatic circumstances;
▶ the death is stigmatised (for example, if the death is a result of suicide, murder, or HIV/AIDS);
▶ the illness has been long, the bereaved is middle-aged, and the illness has overburdened the caregiver's coping mechanisms; or
▶ the death is perceived as having occurred prematurely.

Characteristics of the bereaved

Several key factors of the bereaved have been identified as playing roles in bereavement outcomes. These factors include:
▶ certain stages of the life cycle (for example: an adolescent who has lost a parent and family support perceived as inadequate; a young person who has lost his or her spouse, especially after a long relationship with the deceased; a single mother of a deceased child);
▶ a history of previous losses (such as infidelity, divorce, loss of employment, loss of a pregnancy), particularly if unresolved;
▶ the presence of concurrent stressors (such as: family tension; compromised financial status; dissatisfaction with caregiving; reliance on alcohol and drugs prebereavement);
▶ physical and mental illness (particularly current or past history of mental health problems that have required psychological or psychiatric support or family history of psychiatric disorder);
▶ high predeath distress;
▶ poor initial adjustment to the loss manifested by intense emotional distress or depression;
▶ isolated, alienated individuals;
▶ being a parent of a child who dies;
▶ low levels of internal control beliefs (such as feelings of having no control over life);
▶ inability to use coping strategies (such as: an inability to maintain self-care, an inability to identify or modulate prominent themes of the grief being experienced; an inability to attribute meaning to the loss; an inability to differentiate between letting go of grief and forgetting the bereaved; and an inability to access available support).

Interpersonal relationships

The level of social support, the nature of the relationship between the deceased and the bereaved, and the level of family functioning can all influence bereavement outcomes. If tension within a family is noted, preventive interventions can be instigated (Kissane & Bloch 1994).

Factors that influence complicated bereavement are:

▶ a lack of social support (particularly if people in the immediate environment are unsupportive, unsympathetic, or antagonistic, or if levels of support immediately before the death were good but then subsided after the death);

▶ a lack of a confidant with whom to share feelings, concerns, and other existential issues;

▶ a disturbance in social support systems (such as not seeing old friends as frequently as was the case before the death);

▶ dissatisfaction with the help available during the deceased's illness;

▶ an ambivalent or dependent relationship between the bereaved and the deceased;

▶ the loss of a spouse of a long-term, unusually good, and exclusive marriage; and

▶ lower levels of family cohesion, communication, and conflict resolution.

Characteristics of the deceased

Many of the relevant characteristics of the deceased overlap with risk factors already listed, and are not repeated here. The remaining risk factors associated with the deceased are related to age. The age of the deceased especially influences bereavement outcomes if:

▶ the deceased is a child or an adolescent (especially if the child's death is a result of an inherited disorder, or is sudden or violent); or

▶ the deceased is a parent of children, adolescents, or young adults (particularly if the surviving parent copes poorly and is at increased risk of complicated bereavement outcomes).

Support

The first half of this chapter has focused on assessing families for risk of complicated bereavement in an attempt to improve patient and family care. Such improved care has significant implications for health professionals who are frequently confronted with grief. Grief can involve sadness, anger, helplessness, guilt, and despair (Raphael 1982), can be concentrated in one particular day, and can involve more than one patient and more than one family. Grief can become a constant companion to nurses.

The nurse–patient relationship, especially at the level of physical care, places the nurse in a special position. It is often during routine encounters that trust grows and feelings are expressed in simple and ordinary conversation. Feelings of grief associated with approaching death can find a safe place for expression in this relationship. If the person's feelings of grief are not recognised, an important aspect of care is diminished and unattended. Similar comments apply to families and carers. The nurse is often the person with whom people feel they can talk of their feelings—feelings that they cannot share with the sick person or even with other members of the family. Such feelings of grief might be open and intense, or might remain somewhat hidden. If feelings are not spoken, they might be revealed physically, emotionally, or spiritually in ways that are not overt or easy to understand.

The type of bereavement support offered by the health professional, and the manner in which it is offered, before death and immediately after death, can influence bereavement outcomes (Raphael 1982). It is crucial that nurses, and indeed all health professionals, are given the support they need to feel confident in providing bereavement care.

Four key issues in the provision of bereavement care are discussed here:

▶ personal experience;
▶ education about grief;
▶ understanding the patient and family; and
▶ bereavement support.

Personal experience

If health professionals are to listen to a person's expression of grief appropriately, it is helpful if they are aware of their own personal 'grief story' and attitudes to death, dying, and loss. The personal experience is the place to begin in helping others to express their feelings. It is inevitable that nurses will bring their past experiences into the present encounter, so they need to distinguish between their own way of responding and the other person's way of responding. Having a variety of personal 'gut-level' responses to death is legitimate, and these responses do not preclude nurses doing effective work with the dying and bereaved—so long as they are aware of them (Kavanaugh 1974).

Rando (1984) has suggested two exercises that can assist in reflecting about personal life experiences and preparing for attending to another's grief (see Box, page 295).

In their guidelines for bereavement counsellors, McKissock and McKissock (1998) provide another example of how to reflect on issues of life and death (see Box, page 296).

Self-awareness is very important if nurses are to offer professional support to the dying and bereaved. Keeping a personal journal and regular discussion

Exercises to aid personal reflections on grief

These exercise can assist nurses in personal reflection about life experiences, and can be useful in preparing for attending to another's grief. The exercises can be done privately, in small groups, or with a clinical mentor.

First exercise

The first exercise addresses early life experiences that might influence personal reactions to loss and death. Early experiences with loss and death leave 'imprints' of messages, feelings, fears, and attitudes that can be carried through life. The exercise involves a nurse reflecting on his or her earliest death-related experience—when it was, where it was, who was there, and what happened.

At the time:

- Was the reaction positive or negative?
- Did anyone advise you on what to do? How did you cope?
- What was learnt about death and loss?
- What causes fear and anxiety in present situations of death and loss?
- What makes it easier to cope with death and loss now?
- How does your current thinking about death and loss fit with your present work with the dying and bereaved?

It can be helpful to look at a second experience of loss. Which ideas or feelings were repeated? Which attitudes were maintained?

Second exercise

The second exercise addresses sociocultural, ethnic, religious, and philosophical attitudes to death. This reflection centres on the nurse's personal upbringing and socialisation, and present social and family group. Issues for reflection include: afterlife, burial rites, and expected attitudes to the dying person before and after death. Some of the questions for personal and wider reflection are:

- How do the age and gender of the dying person affect your reaction to death?
- What is the meaning of death during life?
- What is your attitude to children and grief?
- What norms, beliefs, and attitudes have you internalised about death from your present social and family group?

Adapted from Rando (1984)

with a trusted supervisor are also useful aids in the process of developing self-awareness.

Education about grief

Education is an important part of 'being there' for the family in all stages of bereavement. The nurse needs to be able to recognise and facilitate the

Another exercise in self-reflection

McKissock and McKissock (1998) provide another useful exercise in self-awareness. There are 34 questions related to issues of life and death, and eleven questions related to issues of attachment and separation. Questions include:

- What gives meaning to your life?
- What is the most significant contribution you have made to life so far?
- What physical ability would be most difficult for you to lose?
- What would you like your epitaph to say?
- When you think of your own death what are you most afraid of?
- How would you like to be remembered?
- Whose death would affect you most?
- How would you show your grief?

Adapted from McKissock & McKissock (1998)

expression of feelings by the patient or family. For some nurses, having no personal experience or education in grief and loss can leave them feeling 'out of their depth'. For the patient and family, various aspects of the experience of admission to a care facility can trigger significant emotional responses. Some of the triggers can be:

- facing the reality of death and imminent separation;
- hearing the prognosis;
- the physical decline into the dying phase;
- the emotional pain and helplessness of watching the person die; and
- the moment of death itself.

The nurse needs to have at least a basic understanding of normal and abnormal grief reactions. Normal grief behaviours include feelings, physical sensations, thoughts, and behaviours. Knowledge of grief reactions can be gained in the following ways:

- educational courses (for example, courses conducted by the Bereavement CARE Centre in New South Wales or the Centre for Grief Education in Victoria);
- colleagues with experience and training in grief and loss (for example, social workers, pastoral workers, psychologists);
- funeral directors (who often offer bereavement education);
- personal reading and study (libraries and good bookshops);
- newsletters and information from Palliative Care Australia, the National Association for Loss and Grief (NALAG), and state palliative-care bodies. Education is essential if health professionals are to address emotional

responses and identify those at risk of complicated bereavement with a view to offering appropriate support.

Understanding the patient and family

A genogram can be the starting-point of family care. It provides a structured means of documenting the nature of relationships within and between generations, and records a history of loss events, grieving patterns, and coping strategies. It can be an indicator of the nature of relationships and support systems within or around the family. The visual focus of the genogram provides a way of 'seeing' information about a family. Many families (and nurses) have reported suddenly 'seeing' a previously unnoticed connection or being able to recognise that a presumed connection does not really exist.

Information for the genogram needs to be collected in a sensitive manner, and this often requires a certain amount of intuition in recognising the best time to push a person for more detail. It must be remembered that this is a personal story that is being told, and that this demands a non-judgmental respectful attitude to what is being shared.

Family meetings provide an important opportunity to learn about family functioning and coping. Training in conducting family meetings is an essential component of staff development, and a majority of members of the multi-disciplinary team should have skills in this area. If possible, family meetings should involve the patient. The information gathered allows for early planning of bereavement care especially if a risk of complicated bereavement outcomes has been identified. At such meetings, the health professional should be seeking information that will allow assessment of:

▶ How are family members coping with this and previous deaths?
▶ How supported by family or friends do individuals feel?
▶ Will any family member need counselling?
▶ How will the children be prepared for the death?
▶ How well does the family communicate?
▶ How effective is family support of one another?
▶ Are there conflictual relationships within the family?
▶ How does the family resolve conflict?

The nurse will be listening for stories of significant events in the family—especially stories of family distress or breakdown, and of family recovery and growth. This information allows the health professional to identify issues and concerns, and to set an agenda for support of the family. A family approach also avoids stigmatising any individual. Collective responsibility and sharing of problem-solving can be encouraged.

Bereavement support

General bereavement support should begin before death with bereavement risk assessment. The aim is to prepare the person for what lies ahead so the effects of the loss are not overwhelming. Sometimes the health professionals themselves can provide the support, especially if they are part of a cohesive multidisciplinary team. Otherwise a referral can be made.

If children are involved, referral can be made to a suitable service. Centacare Catholic Family Services Victoria can assist with referral to a program called 'Seasons'. This program, which is run through schools, offers assistance for children of all ages who are trying to cope with a dying relative in the home or hospital. This is not a therapy program, but a peer support program guided by a trained adult. Similar programs are run in other states. Health professionals can also become facilitators of the program and run their own groups wherever they are located. There might be more than one family with children involved and these children can be brought together to share experiences.

> 'General bereavement support should begin before death.'

Family gatherings, including the dying person, can be suggested. These meetings can include several families in the same situation. At these gatherings people can be grouped for discussion—for example, sick persons and adult family members in one group and children in another group. Groupings usually depend on the availability of facilitators. All participants then come together to sum up the session. The purpose is to allow for expression of feelings associated with the difficulties of caring for a dying person, and to allow an opportunity for families to become more communicative and cohesive. These sessions last approximately two hours, and can be held approximately every two months. Over time, new families join in and add a different perspective. It is useful to have a specific topic to discuss that encourages participants to remain focused.

In recommending general bereavement support it is important to remember that everyone grieves differently. Some people get the support they need through family, friends, or other networks. However, it is important that the bereaved be aware of the support that is available. This information can be given to the bereaved before they leave the hospice or hospital after the death, or mailed as soon as possible afterwards. In the critical first twelve months after the death, telephone contact from someone on the team might be appreciated. This can be done at appropriate intervals—such as one month, three months, and six months after the death. By then most people will let it be known if they do not wish the contact to continue. Those who have been highlighted as being at risk of complicated bereavement outcomes usually require further support.

The type of bereavement support on offer can be as varied as the individuals who seek it. Some of the different approaches are:

▶ contacting the bereaved after one to two months and offering morning or afternoon tea with the purpose of explaining the bereavement program being offered;
▶ individual counselling and support;
▶ family or couple counselling and support;
▶ age-specific group support across the life span (for example, those 50 and over who have had a partner die, or younger bereaved partners up to 50 years of age);
▶ formal and informal mixed gender group support;
▶ walking groups (providing time to walk and share grief experiences);
▶ support appropriate for children, adolescents, and young adults (usually requiring specific programs with skilled facilitators);
▶ services of thanksgiving and remembrance; and
▶ anonymous support through telephone 'crisis lines' and the Internet.

Conclusion

Nurses are commonly required to provide care to the dying and their families. Bereavement care, in the form of risk assessment, begins before the death, continues through the illness, and persists into the early bereavement phase. If possible, risk assessment should involve the dying person as well as those in a significant relationship with the dying person. People at risk of complicated outcomes can be identified and then supported in the most appropriate manner. Those who are deemed not to be at risk are encouraged to engage their own coping abilities and resources.

> 'Risk assessment should involve the dying person as well as those in a significant relationship with the dying person.'

For those who require and desire general bereavement support, the aim is to assist them in coming to terms with the reality of their loss and, in time, to see movement towards 're-investing in life'. It is up to the health professional to be informed, so that the bereaved can be directed to the support most suitable to them.

For some, especially those at risk of complicated bereavement, the path to life reinvestment can be a long and winding one. As C.S. Lewis wrote in *A Grief Observed* (1961):

> Grief is like a long valley,
> a winding valley,
> where any bend may reveal
> a totally different landscape.

Appendix 20.1
Checklist of risk factors for complicated bereavement outcomes

A. Characteristics of the bereaved

Characteristic	Tick

Predeath
The person is a child or adolescent
The person is a young spouse
The person is an elderly spouse in a long marriage

The person has experienced cumulative multiple losses
The person has experienced multiple stressful situations
The person has experienced mental health problems
The person has experienced a family history of mental illness

The person has few adequate coping mechanisms
The person has high predeath emotional distress

Postdeath
The person demonstrates signs of poor initial adjustment to the death
The person expressed dissatisfaction with their caregiving role during the person's illness

B. Characteristics of the dying person

Characteristic	Tick

The dying person is a child or adolescent
The dying person is the parent of young children

Comments:

C. Character of interpersonal relationships

Characteristic	Tick

Predeath
The person lacks social support
The person feels unsupported
The person feels that support is antagonistic or unsympathetic
The person feels dissatisfied with help available during the illness
The person is isolated
The person has an ambivalent or conflictual relationship with the dying person

The death ends an unusually close or exclusive marriage

The family lacks cohesion
The family has poor communication
The family has difficulty resolving conflict

Postdeath
The bereaved person is isolated after the death
The bereaved person has reduced social support after the death

D. Characteristics of the illness and nature of the death

Characteristic	Tick

Predeath
The person is dying from an inherited disorder
The person is dying from a stigmatised disease
The illness is lengthy and burdensome

Postdeath
The death was sudden or unexpected
The death occurred in traumatic circumstances

Comments:

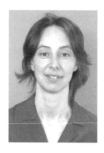 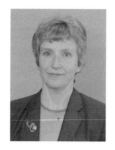

Julie Skilbeck

Julie Skilbeck qualified as a nurse in Newcastle-upon-Tyne (UK) in 1985, and worked in general medicine before specialising in intensive care. After completing a BEd for health-care professionals, she worked as a lecturer practitioner in cardiac care at Kings College University (London, UK). This experience stimulated an interest in end-of-life care for patients with chronic illnesses. She joined the Trent Palliative Care Centre (UK) in 1994 where she has been involved in a variety of projects, including a study of the palliative-care needs of patients with end-stage respiratory disease. Her current research interests involve the development of specialist palliative-care nursing, with a focus on the provision of emotional care to patients and their families. Julie is currently a member of the scientific committee of the Palliative Care Research Society.

Sheila Payne

Professor Sheila Payne is a health psychologist with a background in nursing. She has a research chair with the Sheffield Palliative Care Studies Group, based at the Trent Palliative Care Centre, University of Sheffield (UK), and was formerly director of the Health Research Unit at the University of Southampton (UK), a multidisciplinary group undertaking research in health and social care. Shiela's main research interests are in palliative care, bereavement, and psychosocial oncology, and she has a special expertise in the use of qualitative methodologies. Sheila has undertaken two research fellowships in New Zealand researching aspects of palliative care. She has also been involved in developing a number of British national research organisations in palliative care and bereavement. Sheila has published widely in academic and professional journals and, with Sandra Horn, edits the *Health Psychology* book series published by the Open University Press.

Chapter 21

Palliative Care in Chronic Illness

Julie Skilbeck and Sheila Payne

Introduction

Although most people who receive contemporary palliative care have a diagnosis of cancer, a significant minority are people with one or more of a number of other chronic illnesses. This chapter focuses on the issues involved in the provision of specialist palliative-care services to patients with chronic life-threatening illnesses other than cancer.

The chapter considers the following questions:

▶ What is the focus of specialist palliative care?
▶ Is there a need for service expansion?
▶ What are the issues relating to service expansion?
▶ How should the services be configured and resourced?
▶ What are the implications for the future?

General palliative care can be defined as 'palliative care provided by the patient and family's usual professional carers as a vital and integral part of their routine clinical practice. It is informed by knowledge and practice of palliative care principles' (NCHSPCS 2001, p. 3). The definition goes on to say that it is 'provided for patients and their families with low to moderate complexity of palliative care need, whatever the illness or its stage, in all care settings'. Such general palliative care can be distinguished from specialist palliative care. *Specialist palliative care* is defined as 'palliative care provided by health and social care professionals who specialise in palliative care and work within a multiprofessional specialist palliative care team. The service should be available in all care settings for patients with moderate to high complexity of need' (NCHSPCS 2001, pp 3–4).

The present chapter is concerned with specialist palliative care of people suffering from illnesses other than cancer, and specifically with the provision of specialist palliative care for adults because specialist palliative-care services for children are already predominantly concerned with those experiencing conditions other than cancer.

What is the focus of specialist palliative care?

For more than two decades there has been an increasing acknowledgment that palliative care can be of benefit to patients with life-limiting illnesses other than cancer. It has been recognised that patients dying from these other chronic conditions experience similar physical, psychological, and emotional distress to that suffered by cancer patients. In the United Kingdom, this is reflected in policy documents which advocate that *all* patients who require palliative care should have access to services, irrespective of diagnosis (Addington-Hall 1998). However, referrals to specialist palliative-care units, hospices, and home-care services in Britain are still dominated by patients with a diagnosis of cancer (Cassel & Vladek 1996; Eve, Smith & Tebbit 1997; Maddocks 1998), although some inpatient units have broadened their scope to include patients with HIV/ AIDS and some neurological conditions.

This emphasis on specialist palliative care on the basis of a primary diagnosis of cancer has arisen because, historically, medical diagnostic classifications have pervaded all aspects of health-care services. For example, a patient with breast cancer, diabetes, and osteoarthritis might be required to attend three different clinics in three different locations on three different days. Patients have traditionally been grouped into diagnostic categories by doctors and nurses alike, and specialist palliative-care services have been traditionally associated with a diagnosis of cancer.

'Palliative care can be of benefit to patients with life-limiting illnesses other than cancer.'

But care can be allocated and organised on other parameters of need. For example, many symptoms or problems associated with dying or advanced disease—such as fatigue, breathlessness, pain, and emotional distress—are common to many conditions. It is not necessarily the aetiology of these symptoms that determines nursing interventions. An example of a symptom-based approach (rather than a diagnosis-based approach) is the growth in pain clinics, and many nurses have skills in complex symptom management, such as the skills required to work in these clinics. Similarly, many nurses are skilled in caring for older people in general, irrespective of the precise nature of the various medical problems experienced by these people. These models provide alternative ways of conceptualising the role of specialist palliative-care nursing.

Is there a need for service expansion?
Social needs

Advances in medicine and nursing have led to an increasing number of people now surviving serious illnesses and living longer. As the proportion of older people in the population rises, and as age-associated illness grows, more people are likely to die from diseases that are chronic and have multiple pathology (Murray & Lopez 1997). It is anticipated that, by 2020, the main causes of death in developed countries will be heart disease, cerebrovascular disease, respiratory diseases, and cancer.

The problems facing cancer patients with a limited prognosis are well documented, but much less is known about the palliative-care needs of patients with other chronic life-limiting illnesses. Similarly, the challenges presented by an ageing population are

'More people are likely to die from diseases that are chronic and have multiple pathology.'

under-researched. Nurses already play a crucial role in the care of dying patients with chronic illnesses other than cancer, both in the inpatient setting and the community setting. This role is likely to increase in the future. To ensure that nursing interventions are appropriate, evidence-based, and acceptable to patients and their families, more detailed information about the experience of these people and their families is required.

In most major Western countries, health expectations and service use rose sharply in the latter part of the twentieth century. But these services have been unevenly distributed. Specialist palliative-care services have been a good example of this uneven distribution and, until recently, have not featured prominently in health-care planning. However, planning for the provision of specialist palliative-care services is now receiving attention in several countries, including Australia, the UK, and New Zealand.

Patient needs

People with chronic illnesses other than cancer experience many symptoms and problems that are comparable to those experienced by cancer patients. For example, patients with end-stage chronic obstructive pulmonary disease experience a high level of symptoms, including extreme breathlessness, pain, fatigue, difficulty in sleeping, and thirst. They also suffer reduced physical functioning, psychological morbidity, a low level of social functioning, and an overall poor quality of life (Skilbeck et al. 1998).

People with dementia also suffer pain and breathlessness (Lloyd-Williams 1996), as do people with heart disease (McCarthy, Lay & Addington-Hall 1996; Anderson et al. 2001), stroke (Addington-Hall et al. 1997), motor neurone disease (Barby & Leigh 1995), and kidney failure (Cohen et al. 1995). When comparisons are made with cancer patients, it can be seen that dying patients with other illnesses have physical and psychosocial needs at least as severe as patients with cancer (Edmonds et al. 2001; Skilbeck et al. 1998).

Current services

Current service provision for these people is not always appropriate to the problems identified. For example, symptom control for patients with dementia can be inadequate when compared with current palliative-care practice. There is a reluctance to prescribe adequate doses of opiate analgesia to achieve full symptomatic relief, and a failure to use syringe drivers for those patients unable to take oral medication (Lloyd-Williams 1996).

Services can be geared towards managing acute exacerbations of illnesses. This focus on 'crisis intervention' can result in people experiencing high levels of symptoms most of the time, and can lead to a fragmented service with gaps in community care (Skilbeck et al. 1998).

Uncertainty in being able to provide accurate prognoses appears to influence the level of information that is disclosed to patients and their families, thus potentially affecting access to services. Compared with people with chronic respiratory disease and severe heart failure, people with cancer are more likely to be told their prognoses by hospital doctors, and are more likely to be given information about their illnesses and possible service options by a variety of health-care professionals (McCarthy, Lay & Addington-Hall 1997). The uncertain illness trajectory in some chronic illnesses, and the difficulties in providing an accurate prognosis can prevent these patients receiving palliative care.

Place of death is also an issue to be considered. Almost 60% of cancer patients in the UK now die in a hospice or specialist palliative-care unit, or in the care of community or home-care palliative-nursing teams (Eve, Smith & Tebbit 1997). People with other chronic illnesses are more likely to die in hospital, tend to spend less time in their place of death, and have limited access to specialist palliative-care professionals (Edmonds et al. 2001). Older people are increasingly likely to die in nursing homes (Froggatt 2001; Maddocks & Parker 2001). In 1995, deaths in residential and nursing homes comprised 18% of all deaths in the UK (ONS 1997), and in South Australia the proportion of all deaths occurring in nursing homes increased from 1% in 1960 to 20% in 1990 (Hunt & Maddocks 1997). Considering that older people frequently experience chronic conditions, it is likely that the provision of palliative care to older people in nursing homes will become more prominent in the future.

> 'People dying from chronic, non-malignant illnesses are not receiving the symptom control and psychosocial support that they require.'

It seems that people dying from chronic, non-malignant illnesses are not receiving the symptom control and psychosocial support that they require. Many of these needs could be met by palliative care. However, can the assumption be made that specialist palliative care has the answer? The next section explores whether these patients should receive specialist palliative-care services as part of their care.

What are the issues relating to service expansion?

It is difficult to decide which patients with chronic conditions require specialist palliative care, and difficult to decide the timing of interventions in relation to the illness trajectory. For many people, curative interventions continue to be appropriate treatment. For example, it might be appropriate to continue well-established and broad-based pulmonary rehabilitation programs (Morgan & Singh 1997).

The difficulties in predicting prognosis and life expectancy compound the situation. For those people whose illness trajectory is characterised by acute exacerbations, decisions have to be made about whether to give antibiotics or to make use of life-prolonging technologies. This occurs often in liver disease (Henegan & O'Grady 2001) and in heart disease (Simon & Gibbs 2001). The prediction of life expectancy becomes even more problematic when a diagnosis of a life-limiting disease has not been made. In the case of dementia, for example, Alzheimer's disease is seriously under-reported as a cause of death, and is often not recognised as a 'terminal illness' (Hoyert 1996). It is likely, however, that Alzheimer's disease will become one of the common causes of death in older people (Hanrahan, Luchins & Murphy 2001).

For these reasons, defining the terminal phase of an illness is difficult, and because people are not considered suitable for palliative care until they are in the 'terminal' phase, many people do not receive specialist palliative-care services.

The wishes of the person and his or her family must be taken into account. It is often assumed that all patients would wish to access specialist palliative-care services if they had the opportunity. But it is uncertain whether they would access services that are predominantly used by cancer patients if there is a perception that staff in such services work only with people who are dying. Conversely, personal stories of patients' experiences often illustrate the frustration of not being able to access appropriate services at the end of life (Skilbeck et al. 1997).

How could the services be configured?
Patient needs
Specialist palliative services for cancer patients take a variety of forms, including inpatient units (hospital, hospice), day hospices, hospital and community specialist nursing services, and home-care services. In most instances, apart from inpatient care, specialist palliative-care services work alongside existing services. However, it cannot be presumed that this pattern of service delivery is appropriate to people with other chronic illnesses. Although these people experience similar physical and psychosocial problems, they often experience very different illness trajectories.

In addition, it is not necessarily true that the knowledge and skills developed in the field of cancer care are transferable to people with other diagnoses in different care settings. For example, some symptoms—such as breathlessness (Ahmedzai 1998) and fatigue (Porock 1999)—are difficult to control, even in 'expert' hands. Furthermore, these people are already receiving care from health and social-care professionals with specialist knowledge and skills in their fields.

For many people, a general 'palliative-care approach' applied in their current settings would be sufficient to meet their needs. This would acknowledge the existing knowledge and expertise of nurses working in various fields, and would allow palliative-care specialists to develop collaborative and supportive relationships within which the principles of palliative care could be communicated and practised by those already responsible for caregiving. Such an approach would be more likely to avoid potential conflicts of knowledge and skills—as has occurred in the UK in the relationship between some community nurses and specialist palliative-care nurses (Haste & MacDonald 1992).

There will be some people for whom it is considered necessary to access the services of specialist palliative care. Some people will require specialist palliative inpatient care, where responsibility for care will be assumed by the specialist palliative-care team. The care of other people could be based on the current model of supplementing and complementing existing services—rather than having specialists take over patient care. This would probably involve referral to a hospital or community multidisciplinary palliative-care team, or a specialist nursing service. The challenge is to identify the best management approach for each person.

> 'For many people, a general "palliative-care approach" applied in their current settings would be sufficient to meet their needs.'

Resource use

An expansion in palliative-care services could be achieved by increasing resources or by re-allocating existing resources.

In the UK, current palliative-care resources care for half of all *cancer* deaths per year. If services are to be extended to non-cancer patients, it has been estimated that an expansion of resources to care for half of *all* deaths that occur per year might be required (Addington-Hall, Fakhoury & McCarthy 1998). If a similar increase in responsibility were to occur in other countries, it is unclear where these extra resources would come from, given that such services are currently heavily dependent on private and voluntary sector contributions for finance and personnel

An alternative would be to re-allocate current services—for example, by viewing specialist palliative care as a service for those with complex end-of-life symptoms or problems. Access could be determined by assessment of symptom severity, rather than by a diagnostic label, as is often the case now. However, in many inpatient units, the trend is for increased admissions for acute symptom control followed by discharge home, and this means that some people currently eligible to receive specialist palliative care might be unable to access it if arrangements were changed. Certain patients and families (such as those requiring respite care, those with prolonged dying trajectories and those without carers) might be disadvantaged by changes that re-allocated specialist palliative-care services as an acute medical service. Perhaps there might be a role for innovative nurse-led end-of-life care units to meet these demands.

What are the implications for the future?

Extending palliative care to people with diseases other than cancer will require great effort on the part of all those involved in the care of these people, including nurses.

Issues for consideration include:
▶ new models of working;
▶ collaboration and teamwork;
▶ education; and
▶ research agenda.

New models of working

New models of working with patients and families as 'experts' in managing their chronic diseases are starting to emerge (Nolan, Grant & Keady 1996; Costain Schou & Hewison 1997). According to these models, care should be negotiated between professionals and their clients. Nurses have expertise that they can contribute, but there needs to be a recognition that patients and their families have their own 'lived' experience of chronic illness and skills in self-management.

Collaboration and teamwork

It will be important to establish good working relationships and communication networks with clinicians who have expertise in the care of people with cancer. Such collaboration will acknowledge the strengths and limitations of existing knowledge and skills of both teams, as well as exploring how knowledge developed in the field of cancer can be useful with other patient groups.

Education

It will be necessary to develop specific expertise in applying specialist palliative care to people with other chronic illnesses. Advanced nursing practice skills courses in end-of-life care should not be restricted to those with cancer. The level of knowledge of palliative care among nurses will have to be addressed within preregistration and postregistration education. In particular, educational strategies will need to explore the conceptual confusion that appears to have developed regarding the nursing care of dying patients in general hospitals—confusion that limits a more proactive approach to care (Holmes,

'Advanced nursing practice skills courses in end-of-life care should not be restricted to those with cancer.'

Pope & Lamond 1997). Specific areas of nurse education that will be required include postbasic skills development, and more expertise in recognising and referring complex problems.

Research agenda

Little attention has been given to the effectiveness of specialist palliative-care nursing interventions for different patients in different contexts. More research is needed on what models of care work best, in what conditions, for whom, and under what circumstances (Bonsaquet & Salisbury 1999). It will be important to obtain the views of patients and their families to ensure services are responsive and acceptable. Prospective, longitudinal, and collaborative work is needed to map illness trajectories and to determine obstacles in access and uptake of services.

Conclusion

This chapter has provided a brief overview of some of the issues raised by a consideration of specialist palliative care for people dying from chronic illnesses other than cancer. Nurses working in both general care and specialist palliative care will require creative and novel solutions to the issues raised. These solutions will need to be evidence-based, cost-effective, and collaborative. Most importantly, they will need to recognise the 'lived experience' of the patients and their families.

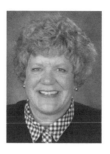

Jenny Abbey

Dr Jenny Abbey trained at St George's Hospital in London (UK), completed her bachelor's degree in nursing at the University of New England (New South Wales, Australia), and gained a PhD in nursing from Deakin University (Victoria, Australia) in 1995. Jenny has also been a hands-on-nurse practitioner, union organiser, and assistant dean in research, at Flinders University (Adelaide, South Australia). She now works with her husband as a health-care consultant and independent researcher. At present they are engaged on a national quality and compliance audit of government contractors in domiciliary nursing. For many years, Jenny has been especially interested in the needs of people with dementia, and has published and lectured widely on the subject. In particular, she has been concerned about the issue of pain management in people with dementia who cannot articulate their needs, and how this issue affects patients, health professionals, and families.

Chapter 22

Ageing, Dementia, and Palliative Care

Jenny Abbey

Introduction

Palliative care for the increasing proportion of frail aged persons is among the biggest challenges facing the health systems of Western nations. Health services must invest more heavily in the study of this issue, and must begin to devise new forms of suitable care, and new means and venues for delivering that care. The challenges for nurses will be immense, and preparations must be made now.

Most of what is known about palliative care comes from work with people suffering from cancer and, to a lesser extent, HIV/AIDS. This knowledge does not easily translate into information that is appropriate to care planning for the broader group of the frail elderly. The stages through which the health status of most elderly people progresses are usually not as well marked as in the 'accepted' diseases requiring palliative care. However, with the development of medical knowledge, diagnostic skills, and investigative technologies, the stages and phases of the illness processes in the aged will become better understood. This knowledge will feed into improved decision-making about the transition from curative care to palliative care. Decisions of this nature will become increasingly common in people in the care of nurses.

This chapter first advances the view that, during the terminal stages of the common illnesses associated with ageing such as chronic cardiac disease, long-standing emphysema, and Alzheimer's disease the care provided needs to be informed by sound palliative practice, just as is now taken for granted in the cases of cancer and HIV/AIDS. Secondly, the chapter argues that the extension of palliative care to these groups will raise distinctive and often novel issues, especially in the case of the frail aged with dementia (because of the specific challenges associated with that disease).

The chapter discusses:

- communication and planning;
- the nurse's role as story-teller;
- whose voice will be heard?;
- problems with communication; and
- when 'enough is enough'.

Communication and planning

Effective, efficient, and timely communication is the keystone of all good nursing care and is also true in the kinds of cases discussed in this chapter. Communication in this context includes, but is not limited to, documentation.

It is likely that the provision of information about the legally available options for a terminally ill person will soon become customary, if not mandatory at the time of admission to a long-term aged-care facility, and for some admissions to an acute-care facility (Madson 1993). Before this happens it will be necessary to encourage thought and discussion on the issue with the people receiving care and their families or significant others. 'Living wills', although still not commonly used in Australia, are being promoted more actively, and popular awareness of the issue will continue to rise.

A 'life-and-health summary' is also valuable. This can be vital if dementia later prevents communication in a conventional manner. Such a summary must be easily accessible to everyone caring for the person.

This documentation ensures that 'personhood' is not lost, and that the progress of any continuing health condition is clearly noted and placed in context. For example, a person might not be able to speak as a result of a stroke, Parkinson's disease, or dementia, but carers should understand that such people have not necessarily lost the capacity to understand how they are being spoken to, or about, in their presence. The kind of documentation being recommended here can help to prevent the sort of unfortunate episode described in the Box below. Incidents such as this demonstrate that an understanding of a person's past is vital if nurses are to assist in shaping a future the person would desire.

'Understanding of a person's past is vital if nurses are to assist in shaping a future the person would desire.'

The nurse's role as story-teller

Nurses are best placed to 'know' the people receiving palliative care. The documentation and reporting of this knowledge in an objective manner is best practice in all nursing care. In palliative care, it is no less important.

The Box on page 316 illustrates an example of a short 'life history' that a nurse could prepare and have available for a case-management discussion about palliative care for this person. A discussion of the implications of this 'life history' follows below.

Note that in keeping with recent amendments to Privacy legislation, extraneous information that is not required for the provision of hands-on care (such as medical and financial details) would be recorded in files elsewhere. The final entry in the sample notes shown in the Box projects a January meeting with Mr S, his family and the multidisciplinary team with a view to seeking broad agreement on the feasible and desirable objectives of future care.

An essential part of the preparation for that meeting will be an awareness of the relevant local legislation pertaining to palliative care. This should be a matter for senior management, with professional legal advice being taken as required. Information and policy decisions need to be presented to nurses clearly and coherently. Nurses need to be aware of the actions that the facility will endorse and support, and the safeguards that it expects to be observed. Individual

---

'That's a good boy, dearie'

The relatives of a former cardiac surgeon, while visiting the man in an aged-care facility, were visibly embarrassed and distressed on hearing a carer say to the man: 'Have one more mouthful, dearie, that's a good boy'.

If the carer had perceived this man as a highly intelligent and respected senior community figure (who now had some failings in his brain's messaging systems), rather than perceiving him as 'an old boy with Parkinson's', the distress caused to the family (and presumably to the man himself), would have been avoided.

nurses need a working understanding of the law, but are not required to be experts. This dimension of care planning is especially important if there are any disagreements among the parties—including the person, the family, or the medical or nursing staff.

An example of a short 'life history'

Mr S.

Age 84

Resident since March 2001

Wife deceased 1965. Partner since 1975, Mr Piers Abraham.

Three children. Eldest son, Jimmy, lawyer, South Africa; daughter, Mary (deceased 1963); daughter, Jane, physiotherapist, lives 80 km away, visits father weekly.

All children communicate comfortably with their father and with each other.

Past occupation: builder in the local area; retired 1988.

Hobbies: Appreciation of Brahms and flying ultra-light planes were his passions.

Medical history:
CVA 1988; left-sided paralysis now resolved; frequent transient ischaemic attacks since then.
Worsening memory loss ascribed to multi-infarct dementia when assessed by Dr White (gerontologist) in December 2000.
Emphysema, worsening since 1998.
Heavy smoker; still wants to smoke.

Living will and advanced directives were discussed on admission. Family and Mr S requested 'no extraordinary measures' but would not formalise any agreement. Jane holds financial power-of-attorney.

August 2001: Mr S reported by staff as saying that he does 'not want to be kept alive'. Comment made while staff caring for Mr S's personal hygiene.

Has had recurrent chest infections since admission.

October 2001: Chest infection. 20 Oct. 2001 Dr Brown discussed with Mr S, Jane, and other family members the use of antibiotics versus the use of aspirin only. All requested that antibiotics be used. Since that time Mr S has had two more chest infections, both treated with antibiotics.

Over Christmas, Mr S's family and partner expressed concern to staff that Mr S seemed depressed and that he repeatedly indicated that he was miserable, in pain, and wanted to die. He was not recognising family members and his requests were increasingly incoherent. Abbreviated Mental Test Score 0/10.

January 2002; Another chest infection. Meeting to be held with Mr S and family members re change of emphasis in care to a palliative approach.

The documentation available in Mr S's case provides a foundation for determining his wishes, but caution is needed. Because Mr S is unable to exercise self-determination, and because there is no record of a health power-of-attorney or living will, decisions will need to be made by consensus between the health-care team and the family as to the best course of action. The nurses' intimate knowledge of Mr S and his story will inform the advocacy and mediation that follows, in association with objective clinical observation to provide inputs to an evidenced-based decision-making process.

For Mr S, changes in care that could be discussed at the forthcoming meeting include the following:

▶ cigarettes only when Mr S can be supervised;
▶ no further antibiotics;
▶ no suction;
▶ sedation and analgesia to relieve discomfort and pain;
▶ making comfort a higher priority than mobilisation;
▶ comfort dressings only for skin tears;
▶ food and fluid only as comfortably tolerated; and
▶ cease food and fluids if any dysphagia or signs of terminal discomfort.

These changes in care differ significantly from the traditional palliative approach in which symptom control and relief of pain are the main focus of care.

Identifying the decisions that need to be made, and obtaining agreement, are not always easy. But the challenges do not stop there. Implementing the decisions is the next challenge.

Whose voice will be heard?

Some parts of the agreed plan can appear to represent the withdrawal of care, and this prospect can be confronting for nurses. Such an approach challenges ingrained notions of the mission of nursing. Implementing these kinds of choices means that members of the nursing team must share trust and a commitment to a palliative approach. Without trust and commitment, and an agreed flexible care plan, many decisions will inevitably be taken at times of crisis. In these circumstances, decisions are likely to depend too heavily on transient factors. Longer-term factors, policy statements, and principles of conduct can be discarded when matters of the moment, personality issues, and subjective judgments take over, and these factors can vary from day to day, or even from shift to shift.

These developments can lead to divisions between nurses and doctors, or between nurses and management. Individual nurses tend to respond differently to 'prn' ('as required') orders, depending on their past experiences and beliefs.

For example, instead of observing a protocol for calling in the person's doctor when nominated 'triggers' occur, the seeking of medical advice can become haphazard and lacking in any consistent rationale. Doctors and nurses alike tend to respond to events in terms of their own beliefs and customary practices, instead of adhering to an agreement to implement what seemed to all involved to be the course of care best suited to the person's needs. Care planning thus gives way to habit or whim at best, and to prejudice at worst.

Research has shown that there are distinct differences between the perceptions of patients regarding good care, and those of caregivers (McCullough & Wilson 1995). Caregivers can be perceived as using 'platitudes and reassurances' (Starck 1992, p. 149) in an effort to comfort clients and families, rather than providing them with objective information and a range of choices.

Platitudes to patients, and unspoken differences of opinion among health professionals are not part of best practice, especially in the last weeks or months of a person's life. A forward-looking plan, including well-documented decisions about care, can avoid this situation.

Conflict or cross-purposes will not disappear, and it is not desirable that they do so entirely. Indeed, such differences can help to identify difficult transitions in the dying process and can reveal alternative thoughts and values in care planning. A mechanism to give vent to these differences, and to allow satisfactory resolutions to be found within the parameters of the agreed care plan, is useful and necessary. The best solution is a system of regular case conferences that allows the care of all clients to be reviewed by a multidisciplinary team on a frequent basis. If some of those involved in care are unable to attend these conferences, the minutes and recommendations of the meeting should be formally conveyed to them. In such conferences, nurses need to ensure that neither the voice of carers nor that of the person receiving care is lost in this process.

For the sake of the person being cared for, nurses must be united in their approach. An example of this breaking down in practice is sometimes seen in the administration of medication. Nurses are often reluctant to give prescribed analgesia (Abbey 1995). The pain relief received can be dependent on a particular nurse's interpretation of the language of the patient, especially if that person has dementia. Communication and explanation with family and friends is vital to ensure that the planned approach can be implemented smoothly.

'For the sake of the person being cared for, nurses must be united in their approach.'

Well-conducted case management, especially with nurses and doctors working closely together in a planned manner, is essential if optimal palliative care is to be offered to elderly people with cognitive impairment and multiple pathologies.

Problems with communication

Problems often arise for nurses caring for elderly and demented people when persons receiving care cannot clearly communicate their unhappiness or pain. This section of the chapter examines some of these difficulties.

Psychological disturbances

Nurses are often asked to make a judgment about whether a person is depressed or anxious. Many older people become depressed or anxious as the losses associated with ageing, organ failure, and dependence on others increase, or as a result of specific conditions such as Alzheimer's disease. In a palliative approach, in assessing medication, it can be difficult to make a judgment between potential side-effects and potential relief of distress. This can be difficult to judge, and can be ascertained only if careful observations are made and documented.

The benzodiazepine group of drugs, such as oxazepam (Serepax) and diazepam (Valium), are anti-anxiety agents that have a sedative effect in association with muscle relaxation. They can cause dizziness and drowsiness. Paradoxically, in some cases, especially in the elderly, they can cause excitement.

Selective serotonin reuptake inhibitor (SSRI) antidepressants, such as sertraline (Zoloft) and fluoxetine (Prozac) can take several days to a week to be effective, and medication should not be discontinued abruptly after long-term use. In the elderly, ataxia and gait abnormality can occur, and confusion can be exacerbated. Gastrointestinal disturbance (diarrhoea, constipation, anorexia, dry mouth, dyspepsia, vomiting, and flatulence) can also occur.

For people who suffer from dementia, agitation and loss of touch with reality can cause distress to the person, family, and staff. Antipsychotic medication such as haloperidol (Serenace), pericyazine (Neulactil), and thioridazine (Mellerill) can be helpful, but these drugs can have marked side-effects, including extra-pyramidal effects, anticholinergic effects, and orthostatic hypotension (with a danger of falls). A person with dementia can be close to death, but still be mobile and agitated. Assisting these people to a dignified, peaceful death might require an increase in antipsychotic medication, with increased risk of side-effects. The use of these drugs in this way can be considered a form of restraint, but their use can be a much kinder way of ensuring safety and providing relief from suffering than the use of physical restraints. However, keeping a person in bed and giving him or her ice-cubes to suck for dry mouth, can help to reduce suffering without drug side-effects. Again, best practice involves working out the best way to provide comfort for an agitated, dying person.

Psychological disturbance in elderly or demented people should be assessed and treated appropriately. It can be a pointer to the need to change to a palliative-care approach.

Pain

It is important to assess and manage pain appropriately in people with dementia or an inability to communicate their suffering. The story related by Glenda (Box, below) shows how an inability to communicate can lead to significant suffering as a result of untreated pain.

This problem of an inability to communicate can be compounded if nursing staff fail to base their decisions on objective assessment of the need for pain relief.

Being aware of pain in those who cannot communicate their suffering

Glenda, an enrolled nurse, had worked for many years in an aged-care facility. She was helping to care for a woman with dementia who showed, by various non-verbal ways, that she was in great pain when she out of bed or when being showered. Glenda reported this to a registered nurse on several occasions, and requested that the problem be identified so that pain relief could be prescribed. Eventually, after some months, the woman's back was X-rayed. This showed significant degeneration of the spine. Pain relief was instituted.

Glenda then faced the same kind of problem with her own father. He was suffering from progressive supra-nuclear palsy. When he became unable to speak or feed himself, and was generally very dependent on care, he was admitted to an aged-care facility where he settled well. After some time, there were changes in the facility and a new resident was admitted to share his room. Glenda's father became distressed, but it was unclear whether his distress was due to the new arrangements, or to some other problem, such as pain. He was not demented, but was unable to verbalise his needs to the nurses caring for him.

Despite Glenda's expressions of concern, no steps were taken to deal with the possibility that her father was in pain. Eventually Glenda took her father out of the facility, and arranged for him to be assessed at a local hospice. There he was assessed as requiring 30 mg of morphine (MS Contin) twice daily. This produced obvious relief from pain, and a marked increase in his ability to enjoy life.

Glenda's father is now being treated as a 'palliative-care patient' rather than as an 'aged-care resident'. The different approach has given him a comfortable and dignified conclusion to his life.

The subjective values and impressions of some nurses can interfere with best practice. The Box below relates such a story.

The point to be noted from the story of Mrs AB is the degree of latitude that the 'as required' order for morphine allowed. A succession of different approaches and attitudes were thus allowed to govern the care given to the woman as she died. It is apparent that there was no planned and united approach. This does not reflect laxity or indifference on the part of any individual. It resulted from a failure to agree upon an openly articulated and universally shared model of care to guide the nursing staff in their care of an elderly lady in the last days of her life.

An uncertain framework results in nursing staff experiencing what is sometimes called 'cognitive dissonance'. Staff should feel confident that they will

---

'If it was me . . . '

Mrs AB, a 90-year-old resident in an aged-care facility, was suffering from dementia and was approaching her death. After family members had contacted their mother's doctor, he wrote in the nursing notes:

'Family requests comfort care only at this stage. Antibiotics ceased. May have morphia 5–10 mg 4 times in 24 hours prn'.

The elderly lady was suffering from quite severe bedsores and was constantly calling out 'Help me, help me'—as she had done for protracted periods during her three years in the facility.

According to the nursing records, only six doses of morphine were given in the last six days of this woman's life—only 25% of the permitted dose. On some days she had received two or three doses of morphine, but on other days she had received none at all. Neither the registered nurses who chose to give the morphine, nor those who did not, gave clear reasons in the nursing notes for their decision. One nursing note read:

'Very quiet evening, no medication given'.

Another nursing note recorded:

'In distress, calling out, needs attended 2-hrly. Accepting small amounts of thickened fluids. IM morphia 10 mg at 1220.'

It is apparent that some nurses accepted the woman's calling out as being her own particular form of 'demented behaviour', whereas others were sure that it represented distress or pain.

When the nurses were asked why they did or did not give morphine, the answers were not based on objective evidence. Rather, it was apparent that decisions were based on subjective values or impressions:

'If it was me I would want it'; 'I would not want to be knocked out and not know what was going on'; 'Morphia is only for pain and I don't think she is in pain now'.

not be criticised for failing to give 'life-preserving curative care'. They should be supported in their role of assisting people to a peaceful death.

Such cognitive dissonance is most often experienced in the provision of pain relief. It can be difficult to recognise pain in a person with dementia who cannot tell nurses that he or she is in pain. The pain scale shown in Figure 22.1 (page 323) has been developed to measure pain in this population. It assists in providing objective evidence for case conferences and well-planned approaches to palliative care.

Such a pain scale allows all nurses in the team to feel confident that pain has been accurately and consistently assessed for people who are unable to communicate their pain by conventional means.

Objective measures such as this scale and other assessment tools assist in assessing pain and prescribing pain relief. Drug therapy is not the only way to relieve pain. Table 22.1 (page 324) presents suggestions for other nursing interventions as alternatives or adjuncts to drug treatment.

A planned and well-documented regimen for pain relief is an essential part of palliative care. Nurses who are implementing 'prn' ('as required') orders need objective measures to judge when pain relief is needed, rather than relying on their own personal views. In palliative care, the balance between drug side-effects and relief of suffering needs to be carefully considered.

When 'enough is enough'

The accepted indicators of the terminal stage of an illness are 'poor appetite, weight loss, recumbency, lassitude, failure of physiological systems and progression of the disease' (Ashby & Stoffell 1991). However, these signs and symptoms are often conceptualised by nurses as merely being indicators that an elderly person or a person with dementia is 'deteriorating', rather than indicators that the person has reached a stage where palliative care is appropriate

It is now accepted that there are occasions when it is appropriate to withdraw mechanical life support in critically ill people who will not recover. But it is difficult to gain acceptance for the notion that this situation is similar to that which often arises in the care of seriously ill elderly and/or demented people, especially when this touches on emotionally charged issues of nourishment, mobilisation, the use of antibiotics, and so on. Polarised positions are usually taken. Some nurses understand the 'respirator metaphor', and are prepared to tackle the difficult questions raised by such a metaphor. Others want no part of such a debate, believing that any change to the present paradigm of care would turn staff into 'death squads'.

Abbey Pain Scale
For measurement of pain in people with dementia who cannot verbalise

How to use scale: While observing the resident, score questions 1 to 6.

Name of resident: ....

Name and designation of person completing the scale: ....

Date: ....   Time: ....

Latest pain relief given was .... at .... hrs.

01. Vocalisation
e.g. whimpering, groaning, crying   Q1 ☐
Absent 0   Mild 1   Moderate 2   Severe 3

02. Facial expression
e.g. looking tense, frowing, grimacing, looking frightened   Q2 ☐
Absent 0   Mild 1   Moderate 2   Severe 3

03. Change in body language
e.g. fidgeting, rocking, guarding part of body, withdrawn   Q3 ☐
Absent 0   Mild 1   Moderate 2   Severe 3

04. Behavioural Change
e.g. increased confusion, refusing to eat, alteration in usual patterns Q4 ☐
Absent 0   Mild 1   Moderate 2   Severe 3

05. Physiological change
e.g. temperature, pulse or blood pressure outside normal limits,   Q5 ☐
perspiring, flushing or pallor
Absent 0   Mild 1   Moderate 2   Severe 3

06. Physical changes
e.g. skin tears, pressure areas, arthritis, contractures,   Q6 ☐
previous injuries
Absent 0   Mild 1   Moderate 2   Severe 3

Add scores for 1–6 and record here   Total Pain Score ☐

Now tick the box that matches the Total Pain Score

0–2	3–7	8–13	14+
No pain	Mild	Moderate	Severe

Finally tick the box that matches the type of pain

Chronic	Acute	Acute on Chronic

Figure 22.1 Abbey Pain Scale
Abbey et al. (2001)

Table 22.1 Pain relief: alternatives to drug therapy

Intervention	Indications and effects
Heat (bath, hot-water bottle, heat pads)	Decreases muscle stiffness; relieves muscle spasms; increases circulation
Cold (covered ice pack gently rubbed on painful area)	Helps restore mobility and function to a joint; relieves pain and prevents complications of acute injuries
Remove or adjust sensory stimulation (TV, radio, check mirrors, hearing aid)	Decreases agitation and sensory overload (but might need substitution with comforting sensory stimuli such as pet, soft animal, doll)
Massage	Comforting and relaxing; aids circulation; alleviates rheumatic pain and stiffness
Counselling, reminiscence therapy, and conversation	Can relieve anxiety, boredom, feelings of being a nuisance, and feeling unimportant

This question is best understood as a balance between conflicting perceptions, value systems, and nursing habits. It is a fine line between, on the one hand, withdrawing food and water consistent with providing optimum comfort and, on the other hand, being neglectful and allowing a person to suffer from hunger and thirst. When is it appropriate to cease antibiotics, and merely give aspirin or other analgesia for comfort? When is it appropriate to stop suction? When should nurses cease the established practice of getting people out of bed, and accept that 'dying' has commenced? In many cases, no one knows the precise answers to these questions. Judgments are not easy. However, it must be remembered that the comfort of the person, rather than nursing tradition, is paramount.

Accepted nursing practice states that getting people out of bed for mobilisation assists in preventing pneumonia, contractures, and pressure sores. Nurses and relatives alike perceive this sort of practice as providing 'care'. But these activities can cause distress for a person with dementia, severe arthritis, or chronic emphysema. In contrast, such a person might be much more comfortable if left in bed, as long as the person is not simply left alone. He or

> 'Judgments are not easy . . . [but] . . . the comfort of the person, rather than nursing tradition, is paramount.'

she should be moved gently if apparently stiff or sore from being in one position.

In this scenario, the avoidance and management of skin breakdown—in the form of skin-tears, decubitus ulcers, or non-healing wounds—needs careful consideration. Breakdown of skin exemplifies 'failure' for nurses. Nurses have to balance the comfort of the person against their own feelings that they must go on treating and healing up to a person's death. There comes a time when pain relief and simple comfort cover to wounds are less traumatic than changing wound dressings, moving a person every two hours, and so on.

Similar difficulties arise with the question of withdrawing food and fluids. Eating and drinking have important symbolism in life (see Chapter 13, page 187). However, as McCue (1995, p. 1039) has observed: 'very elderly patients eventually undergo a process of functional decline, progressive apathy and loss of willingness to eat and drink that culminates in death'. Many people with late-stage dementia reject food. They might refuse to open their mouths, spit food out, allow food to drop out of their mouths, or refuse to swallow (Watson 1994).

The act of nourishment can become confused with issues of care. Keeping people alive can become important for nurses to feel 'connected with' (rather than 'alienated from') their work. However, if it is appropriate to discontinue food and fluids, such a policy must be undertaken by all staff. If not, a person might suffer from being forced or pressured to eat on one shift, but being starved on another shift. Spitting out food, pushing it away, and refusing to swallow might all be indications that the person simply does not want to eat any more. Family and nurses can find this hard to cope with. But entrenched values, moral positions, and platitudes should give way to objective evidence, clinical observation, and insightful knowledge in these situations.

Billings (1985, p. 109) has made some interesting observations on the nature of salt and water metabolism in these patients. Eventually, terminally ill patients develop mixed disorders of salt and water depletion such that:

> Disorders of thirst and the mental status changes that foster and perpetuate salt and water deficiencies may protect against discomfort or obliterate the awareness of suffering. Indeed, patients who become dehydrated may be too lethargic to be troubled by symptoms potentially produced by fluid deprivation.

Billings (1985) concluded that fluid depletion in dying patients is best dealt with by mouth care only, and noted that the administration of fluids is more often 'determined by the symbolic or emotional meanings of such measures'.

Conclusion

Providing dignity to the older population requires knowledgeable, observant, caring, and courageous nurses who work as equal partners in a multidisciplinary team. Government guidelines for effective and safe palliative care in residential settings are now being developed, and government will be spending more money in future to ensure that appropriate palliative care is available to our elderly citizens. Nurses have to ensure that they carefully consider the issues involved, and that they are prepared to meet the challenges ahead with an educated and mature approach.

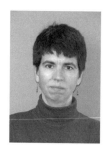

Jane Seymour

Dr Jane Seymour is a nurse and sociologist, and a research fellow in the Sheffield Palliative Care Studies Group (UK), which is comprised of the Department of Palliative Medicine in the University of Sheffield and the Trent Palliative Care Centre. Jane has worked in palliative-care research and education since 1994, before which she pursued a career in clinical nursing. Her PhD was an ethnographic study of the management of death, dying, and end-of-life decision-making in intensive-care units. Her current research focuses on the understandings and preferences of older people with respect to end-of-life care technologies.

Chapter 23

Caring for Dying People in Critical Care

Jane Seymour

Introduction

Although critical care and palliative care might appear to be at opposite ends of a spectrum, closer inspection reveals many similarities. Historically, the two specialities developed at similar times, and both care for patients and their families at moments of extreme vulnerability and need. Staff in both specialities frequently face the deaths of those in their care, and must manage the implications of these deaths for patients, families, and themselves. Both specialities rely on models of nursing care in which the 'total' care of patients and their families is paramount, and in which recognition of the inter-dependency of medicine and nursing, and the importance of team integrity, are highly developed (Randall-Curtis & Rubenfeld 2001).

These similarities are obscured somewhat by the technological scene that critical care presents. Noise, bright lights, and machinery can give the impression that technology operates to obscure the identities of patients and, indeed, to obscure everything that is human and compassionate. There can appear to be little space for a philosophy of palliative care in which dying people and their families can 'draw meaning and solace from their personal lives and culture in the face of death' (Miles 2001, p. 207). In the critical-care context, one of the central tenets of palliative care—that people have an awareness of dying—is usually absent (Seymour 2001).

Certain features of critical care have been identified as contributing to an 'overwhelming' culture (Miles 2001) in which it can be difficult to accommodate practices that facilitate a 'good death' for patients, families and staff (see Box, below). All of these features are likely to become more marked with the growing sophistication of medical technologies:

This chapter explores these issues through interviews with doctors and nurses in general adult critical-care units in the United Kingdom (Seymour 2001). The chapter concludes with some recommendations for the care of dying people in the challenging environment of critical care.

Caring and coping with death in critical care

'Integrity' is a term often used to describe an ideal relationship between dying people and their professional carers (de Raeve 1996; Saunders & Valente 1994). When caring for dying people and their families, nurses and other critical-care staff strive to create a sense of 'occupational integrity', both personally and in a team context, in which they:

Difficulties in managing death in critical care

Certain features of critical care make it difficult to manage a 'good death'. These include the following.
- A growing proportion of critical-care patients are elderly and suffering from an acute exacerbation of a long-term chronic illness, rather than from the effects of infectious disease or sudden trauma.
- 15–35% of patients die during critical therapy and a significant proportion die shortly after discharge.
- Approximately 90% of patients who die in critical care do so following a non-treatment decision involving withholding or withdrawal of life-prolonging therapies.
- Non-treatment is an unfolding process and is marked by significant ethical and diagnostic complexity, and staff are at the 'sharp end' of resolving potentially irreconcilable interests.

Adapted from Seymour (2000, 2001); Audit Commission (1999); Prendergast & Luce (1997)

- attempt to separate professional and personal identities;
- emphasise the comfort of the dying person and the presentation of his or her body;
- attempt to disclose appropriate information to patients' families in a compassionate manner; and
- protect the 'team' by balancing the different orientations of medicine and nursing.
  Each of these is discussed below.

Separation of personal and professional self

Critical-care staff consciously deploy certain strategies or 'rules' to ensure that distressing emotions and feelings are controlled. This is particularly the case with nurses, for whom intimacy with patients and their families is a defining feature of their work. Nurses have a definite sense of 'involvement' and of emotional investment. They describe incidents that might be interpreted as formative 'rites of passage', in which they over-stepped the invisible line between self and professional. Such experiences led to subsequent efforts to ensure that

> 'Staff consciously deploy certain strategies or "rules" to ensure that distressing emotions and feelings are controlled.'

their emotions are 'managed' and that separation between personal and professional selves is achieved. This process of separation is, however, complex and difficult to sustain because such involvement and expression of emotion is integral to their professional identity. One junior staff nurse put it this way:

> I think it's because we are all human, you do get close . . . I try to think of my patients as family, like when you're a student nurse and you're taught to think: 'That's my granny there'. So you try to look after them as well as you would your granny.

A more experienced nurse described how she had once become 'over-involved' with a young patient who had eventually died from severe injuries. She likened this experience to:

> . . . getting my fingers burnt . . . it was so painful, I decided I wasn't ever going to do that again.

Another nurse recalled her feelings of extreme anxiety and stress while caring for a young man who eventually survived. She described a high level of personal involvement which was personally exhausting and which constituted a threat to her 'professional self':

> . . . he was only 28 and I was determined that he wasn't going to die . . . I was so wound up. If he had died I would have probably just not wanted to come back to work again. I'd put so much of myself into making him better . . . it just drained me.

In their emphasis on the precarious nature of the separation between 'personal' and 'professional' selves, nurses are very much aware that the nature of nursing as a caring occupation is the root cause of such difficulties. In contrast to the lay perception of critical-care nurses as 'technical experts', critical-care nursing is perceived by nurses as demanding intimate interpersonal relationships with patients and their families. Although the opportunity to become emotionally involved is welcomed, nurses are conscious of the personal tensions that can emerge in such caring work. Nurses who are more experienced describe strategies of 'depersonalisation' which they employ to manage these tensions and protect their 'personal' selves. However, such strategies are only partially successful, and require high levels of energy. A nurse expressed it in these terms:

> I can still do it [caring] on a partially impersonal [level] . . . I hope they never get the impression of this, but because you're dealing with so many people all of the time you can't get totally involved all of the time . . . you put a bit of a mask on . . . you've got to say: 'This is a nurse doing her job'. I think that the reason you're successful is the family thinking that you are wonderful . . . [laughter] . . . that's the impression they get, when really it's . . . just acting a part, being a nice person who cares.

But nurses can find this emotionally tiring. A staff nurse explained:

> I feel quite exhausted after each shift . . . I try to use the time from leaving work to coming home and then back again to get rid of it. I try not to think about it too much. It makes me sound very automated, I suppose, but I have to cut off . . . it's very busy and people die. And they die young. It can all get too much sometimes.

In certain circumstances this strategy becomes untenable. These are situations in which a particular sense of identity develops between a nurse and a patient or a patient's family. Nurses describe how some patients evoke such strong feelings within them that they cannot 'let go' of these individuals. A common pattern is that care can be delivered over many weeks or months without undue distress being experienced, but then close contact with a particular patient or a particular family suddenly engenders powerful feelings of almost familial identification that are extremely hard to contain. This does not occur in a predictable way, and does not apply only to the 'tragic' deaths of previously fit, young, attractive people. Such experiences are not confined to nurses. A female doctor recalled:

> . . . sometimes you can remain relatively emotionless, surprisingly so, and at other times, completely out of the blue, you can be 'hit for six' by a certain patient . . . goodness knows what reasons, but you are. One of the things I find difficult is if there is somebody that you relate to . . . some people, they could almost be your friend . . . you understand where they're coming from, and if they try to explain their emotions to you and why it is that they're upset, and you internalise that, then you get upset as well . . . [it is] a deep emotional feeling, [but] it doesn't actually detract from the job. In some ways it's almost a relief that you still *do* feel every now and again.

Comfort for the dying person

Nursing staff report high levels of satisfaction from giving what they term 'basic nursing care' to their patients. Such care is referred to frequently, but in terms that appear to marginalise its role as compared with the overall management of patients. The expressions 'little things' or 'just basic care' are used in many instances when nurses describe their daily work:

> I care for one patient per shift . . . I provide all their care for them, just basic care, mouth care, pressure area care, washing . . . things like that.

> I get satisfied when . . . somebody says: 'Oh, they look really comfortable' or 'They look well looked after'. And it might have been that you've just shaved somebody that you've not managed to shave before . . . the little things we do like that matter.

The status of such care is heightened when a patient is known to be approaching death. In such instances, physical care and careful presentation of the body becomes a means of affirming the individuality of the dying person. Such bodily attention appears to be central to nurses' attempts to portray to families the social worth of dying people—even

'Physical care and careful presentation of the body becomes a means of affirming the individuality of the dying person.'

in the case of people whom nurses often never knew as conscious beings. It is also the means by which nurses themselves relate to their patients as individuals, and the way in which their relationships with families are sustained. The following comments of nurses all refer to their care of unconscious patients:

> I looked after him the previous week on nights and came back onto days and looked after him again. That was my choice. I wanted to do it because I felt like he knew me, because now and again he would open his eyes. I just wanted to be there for him, I wanted him to know I was there.

> You don't know the patients at all. You don't know what sort of person you have on the unit, what sort of people they are, what they've done in their life or anything like that . . . it's just looking after their body until they die and looking after their relatives. It's only by talking to their relatives that you piece together a picture of what this person might be like . . . you have to go on photographs and then you can see what the person might be like.

> . . . sometimes [relatives] watch you do things and that's enough, that you're doing something whether it's to help [the patient] get better or to help them die. Just that, in a way, is enough.

Nurses try to discover details of patients' lives, family relationships, personalities, and usual appearances. This strengthens the sense of 'person' within the body of each dying individual, and it creates a bond with their families, because the families are the providers of such information. Bodily attention given in this way is an expression of respect for personhood and a means of portraying 'doing' in a situation where hope of recovery has gone. In some circumstances, however, such bodily care becomes problematic for nurses. This is especially the case in those situations in which death is sudden and traumatic, or when the process of dying is prolonged.

Disclosure of information to patients' families

A major issue for all staff in critical care is that of achieving a balance between the delivery of nursing care to their patients and the preparation of their families for the possibility of the person's death. One nurse reflected:

> You had to watch what you said to her because she sort of clung to every piece of hope and she wanted to know exactly everything, which was fine, but it took up a lot of your time. You had to be with her and not with [the patient] . . . you had to go into every tiny thing and if one nurse said a

slightly different thing she would ask you to make sure, [but] then she couldn't take it in because she was really upset . . . she had so much faith that he was going to pull through . . . you couldn't *not* encourage her faith, because without that she would have had nothing, so you couldn't be too pessimistic and you couldn't be too optimistic. But he was very ill.

As this illustrates, nurses are very much aware of tensions in their relationship with families and struggle to ensure that they achieve a balance between the delivery of patient care and the disclosure of information. The informal way in which nurses give information sometimes creates difficulties in achieving consistency with the disclosures of other team members. Although it is accepted that the nurse's role in disclosing information is to prepare families for the likelihood of the person's death, nurses feel anxious about the extent and form that such disclosure should take. Of particular concern among nurses is the possibility of encroachment on the 'formal' disclosure of bad news or of critical decisions concerning treatment withdrawal. These are seen to be the province of medical staff. One nurse observed:

> 'Nurses struggle to ensure that they achieve a balance between the delivery of patient care and the disclosure of information.'

I'll always remember my first death on critical care, I think more so than on the general wards, I hadn't been on the unit long and they'd decided to withdraw treatment on a chap . . . the doctors decided this but felt that they couldn't speak to his wife who was sitting out in the waiting room on her own. They thought they had to wait for her family to come in. But she knew what was going on. She knew that he had deteriorated and that we would be discussing it. It was inevitable. I remember going out to see her and I was just going to say: 'He's not doing well and the doctors will probably have a talk with you later on'—knowing at the back of my mind that they were going to see her when the son came in, and that they were going to withdraw treatment. But when she came in beside the bed . . . and she was asking questions, I couldn't lie . . . I didn't know where to stop or how far to go.

Sometimes, in circumstances in which no 'formal' decision has been agreed regarding the continuation of treatment, nurses find themselves having to forestall the enquiries of patient's families. This can lead to extreme feelings of discomfort and can create a barrier between the nurse and the patient's family at a time when the families are very vulnerable.

Doctors assume a more formal relationship with patients' families and have a more clearly delineated view of their responsibilities regarding the disclosure of information and their role in patient care. Their concerns are to consolidate in a clear way the preparatory 'groundwork' that nurses have undertaken with families. Doctors want to ensure that they have been seen to do all that was possible with regard to treatment. These concerns are associated with a belief that responsibility for critical treatment decisions should not be assumed by families. A consultant doctor commented:

> We did what we could and there was nothing more that could be done. You can only do your best . . . it was pushing our knowledge and expertise forward and that's what we are here for . . . you can only reassure [families] that what you are doing is right, that you are doing everything that you possibly can . . . I'm very keen for relatives to be informed of decisions but . . . not to actually put the burden on them of making the decision . . . it's *not* their decision. There must be a lightening of that load. [They should be told] we've done our best and do you agree with what's happening?

These extracts reveal clearly the division of labour that exists between doctors and nursing staff in critical care with regard to the care of dying patients and the support of families. The roles that each assume during the process of patient care are interdependent, but enacted according to clearly defined boundaries.

Protecting the team

Medical and nursing staff alike emphasise the importance of teamwork in their management of dying people. The 'team' offers informal staff support as well as a means of 'getting through the work' of caring for dying people. It is seen as a means of defusing some of the more extreme pressures associated with such care. As a staff nurse observed:

> I think that it's teamwork that we have here . . . a good rapport with everybody and we're all able to help one another. We have dinner time when we laugh about stupid things . . . you can laugh about things even though they're not laughable, even though they're deadly serious. You have to laugh at them because otherwise you'd just go silly. You'd go mad.

In critical care, nurses and doctors work closely together in the delivery of care to seriously ill and dying people. Some nurses ascribe a more 'respectful' attitude to nurses among critical-care doctors as being the basis for teamwork in critical care. Doctors also tend to emphasise their cooperation and consultation with nurses in this setting.

However, there is some doubt regarding the extent to which nurses are actually able to influence the management of particular patients, and the organisation of medical work (both within critical care and within the wider hospital) operates to reinforce doctor-to-doctor collegial consultation, rather than multidisciplinary teamwork. From the nurses' perspective, this style of working adds an element of unpredictability in patient management, and ensures that many aspects of the care of dying patients are outside the influence of nursing staff.

Nurses frequently voice concerns about the extent to which they can participate in, or question, 'medical' decisions about patients. Their anxieties seem to centre upon their rather ambiguous relationship with doctors. Much of the medical work involved in caring for patients in critical care is shared between nurses and doctors—for example, in nurses' assuming a great deal of responsibility for the assessment of blood results, and for the adjustment of analgesia and sedation given to patients. One nurse described how she spent part of her time 'prompting doctors without telling them', and how she was aware that many medical decisions concerning patients were based on observations reported by nurses.

'Many aspects of the care of dying patients are outside the influence of nursing staff.'

Nurses are expected to play an important role in ward rounds—a central feature of critical-care work. However, nurses report a lack of confidence in questioning doctors. It is commonly felt that doctors are in a position to 'veto' the opinion of nurses by setting the agenda for acceptable, 'sensible' knowledge. Two nurses described this in the following terms:

> If you think one thing and the doctors think another . . . although they'll listen to you, they'll then tear what you've got to say to shreds if they don't agree with it . . . it can be quite frustrating.

> I do find it difficult when they're pulling all the stops out on somebody and then, within half an hour, they will say: 'Let's just stop everything'. I find it difficult to take in sometimes . . . I think its up to me to stand up and get a bit more confidence and ask questions. [But] . . . I don't want to appear stupid. I don't want to be seen as being silly.

Experienced nurses report a greater role in treatment decisions, but are still aware that the extent to which they can influence decision-making is determined by the willingness of each particular doctor to allow nursing participation, and by the personality of the nurse. A nurse observed:

> ... the nurses ... would welcome a bit more notice of what they feel. [But] really, to be honest, I think it depends very much on which particular consultant it is and I think it also depends on how assertive the nurse is, what sort of personality she has, and how she makes her general feelings known.

Nurses are aware that much medical decision-making takes place 'behind the scenes' and effectively excludes the influence of other disciplines. Nurses also feel constrained by a need to remain at the bedside of the patient. This means that they cannot fully participate in negotiations taking place elsewhere that affect medical decision-making. Doctors acknowledge that their relationships with other doctors determine, in large part, the outcome of deliberations about the treatment of patients. As a consultant doctor observed:

> Basically the decision ... with most people is that the critical-care doctors come to an opinion ... once we come to that opinion, and before we talk to the relatives, we ask the nurses and they usually unanimously agree ... and then, depending on which admitting team it is, we inform them or discuss it with them. It very much depends on the admitting surgeon [and whether] we have a good rapport with him ...

Conclusion

This chapter has highlighted some of the special difficulties that critical-care staff face when caring for dying patients and their families. The delicate balance between personal and professional selves is of critical importance in coping with work that demands high levels of intimacy in a series of relatively short-term, intense exchanges. Staff members learn to manage the demands of caring for dying people through exposure to profoundly disturbing and painful experiences of dying and death that can be likened to formative 'rites of passage'. The nature of 'teamwork' in critical care has been briefly explored, with reference to the varying influence of medical and nursing staff on aspects of the management of dying patients.

Care for the caregivers must be afforded a high priority (Puntillo 2001). In critical care, there are few opportunities to reflect on the experiences of caring for dying people, and often the dying process is telescoped into a few days and hours. These are critical moments in which staff risk emotional exhaustion as they strive to provide good care to their patients while putting their own fears and feelings 'on hold'. It is possible to create time and space for reflection and case discussion, but this requires a commitment from management and from all team members. Such discussion should involve doctors and nurses—perhaps by way of a regular 'separation review', in which the circumstances of the illness, care, and death of a patient can be discussed (McNamara 2001, p. 112).

Structured opportunities such as these can provide a valuable opportunity for doctors and nurses to share their 'narratives of care' (Hall 2002) and develop a shared understanding of the goals and constraints that fashion their work and influence their perspectives (Johnson et al. 2000).

'Care for the caregivers must be afforded a high priority. In critical care, there are few opportunities to reflect on the experiences of caring for dying people.'

Critical-care nurses should, together, explore how their patients' dignity can be maximised (Block 2001). This can refocus attention on the 'little things' that are so important to nurses, patients, and families, but which are devalued by the manner in which they are described by nurses themselves. Developing models of bereavement care and family support by drawing on the expertise of colleagues in specialties such as palliative care and psychiatry can enable nurses to 'broaden their definitions of success to include both rescue and an appropriate, dignified death' (Block 2001, p. 187). In turn, this can lead to a change in culture, such that critical care is better suited to give care to those who die and those who are bereaved within its confines.

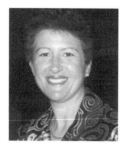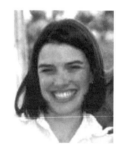

Leanne Monterosso

Dr Leanne Monterosso holds a joint appointment with Edith Cowan University (Perth, Western Australia) as a paediatric postdoctoral research fellow in cancer and palliative care, and with Princess Margaret Hospital for Children, Perth, where she is a senior health researcher. Before taking up this appointment, Leanne worked for many years in neonatal intensive care. The current focus of Leanne's work is in paediatric oncology and palliative-care nursing research. Leanne is committed to building collaborative and multidisciplinary research teams, and is currently involved in a number of clinically focused paediatric cancer and palliative-care studies. She is a board member of the Children's Hospice Association in Western Australia.

Sharon De Graves

Sharon De Graves is a registered nurse on the haematology and oncology unit at the Royal Children's Hospital, Melbourne (Victoria, Australia). For several years she has been caring for children with cancer, and their families, and has a particular interest in the families' experience of childhood cancer and end-of-life issues. Sharon's master's degree in nursing explored the issues faced by health professionals when caring for children with cancer during the shift from cure to palliation. This study has since been expanded and converted to a PhD thesis, and Sharon is currently involved in research exploring the experiences and decision-making processes of families when a child with cancer relapses.

Chapter 24

Paediatric Palliative Care

Leanne Monterosso and Sharon De Graves

Introduction

Paediatric palliative care can be an emotive clinical issue. Although some issues in palliative care are similar in adults and children, there are several striking differences. These differences pose distinctive challenges to nurses who care for children with life-threatening conditions and their families.

This chapter provides an overview of the issues involved in paediatric palliative care, and the strategies that can be used in a comprehensive approach to care.

Features of paediatric palliative care
Life-threatening illnesses in children

Paediatric care has traditionally been limited to investigation, diagnosis, treatment, and cure. In recent decades, advances in medical science and technology have been rapid and have contributed to improved survival rates for children with life-threatening illnesses. However, despite improved survival rates, there can be no assurance of cure. Rather, the imminence of death has been replaced by uncertain survival. The Box below provides a list of the major types of life-threatening illnesses from which children can suffer.

Perceived barriers to paediatric palliative care

The growth of palliative care for adults has not been parallelled in paediatrics. There is an increasing awareness of the need for comprehensive care for dying children and their families. However, there is a lack of evidence-based research to guide paediatric palliative care.

> 'The growth of palliative care for adults has not been parallelled in paediatrics.'

Despite changes in thinking about what palliative care means, and to whom palliative care should be directed, outdated perceptions of palliative care—as 'failed' attempts at cure—remain prominent in the minds of many people in health care and in the general public (Frager 1996). This belief is even more prominent in the paediatric setting in which the assumed goal of medical treatment is to achieve a cure.

Perceived barriers to provision of paediatric care can be divided into those that relate mainly to parents and those that relate mainly to caregivers.

In relation to parents, the following barriers are perceived.

▶ Parents might be unwilling or unable to make a formal transition to a state of care that is labelled 'palliative' (Stevens, Jones & O'Riordan 1996).

▶ Parents can find themselves forced to make a difficult choice when interventions directed to cure and those directed to comfort are presented as being mutually exclusive (Frager 1996).

Life-threatening illnesses from which children can suffer

The major types of life-threatening illnesses from which children can suffer include:

• *conditions such as cancer*—for which curative treatment is available, but can fail;

• *conditions such as cystic fibrosis or HIV-1 infection*—for which prolonged and intensive therapy can provide a good quality of life, but might not prevent premature death;

• *progressive conditions such as mucopolysaccharidoses*—for which treatment is exclusively palliative from the time of diagnosis and might extend over many years; and

• *severe disabilities such as congenital anomalies or neurological disabilities (such as cerebral palsy)*—which are neither progressive nor immediately life-threatening, but which can lead to complications with a risk of premature death.

Adapted from Liben & Goldman (1998)

▶ Parents prefer the child's practitioner to be a person who knows their child and his or her history, and prefer this person to provide care throughout their child's life including the terminal phase (Kane & Primomo 2001). In relation to caregivers, the following barriers are perceived.

▶ There can be a lack of knowledge among caregivers of children of the potentially fatal diseases of childhood (Colleau 2001).

▶ Carers might be unfamiliar with pain and symptom management and might be uncomfortable in addressing personal and professional psychological stress (Colleau 2001; Liben 1996).

▶ The uncertainty inherent in most life-threatening childhood illnesses makes prognostication difficult and complicates end-of-life decision-making (Frager 1996; Levetown 1996; Sahler et al. 2000).

▶ Children who do receive palliative care in the community are sometimes cared for by community-based health professionals who have training and experience in palliative care in general, but little in the way of specific paediatric experience.

Palliative care needs of children and their families

The death of a child is one of the most traumatic events that families can be called upon to endure, and a child's progressive, life-threatening illness has a profound effect on all dimensions of family life. Families are affected physically, psychologically, and financially, and the family structure is permanently altered. Although there is a considerable body of qualitative research into the needs of families caring for a child with a life-threatening condition, the palliative-care needs of children and their families have been less well recognised. The needs of dying children and their families differ somewhat from those of adults and require special consideration, as indicated in the Box on page 344.

'The needs of dying children and their families differ from those of adults and require special consideration.'

The aims of palliative-care interventions are to optimise the quality of life of the dying child, and to enable families to care for the child, individual family members, and for the family unit as a whole. Family interventions seek to sustain and improve family cohesion, communication, and family support.

Communicating with children about death and dying

Communicating with children is an essential and challenging aspect of paediatric care. When a child is diagnosed with a life-threatening illness, good

Needs of dying children and their families

The needs of dying children and their families differ somewhat from those of adults. These include the following.

- Traditional hospital care is not necessarily the most appropriate model for the provision of palliative care for children, and most families of children with life-threatening diseases choose home care if given the opportunity (Vickers & Carlisle 2000).
- The age of the child affects the child's understanding of illness and death, his or her ability to communicate and participate in decision-making, and the response to pain.
- Children are physiologically and pharmacodynamically different from adults.
- Paediatricians often develop longstanding relationships with children and their families and are less likely to hand over care (Wolfe et al. 2000).
- Grief is often more prolonged following the loss of a child (Rando 1983).

communication becomes even more important. When the focus of treatment shifts from cure to palliation, nurses are faced with additional challenges. Questions from children can be confronting: 'Am I dying?'; 'Is there a heaven?'; 'What happens when you die?'. Such questions must be answered with care and consideration of the child's developmental understanding and individual circumstances, including his or her past experiences, religion, and culture. It is equally important to prepare families for such questions. Parents will often ask questions such as: 'How do we know when to tell her that she is dying?', 'What do we tell her?', or 'What do we tell our other children?'. Children cannot be protected from death. Limiting communication about death and dying hinders their understanding and ability to cope, and can lead children to develop inaccurate and inappropriate beliefs and ideas (Faulkner 1997; Schonfeld 1993).

An understanding of the concepts that children can understand at different developmental stages can be helpful when confronted with questions such as these. However, it is important to recognise that each child's development is influenced by individual circumstances and life experiences. It is significant that most children with a life-threatening illness have a greater understanding of death than do other children their age, and are usually more aware of their condition than their parents and carers expect (Faulkner 1997).

Some useful guidelines for communicating with children about death and dying can be found in the Box on page 345.

Guidelines for communicating with children about death and dying

The following practical guidelines can be useful when communicating with children about death and dying.
- Be flexible.
- Recognise that children communicate best through non-verbal means such as artwork, music, and play.
- Respect the need for children to be alone, as well as their desire to share. Be there to provide support, but do not force communication.
- Be receptive when children initiate a conversation. They often take great care in choosing the person to whom they will direct questions.
- Be specific and literal in explanations.
- Remember that euphemisms about death, such as 'going to sleep', can be confusing for children.
- Acknowledge that a child's life can be complete, even if it is brief, and that he or she will always be loved and remembered.
- Empower each child as much as possible regarding the circumstances of his or her own death. Involve the child in decision-making whenever possible, including where the child wishes to die, and (perhaps) planning the funeral.

Adapted from Faulkner (1997)

Paediatric symptom management
General comments

The key to palliation for any age group lies in the delivery of appropriate and effective symptom management. Although there is little variation between the symptoms that children and adults experience towards the end of life, the clinical focus of caring for children with life-threatening conditions has been on cure. However, the research and clinical focus has now shifted somewhat to include symptom management, and this has led to more sensitive standards of care.

Despite this change in focus, the symptom of fatigue has yet to receive the same degree of attention. The subjective nature of fatigue makes fatigue one of the most difficult paediatric symptoms to manage. Developmental differences between age groups can mean that young children are sometimes unaware of changes in their physical stamina and the activities of daily living, and older children might simply accept their lack of energy as being a natural consequence of being ill.

'Young children are sometimes unaware of changes in their physical stamina and the activities of daily living.'

Pain, fatigue, and dyspnoea have been identified by parents as the most common symptoms experienced by children with cancer in their last month of life (Wolfe et al. 2000). Other symptoms that can cause distress include dyspnoea, nausea and vomiting, excess secretions, agitation, dysphagia, psychological distress, anorexia, seizures, and skin changes (Hunt 1990).

Delivery of developmentally appropriate symptom management is essential, as is effective communication and shared goals among members of the care team. It is important to regard the child and family as a unit that is involved in planning the goals of care and making decisions regarding the management of symptoms.

The Box below lists some important factors to be considered in symptom management in children.

As noted above, the age and development of a child is very important in symptom assessment. Table 24.1 (page 347) provides developmental guidelines for symptom assessment and management in children of various ages.

Pain management

Pain is a multifaceted, individual experience which is influenced not only by the

---

Important factors in symptom management in children

- Assessment and management should consider the child's physical, cognitive, and emotional status.
- Signs and symptoms tend to develop more quickly in children and can be more difficult to localise.
- Children absorb, distribute, metabolise, and eliminate drugs differently from adults.
- The doses of most drugs are based on a milligram per kilogram calculation.
- Painful injections should be avoided. Oral drugs should be used whenever possible.
- It is important to distinguish between symptoms that are distressing the parents and carers and those that are distressing the child. Management should be focused on the needs of the child.
- Unconventional assessment techniques (such as play, drawing, and story-telling) and observation of behavioural changes are very important in symptom management.
- The role of the family should be acknowledged by treating family members as part of the team caring for the child, and by including the child and the family in decision-making.
- There is a lack of formal assessment tools for most symptoms except pain.

Adapted from Goldman (1998); McQuillan & Finlay (1996); Sahler et al. (2000); Whaley & Wong (1997)

Table 24.1 Developmental guidelines for assessment of symptoms in children

Age	Guidelines
0–2 years	Taking a comprehensive history from caregiver is essential.
	The needs of an infant are often communicated through non-verbal behaviour and vocalisations that might require interpretation from family.
	Crying can be a way of communicating unpleasant stimuli (hunger, pain, loneliness). Parents can often help in interpreting an infant's cry.
	Separation anxiety can occur when an infant is taken from his or her parents' arms or put in a position where the infant can no longer see a familiar face. Assessment of an infant should, as much as possible, be performed without disturbance. Observation is an essential skill in assessing children of all ages, but is especially so with infants.
	Be calm, talk quietly, and use firm, gentle handling.
	Be aware that an infant who is quiet might be too unwell and lethargic to exhibit any behaviour.
	Pain or discomfort might be manifested as a generalised body response (thrashing or rigidity with or without 'expected' facial expressions).
	There is no association between approaching stimulus and discomfort.
	Physical assessment is important in the assessment and management of symptoms at all ages (for example, increased blood pressure might be associated with pain).
2–7 years	Do not use euphemisms or analogies to explain what is happening during the examination. Children this age are very literal and require concrete, direct communication. (For example, a five-year-old child might misinterpret 'the dog has been put to sleep' as meaning that the dog has been put in its kennel to rest).
	Use words that are developmentally appropriate and familiar to the child. Allow the child to touch, feel, and play with articles used in any assessment.
	Be aware of non-verbal communication, especially in play and drawing.
	Pain or discomfort might be manifested as loud crying, screaming, verbal expressions ('ouch'; 'it hurts'), thrashing, pushing away painful stimuli, lack of cooperation, or clinginess.

(Continued)

Table 24.1 Developmental guidelines for assessment of symptoms in children (*Continued*)

2–7 years	A child of this age might have difficulty in describing the character of pain or its exact location. Using a doll or drawing can help in locating the site of pain. A child this age might be comforted by emotional support from a parent or other significant person.
7–11 years	It is important to provide clear explanations and reasons for any intervention. Create an atmosphere that is encouraging and permissive of questioning and participation. Communicate on an individual level with the child (ask how he or she is feeling; ask if he or she has any pain, feels sick, and so on). Utilise play to assist in assessments and aid communication. Ask a child to say how a doll is feeling and to point to where the doll hurts. Pain or discomfort is displayed in similar ways as younger children. A child of this age might use stalling tactics before a painful procedure.
11 years and over	Behaviour can regress to a younger level when in distress. Be willing to use a variety of approaches during communication and assessment, and be prepared for a variety of responses (cooperation, hostility, anger, bravado, and so on). Be genuine and respectful of an adolescent's thoughts and beliefs. Listen actively. Pain will be described with more precise verbal expressions. Increased muscle tension and body control may also be seen. However note that a child of this age might 'conceal' pain by less vocal protest and less motor activity.

Adapted from Whaley & Wong (1997)

degree of physical damage, but also by developmental age and understandings, past experiences, and cultural and social factors. The management of pain in children has, in the past, been handicapped by certain misconceptions that some people have about children and pain. Such misconceptions can lead to suboptimal symptom management and unnecessary suffering for children (McGrath 1996; Sahler et al. 2000). Some of these misconceptions include the following:

▶ that infants and children do not feel pain or feel less pain than adults do;

▶ that children cannot tell where they are experiencing pain;
▶ that children respond honestly when questioned about their level of pain;
▶ that behavioural expressions of pain reflect pain intensity; and
▶ that opioids are addictive and have more side-effects in children.
  These misconceptions are discussed below.

That infants and children feel less pain than adults do

Infants and children of all ages can experience pain. Failure to relieve pain results in needless suffering and might cause adverse physiological problems.

That children cannot tell where they are experiencing pain

Children can describe their pain and asking children about their pain should be a central part any assessment. However, it is important to use words that are appropriate to the child's stage of development (such as 'hurt' or 'sore'). Assessment tools are also useful. Combining verbal assessment with physical assessment and observation is essential, especially with preverbal children.

That children respond honestly when questioned about pain

Children respond differently when asked about their pain—depending on who is asking the questions. In addition, they might deny having pain because they know that an injection or unpleasant medicine is likely to follow any admission of their having pain.

'Children respond differently when asked about their pain— depending on who is asking the questions.'

That behavioural expressions of pain reflect pain intensity

Behavioural responses are influenced by developmental age, past experiences, and coping strategies, and might therefore fail to reflect the intensity of pain. Children might or might not cry when in pain. Some withdraw and stiffen their bodies, whereas others thrash about wildly. It is important to observe behaviour and ask parents how their child normally responds to pain.

That opioids are addictive and have more side-effects in children

Children are not more easily addicted to narcotics (Goldman 1998). However, as with adults, physiological tolerance can develop, necessitating increased opioid dosages (McGrath 1996). Parents should be reassured that a decision to start treatment with morphine does not mean that there is nothing more that can be done if their child's pain increases. It should be explained that doses can be safely increased if required. Concerns about side-effects, especially respiratory depression, should be allayed by the knowledge that there is a significant difference between dosages required for pain relief and dosages that might cause respiratory depression. Moreover, pain decreases the chances of respiratory depression occurring with morphine administration (Goldman 1996).

Accurate assessment of a child's pain relies on four key components:

▶ obtaining an accurate history including details of the nature, severity, time, and influencing factors;

▶ identifying the location of pain and its severity using developmentally appropriate, standardised assessment tools (such as facial pain scales for ages 3–7, and visual analogue scales for 7 years and older) (Sahler et al. 2000); the use of dolls to point at, and draw on, or getting the child to 'colour in' a drawing of a body with different colours indicating the severity of pain can assist in determining the site and intensity of a child's pain;

▶ conducting a physical assessment; and

▶ observation of behaviour (especially in preverbal children).

The World Health Organization has developed guidelines for the management of cancer pain in children. The guidelines encourage the administration of 'appropriate analgesics in effective doses at regular intervals by the least painful route; regularly incorporating non-drug therapies into all treatment protocols; managing opioid-related side-effects; and using adjuvant drugs' (McGrath 1996, p. 88). The three-step analgesic ladder provided with the guidelines provides a useful framework for the pharmacological management of pain (McGrath 1996). However, non-pharmacological approaches to pain management should not be overlooked. Techniques such as explanation, reassurance, distraction, relaxation, music therapy, and visual imagery can work well, either on their own or as an adjunct to medication, and can provide a child with a sense of control and mastery (Goldman 1996; Sahler et al. 2000).

Loss, grief, and bereavement
The effect on the family

The death of a child can be especially difficult to cope with. Most industrialised societies have a 'death-defying' culture in which the death of a child is a 'foreign', socially unacceptable event. In the past, when childhood death was part of neighbourhood life, communities would pull together, providing support and acknowledging the death of loved ones. Improved living conditions and the breakdown of extended family have led to a society that is unfamiliar with death

(Dominica 1998). Advances in modern medicine and public health have meant that the death of a child is relatively rare, and that nurses are less prepared when they encounter a child who is dying. The 'natural' reaction is to fight for a child's life, and it can seem 'unnatural' for that child to die.

Parents of children who die can feel *cheated* (of the life no longer possible for their child), *punished* (for failing to be 'good-enough' parents), and *isolated* (in a society unprepared for a child's death). Parents and grandparents can feel guilty to have survived their offspring, and require support in their grief reactions. Good palliative care assists parents, siblings, and grandparents to prepare for the loss of a child, and extends into bereavement support after the child's death.

The grief associated with the death of a child is painful and enduring, and is associated with a higher risk of pathological grief reactions (Black 1998; Goldman 1998). Parents can experience multiple losses when facing the death of their child. In addition to the physical loss of the child, they also lose their dreams and hopes for the child, and their role as parents (Goldman 1998). Furthermore, grief can be prolonged with each milestone the child would have experienced, and each milestone can renew feelings of loss and sadness.

> 'Parents of children who die can feel cheated . . . punished . . . and isolated.'

However to grieve is normal, and most families will benefit from the knowledge and reassurance that their thoughts and feelings are not abnormal Goldman (1998).

Grief is an individual experience and progression through the phases of grief is never uniform (Black 1998). Many parents feel that they never recover from the loss of a child. These parents find that, although they can move on with life, they remain vulnerable and are no longer the same person. Such a profound experience has the potential to affect all areas of family life, including marital relationships, the parenting of other children, and the reactions of siblings. All of these issues should be considered when providing bereavement care.

The effect on the siblings

The needs of siblings are often overlooked. Siblings are often poorly prepared for death and can find it difficult to accept death if they were prohibited from visits or being involved in care (Black 1998). Siblings might not feel that they can talk to their parents about how they are feeling for fear that they will increase their parents' distress, or they might think that their parents do not have any time for them because the sick child is taking all of their energy and time. These factors can lead to a sibling feeling rejected and isolated (TG 2001).

The Box below presents some useful thoughts to help siblings cope with the death of their brother or sister.

The effect on children

The way in which a child responds to the prospect of his or her own death, or to the death of a loved one, is influenced by the child's developmental under-standing and conceptualisation of death. For example, a young child might create fantasies about a sibling's death and might believe that he or she caused it to happen.

Involving children in end-of-life care can give them a sense of control and provide opportunities for them to discuss their fears and anxieties surrounding death. Some children want to talk about their death and might even benefit from planning their funerals and writing their wills, whereas others apparently ignore impending death, perhaps trying to protect their parents from the pain. It is important to encourage families to take their child's lead, supporting them through their journey while providing simple, factual, and age-appropriate information when asked. Kindergartens and schools also play an important supportive role for both the child who is dying, and for his or her fellow students. To facilitate this supportive role it is essential that health carers liaise with a child's teacher and participate in classroom activities if appropriate (for example, through role-playing). Ways in which kindergartens and schools can provide

---

Helping siblings

The following points adapted from *Therapeutic Guidelines: Palliative Care* (2001) can help guide the care of siblings leading up to, and following, the death of a brother or sister.

- Involve siblings in the care of the child.
- Encourage siblings to visit their brother or sister in hospital and maintain normal relationships.
- Provide siblings with accurate and simple explanations of what is happening.
- Encourage parents to allocate time to spend with their sick child's sibling.
- Reassure siblings that they have not caused their brother or sister's illness or death and, where appropriate, reassure them that they cannot catch the disease.
- Liaise with the sibling's school and provide access to age-appropriate support groups.
- Help siblings to create memories of their brother or sister—for example a memory book with photographs, stories, and drawings.

Adapted from TG (2001)

support include providing continuing education to fellow students about the dying child's progress, encouraging a philosophy of normality for the dying child and fellow students, providing a stable support network, and encouraging socialisation among peers.

Conclusion

The provision of palliative and supportive care for children with life-threatening conditions, and for their families, is complex and challenging. Although the traditional adult-focused principles of palliative care can be applied to children with life-threatening illnesses, the needs of dying children and their families are distinctive and require special consideration.

The aims of palliative care should be to optimise the quality of life of the child and the quality of family functioning. Good care should assist families to care for the ill child, for individual family members, and for the family unit itself.

The developmental stage of the child must be considered when planning or delivering palliative care for children. Each child's understanding of illness, pain, and death must be considered. Children suffering from a

'The needs of dying children and their families are distinctive and require special consideration.'

life-threatening illness, and their families, need a supportive presence that is active, easily accessible, responsive, flexible, and collaborative—but discreet and sensitive to individual needs. The needs of siblings, grandparents, and extended family should be considered when providing care and support.

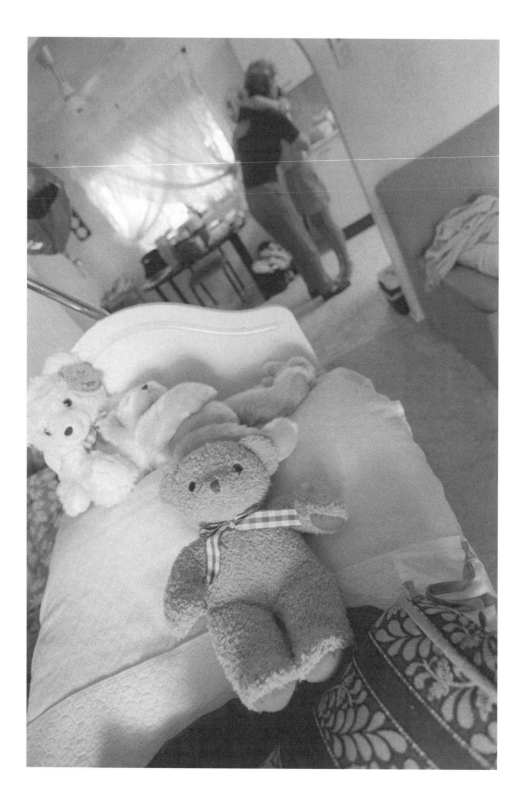

References

Foreword
World Health Organization (WHO) 2002, *National Cancer Control Programmes: policies and managerial guidelines*, 2nd edn, Geneva.

Preface
Palliative Care Australia (PCA) 1999, *Standards for Palliative Care Provision*, 3rd edn, PCA, Australian Capital Territory.

Chapter 1 Framing Palliative Care
Finlay, I.G. & Jones, J.V.H. 1995, 'Definitions in Palliative Care', *British Medical Journal*, 311, p. 754.

Chapter 2 Evidence-Based Practice in Palliative Care
Cochrane, A. 1979, '1931–1971: a critical review with particular reference to the medical profession', in *Medicine for the Year 2000*, Office of Health Economics, London.

Commonwealth Department of Health, Housing and Community Services (DHHCS) 1992, Review of Professional Indemnity Arrangements for Health Care Professionals, *Compensation and Professional Indemnity in Health Care—a discussion paper*, AGPS, Canberra.

DHHCS, *see* Commonwealth Department of Health, Housing and Community Services.

Fitch, M., Bolster, A., Alderson, D., Kennedy, G. & Woermke, D.H. 1995, 'Moving towards research-based cancer nursing practice', *Canadian Oncology Nursing Journal*, 5(1): 5–8.

Gerson, L.B. & Triadafilopoulos, G. 2000, 'Palliative care in inflammatory bowel disease: an evidence based approach', *Inflammatory Bowel Disease*, 6(3): 228–43.

Grande, G.E., Todd, C.J., Barclay, S.I.G. & Farquhar, M.C. 1999, 'Does hospital at home for palliative care facilitate death at home? Randomised controlled trial', *British Medical Journal*, 319: 1472–5.

Green, J. & Britten, N. 1998, 'Qualitative research and evidence based medicine', *British Medical Journal*, 316: 1230–2.

Higginson, I.J. 1999, 'Evidence based palliative care', *British Medical Journal*, 319: 462–3.

Keeley, D. 1999, 'Rigorous assessment of palliative care revisited', *British Medical Journal*, 319: 7223, 1447–8.

Lemmer, B., Grellier, R. & Steven, J. 1999, 'Systematic review of nonrandom and qualitative research literature: exploring and uncovering an evidence base for health visiting and decision making', *Qualitative Health Research*, 9: 315–28.

Pearson, A. 1998, 'Excellence in care: Future dimensions for effective nursing', *Nursing Times Research*, 3: 1, 25–7.

Popay, J. & Williams, G. 1998, 'Qualitative Research and Evidence Based Health Care', *Journal of the Royal Society of Medicine*, 91 (Suppl. 35): 32–7.

Qualitative Methods Network 1999, Report on Rome Workshop, November, <www.salford.ac.uk/jhr/cochrane/homepage.htm>; and Draft Methods Group Module.

Sackett, D.L. & Rosenberg, W.M.C. 1995, 'On the need for evidence-based medicine', *Health Economics*, 4: 249–54.

Sackett, D.L., Rosenberg, W.M.C., Gray, J.A.M., Haynes, R.B. & Richardson, W.S. 1996, 'Evidence-based medicine: what it is and what it is not', *British Medical Journal*, 312: 71–2.

Sandelowski, M., Docherty, S. & Emden, C. 1997, 'Qualitative metasynthesis: Issues and techniques', *Research in Nursing and Health*, 20: 365–71.

Chapter 3 Communication Skills in Palliative Care

Breitbart, W. & Passik, S.D. 1997, 'Psychiatric aspects of palliative care,', in Doyle, D., Hanks, G.W. & Macdonald, N. (eds), *Oxford Textbook of Palliative Medicine*, Oxford University Press, Oxford.

Breitbart, W., Rosenfeld, B., Pessin, H., Kaim, M., Funseti-Esch, J., Galietta, M., Nelson, C. & Brescia, R. 2000, 'Depression, hopelessness and desire for hastened death in terminally ill patients with cancer', *Journal of the American Medical Association*, 284, 2907–11.

Derogatis, L.R., Marrow., G.R., Fetting, J., Penman, D., Paitsetsky, S., Schmale, A.M., Henrichs, M. & Camicke, C.L.M. 1983, 'The prevalence of psychiatric disorders in cancer patients', *Journal of the American Medical Association*, 249, 751–7.

Devlen, J., Maguire, P., Phillips, P., Crowther, D. & Chambers, H. 1987, 'Psychological problems associated with diagnosis and treatment of lymphomas', *British Medical Journal*, 295, 953–7.

Egan, G. 1998, *The skilled helper: A problem-management approach to helping*, 6th edn, Brooks-Cole Publishers, Pacific Grove, USA.

Fallowfield, L., Hall, A., Maguire, G. & Baum, M. 1990, 'Psychological outcomes of different treatment policies in women with early breast cancer outside a clinical trial', *British Medical Journal*, 301, 575–80.

Fallowfield, L., Saul, J. & Gilligan, B. 2001, 'Teaching senior nurses how to teach communication skills in oncology', *Cancer Nursing*, 24, 185–91.

Faulkner, A. & Maguire, P. 1994, *Talking to Cancer Patients and Their Relatives*, Oxford University Press, Oxford.

Fielding, R. & Hung, J. 1996, 'Preferences for information and involvement in decisions during cancer care among a Hong Kong Chinese population', *Psycho-Oncology*, 5, 321–9.

Heaven, C. & Maguire, P. 1997, 'Disclosure of concerns by hospice patients and their identification by nurses,' *Palliative Medicine*, 11, 283–90. .

Heaven, C. & Maguire, P. 1998, 'The relationship between patients' concerns and psychological distress in a hospice setting', *Psycho-Oncology*, 7, 503–7.

Jeffrey, D. 1998, 'Communication skills in palliative care', in Faull, C., Carter, Y. & Woof, R. (eds), *Handbook of Palliative Care*, Blackwell Science Ltd, Oxford.

Jenkins, V. & Fallowfield, L. 2002, 'Can communication skills training alter physicians' beliefs and behaviour in clinics?', *Journal of Clinical Oncology*, 20, 765–9.

Lugton J. & Kindlen, M. 1999, *Palliative Care: the Nursing Role*, Churchill Livingstone, Edinburgh.

Macleod-Clark, J. 1982, 'Nurse/patient verbal interaction', unpublished PhD thesis, University of London, London.

Maguire, P. 1999, 'Improving Communication with Cancer Patients', *European Journal of Cancer*, 35, 14, 2058–65.

Maguire, P. Booth, K., Elliott, C. & Jones, B. 1996, 'Helping health professionals involved in cancer care acquire key interviewing skills—the impact of workshops', *European Journal of Cancer*, 32A, 1486–9.

Maguire, P., Faulkner, A., Booth, K., Elliott. C. & Hillier, V. 1996, 'Helping cancer patients disclose their concerns', *European Journal of Cancer*, 32A, 78–81.

McCorkle, R., Frank-Stromberg, M. & Pasacreta, J.V. 1998, 'Education of Nurses in Psycho-Oncology', in Holland, J.C. (ed.), *Psycho-Oncology*, pp 1069–73, Oxford University Press, New York.

Parle, M., Maguire, P. & Heaven, C. 1997, 'The development of a training model to improve health professionals' skills, self-efficacy and outcome expectancies when communicating with cancer patients', *Social Science and Medicine*, 44, 231–40.

Parle, M., Jones, B. & Maguire, P. 1996, 'Maladaptive Coping and Affective Disorders in Cancer Patients', *Psychological Medicine*, 26, 735–44.

Razavi. D. and Delvaux. N. 1997, 'Communication Skills and Psychological Training in Oncology', *European Journal of Cancer*, 33, S15–S21.

Razavi, D., Delvaux, N., Farvacques, C. & Robaye, E. 1990, 'Screening for adjustment disorders and major depressive disorder in cancer care', *British Journal of Psychiatry*, 156, 79–83.

Rothenbacher, D., Lutz, M.P. & Porsolt, F. 1997, 'Treatment decisions in palliative care: patients preferences for involvement and doctors' knowledge about it', *European Journal of Cancer*, 33, 1184–9.

Roter, D. & Fallowfield, L. 1998, 'Principles of Training Medical Staff in Psychosocial and Communication Skills', in Holland, J.C., *Psycho-Oncology* (eds), Oxford University Press, New York.

Speigel, D. 1994, *Living Beyond Limits: New Hope for People Facing Life-Threatening Illness*, Random House, New York.

Stewart, M.A. 1995, 'Effective physician–patient communication and health outcomes: A review', *Canadian Medical Association Journal*, 152, 1423–33.

Stewart, F., Walker, A. & Maguire, P. 1988, 'Psychiatric and social morbidity in women treated for cancer of the cervix', report to the Cancer Research Campaign.

Weisman, A, D. & Worden, J, W. 1997, 'The existential plight in cancer: Significance of the first 100 days', *International Journal of Psychological Medicine*, 7, 1–15.

Wilkinson, S. 1991, 'Factors which influence how nurses communicate with cancer patients', *Journal of Advanced Nursing*, 16, 677–88.

Wilkinson, S., Roberts, A. & Aldridge, J. 1998, 'Nurse patient communication in palliative care: an evaluation of a communication skills program', *Palliative Medicine*, 12, 13–22.

Chapter 4 Occupational Stress in Palliative Care

Amenta, M.M. 1984, 'Traits of hospice nurses compared with those who work in traditional settings', *Journal of Clinical Psychology*, 40: 414–19.

Barnard, D. 1995, 'The promise of intimacy and the fear of our own undoing', *Journal of Palliative Care*, 11(4): 22–6.

Barnard, D., Towers, A., Boston P., Lambrinidou, Y. 2000, *Crossing Over: Narratives of Palliative Care*, Oxford University Press, New York.

Bené, B, Foxall, M.J. 1991, 'Death anxiety and job stress in hospice and medical-surgical nurses', *Hospice Journal*, 7(3): 25–41.

Boston, P., Towers, A. & Barnard, D. 2001, 'Embracing vulnerability: risk and empathy in palliative care', *Journal of Palliative Care*, 17: 248–53.

Cho, C. & Cassidy, D.F. 1994, 'Parallel processes for workers and their clients in chronic bereavement resulting from HIV', *Death Studies*, 8: 273–92.

Copp, G. & Dunn, V. 1993, 'Frequent and difficult problems perceived by nurses caring for the dying in community, hospice and acute care settings', *Palliative Medicine*, 7: 19–25.

Coyle, N. 1997, 'Focus on the nurse: ethical dilemmas with highly symptomatic patients dying at home', *The Hospice Journal*, 12(2): 33–41.

Cumes, D. 1999, *The Spirit of Healing*, Llewellyn Publications, St Paul, USA.

Florio, G.A., Donnelly, J.P. & Zevon, M.A. 1998, 'The structure of work-related stress and coping among oncology nurses in high-stress medical settings: a transactional analysis', *Journal of Occupational Health Psychology*, 3: 227–42.

Graham, J., Ramirez, A.J., Cull, A., Gregory, W.M., Finlay, I., Hoy, A. & Richards, M.A. 1996, 'Job stress and satisfaction among palliative physicians: a CRC/CRF Study', *Palliative Medicine*,10: 185–94.

Guggenbühl-Craig, A. 1971, *Power in the Helping Professions*, Spring, Texas.

Hart, G., Yates, P., Clinton, M. & Windsor, C. 1998, 'Mediating conflict and control: practice challenges for nurses working in palliative care', *International Journal of Nursing Studies*, 35: 252–8.

Heim, E. 1991, 'Job stressors and coping in health professions', *Psychotherapy and Psychosomatics*, 55: 90–9.

Heming, D. 1988, 'The Titanic truimvirate: Teams, teamwork and teambuilding', *Canadian Journal of Occupational Therapy*, 55: (1): 15–20.

Kash, K.M., Holland, J.C., Breitbart, W., Brenson, S., Dougherty, J. & Ouellette-Kobasa, S. 2000, 'Stress and burnout in oncology', *Oncology*, 14: 1621–9.

Kearney, M. 1996, *Mortally Wounded*, Scribner, New York.

Kearney, M. 2000, *A Place of Healing: Working with Suffering in Living and Dying*, Oxford University Press, Oxford.

Kearney, M. & Mount, B. 2000, 'Spiritual care of the dying patient',in Chochinov, H.M. & Breitbart, W. (eds), *Handbook of Psychiatry in Palliative Care*, pp 357–73, Oxford University Press, New York.

Maslach, C. & Jackson, S. E. 1986, *Maslach Burnout Inventory Manual*, Consulting Psychologists Press, Palo Alto.

Nouwen, H. 1972, *The Wounded Healer*, Doubleday, Garden City, NJ, USA.

Papadatou, D. 2000, 'A proposed model of health professionals' grieving process', *Omega*, 41: 59–77.

Payne, N. 2001, 'Occupational stressors and coping as determinants of burnout in female hospice nurses', *Journal of Advanced Nursing*, 33: 396–405.

Pines, A.M. 2000, 'Treating career burnout: a psychodynamic existential perspective', *Psychotherapy in Practice*, 56: 633–42.

Remen, R.N. 1996, *Kitchen Table Wisdom*, Riverhead Books, New York.

Remen, R.N. 2000, *My Grandfather's Blessings*, Riverhead Books, New York.

Schneider, R. 1997, 'The effects on nurses of treatment-withdrawal decisions made in ICUs and SCBUs', *Nursing in Critical Care*, 2: 174–85.

Speck, P. 1996, 'Unconscious communications' (editorial), *Palliative Medicine*, 10: 273.

Sulmasy, D.P. 1997, *The Healer's Calling*, Paulist Press, New York.

Taylor, E.J., Highfield, M.F. & Amenta, M. 1999, 'Predictors of oncology and hospice nurses' spiritual care perspectives and practices', *Applied Nursing Research*, 12(1): 30–7.

Vachon, M.L.S. 1987, *Occupational Stress in the Care of the Critically Ill, the Dying and the Bereaved*, Hemisphere Press, New York.

Vachon, M.L.S. 1995, 'Staff stress in palliative/hospice care: a review', *Palliative Medicine*, 9: 91–122.

Vachon, M.L.S. 1996, 'What makes a team?', *Palliative Care Today*, 5(3): 34–5.

Vachon, M.L.S. 2001, 'The nurse's role: the world of palliative care nursing', in Ferrell, B. & Coyle, N. (eds), *The Oxford Textbook of Palliative Nursing*, pp 647–62, Oxford University Press, New York.

Vachon, M.L.S. 2002a, 'Staff stress and burnout', in Berger, A.M., Portenoy, R.K. & Weissman, D.E. (eds), *Principles and Practice of Palliative Care and Supportive Oncology*, , 2nd edn, Lippincott Williams & Wilkins, Philadelphia.

Vachon, M.L.S. 2002b, 'Stress of caregivers', in Doyle D. Hanks, G., Cherny, N. & Calman, K. (eds), *Oxford Textbook of Palliative Medicine*, 3rd edn, Oxford University Press, Oxford.

van Staa, A.L., Visser, A. & van der Zouwe, N. 2000, 'Caring for caregivers: experiences and evaluation of interventions for a palliative care team' *Patient Education and Counseling*, 41: 93–105.

Watson, J. 1989, 'Human caring and suffering: a subjective model for health sciences', in Taylor, R.L. & Watson, J. (eds), *They Shall Not Hurt: Human Suffering and Human Caring*, pp 125–35, Colorado Associated University Press, Boulder.

Chapter 5 Ethical Decision-making

AMA, *see* Council on Ethical and Judicial Affairs, American Medical Association.

Council on Ethical and Judicial Affairs, American Medical Association 1992, 'Decisions Near the End of Life', *Journal of the American Medical Association*, 267 (16), 2229–33.

Cassell, Eric, J. 1991, *The Nature of Suffering and the Goals of Medicine*, Oxford University Press, New York.

Cherney, N.I. & Portenoy, R.K. 1998, 'Sedation in the Management of Refractory Symptoms: Guidelines for Evaluation and Treatment', *Journal of Palliative Care*, 10: 2, 31–8.

Fins, J.J. & Bacchetta, M.B.A. 1995, 'Framing physician assisted suicide and voluntary active euthanasia debate: the role of deontology, consequentialism, and clinical pragmatism', *Journal of the American Geriatric Society*, vol. 43: 563–8.

Mount, B. 1996, 'Morphine Drips, Terminal Sedation and Slow Euthanasia: Definitions and Facts, Not Anecdotes', *Journal of Palliative Care*, 12: 4, 31–7.

O'Connor, M., Kissane, D. & Spruyt, O. 1999, 'Sedation in the "Terminally Ill" — a clinical perspective', *Monash Bioethics Review*, 18(3), pp 17–27.

Senate 1997, Euthanasia Laws Bill 1996, Senate Legal and Constitutional Legislation Committee, Submission No 4036 (Michael Ashby).

Syme, R. 1999, 'Pharmacological oblivion contributes to and hastens patients' deaths', *Monash Bioethics Review*, 18: 2, 40–4.

WHO, *see* World Health Organization.

World Health Organization 1990, 'Cancer pain relief and palliative care', Technical report series 804, WHO, Geneva.

Chapter 6 Spiritual Care

Burns, S. & Bulman, C. (eds) 2000, *Reflective practice in nursing: the growth of the professional practitioner*, Oxford, Blackwell.

Center to Improve Care of the Dying (CICD) 2001, <www.gwu.edu/~cicd/toolkit/toolkit.htm>.

CICD, see Center to Improve Care of the Dying (CICD).

Cobb, M. 1998, 'Assessing spiritual need: an examination of practice', in Cobb & Robshaw 1998 (op. cit.).

Cobb, M. 2001, *The dying soul: spiritual care at the end of life*, Open University Press, Buckingham.

Cobb, M. & V. Robshaw (eds) 1998, *The spiritual challenge of health care*, Churchill Livingstone,Edinburgh.

Fook, J., Ryan, M. & Hawkins, L. 1997, 'Towards a theory of social work expertise', *British Journal of Social Work*, 27, 399–417.

Hudson, R. 1997, 'Documented life and death in a nursing home', in *Nursing Documentation: writing what we do*, J. Richmond, pp 29–38, Ausmed Publications, Melbourne.

Johns, C. & Freshwater, D. (eds) 1998, *Transforming nursing through reflective practice*, Blackwell, Oxford.

Johnston Taylor, E. 2001, 'Spiritual Assessment', in *Textbook of Palliative Nursing*, B. Ferrell & N. Coyle, Oxford University Press, Oxford.

Kaufmann, W. 1970, 'I and You: a prologue' in *I and Thou*, pp 9–48, T&T Clark, Edinburgh.

Kellehear, A. 2000, *Eternity and me: the everlasting things in life and death*, Hill of Content, Melbourne.

Kemp, C. 2001, 'Spiritual care interventions', in *Textbook of Palliative Nursing*, pp 414–17, B. Ferrell & N. Coyle, Oxford University Press, Oxford.

Lartey, E. 1997, *In living colour: an intercultural approach to pastoral care and counselling*, Cassell, London.

McGrath, P. 2002, 'New horizons in spirituality research', in *Spirituality and Palliative Care: social and pastoral perspectives*, Chapter 12, B. Rumbold (ed), Oxford University Press, Melbourne.

McSherry, W. 2001, 'Spiritual crisis? Call a nurse', in *Spirituality in Health Care Contexts*, H. Orchard, pp 107–17, Jessica Kingsley Publishers, London.

Neuhaus, R. 2000, 'Born toward dying', *First Things*, February, 15–22.

Nuland, S. 1994, *How we die: reflections on life's final chapter*, Alfred A Knopf, New York.

Palliative Care Australia (PCA) 1999, *Standards for Palliative Care Provision*, 3rd edn, October, <www.pallcare.org.au>.

PCA, *see* Palliative Care Australia.

Polanyi, M. 1969, *Knowing and being*, University of Chicago Press, Chicago.

Rumbold, B. 1986, *Helplessness and hope: pastoral care in terminal illness*, SCM Press Ltd, London.

Chapter 7 A Framework for Symptom Assessment

Aranda, S, Kissane, D. & Long, C. 2000, *Quality in Community-Based Palliative Care (QUIC-PC)*. *QUIC-PC Project Report—Stage 3*, Centre for Palliative Care, Melbourne.

Bruera, E. 1998, 'Research into symptoms other than pain', in Doyle, D., Hanks, G.W.C. & MacDonald, N., *Oxford Textbook of Palliative Medicine*, 2nd edn, Oxford University Press, Oxford.

Bruera, E. & Neumann, C.M. 1998, 'Management of specific symptom complexes in patients receiving palliative care', *Canadian Medical Association Journal*, 158, 13: 1717–26.

Estes, M.R.Z. 1998, *Health Assessment & Physical Examination*, Delmar Publishers, New York City.

Heaven, C.M. & Maguire, P. 1996, 'Training hospice nurses to elicit patient concerns', *Journal of Advanced Nursing*, 23: 280–6.

Heaven, C.M. & Maguire, P. 1997, 'Disclosure of concern by hospice patients and their identification by nurses', *Palliative Medicine*, 11 4: 283–90.

Higginson, I., Priest, P. & McCarthy, M. 1994, 'Are bereaved family members a valid proxy for a patient's assessment of dying?', *Social Science and Medicine*, 38: 553–57.

McDaniel, R.W. & Rhodes, V.A. 1995, 'Symptom Experience', *Seminars in Oncology Nursing*, 11 4: 232–4.

National Council for Hospice and Specialist Palliative Care Services (NCHSPCS) 1998, *Reaching out: specialist palliative care for adults with non-malignant disease*, occasional paper 14.

NCHSPCS, *see* National Council for Hospice and Specialist Palliative Care Services (NCHSPCS).

Rhodes, V.A. & Watson, P.M. 1987, 'Symptom Distress—the Concept: Past and Present', *Seminars in Oncology Nursing*, 3 4: 242–7.

Roberts, A. & Bird, A. 2001, 'Assessment of symptoms', in Kinghorn, S. & Gamlin, R., *Palliative Nursing: Bringing Comfort and Hope*, pp 35–41, Bailliere Tindall, Edinburgh, in association with the Royal College of Nursing.

Street, A.F. & Kissane, D.W. 2001, 'Constructions of dignity in end-of-life care', *Journal of Palliative Care*, 17(2): 93–101, Summer.

Wilkinson, S.M. 1991, 'Factors which influence how nurses communicate with cancer patients', *Journal of Advanced Nursing*, 16: 677–88.

Wilkinson, S.M., Roberts, A. & Aldridge, J. 1998, 'Nurse–patient communication in palliative care: an evaluation of a communication skills programme', *Palliative Medicine*, 12: 13–22.

Chapter 8 Pain Management

Agency for Healthcare Policy and Research (AHCPR) 1994, *Management of Cancer Pain*, United States Department of Health and Human Services, Rockville, USA.

AHCPR, *see* Agency for Healthcare Policy and Research (AHCPR).

American Pain Society (APS) 1999, *Principles of Analgesic Use in the Treatment of Acute Pain and Cancer Pain*, 4th edn, American Pain Society, Glenview, USA.

American Pain Society Quality of Care Committee (APSQCC) 1995, 'Quality improvement guidelines for the treatment of acute pain and cancer pain', *Journal of the American Medical Association*, 274: 1874–80.

APS, *see* American Pain Society (APS).

APSQCC, *see* American Pain Society Quality of Care Committee (APSQCC).

Britton, C.B. & Miller, J.R. 1984, 'Neurologic complications in acquired immunodeficiency syndrome (AIDS)', *Neurology Clinics*, 2: 315.

Bruera, E., Brenneis, C., Paterson, A.H. & MacDonald, N. 1989, 'Use of methylphenidate as an adjuvant to narcotic analgesics in patients with advanced cancer', *Journal of Pain and Symptom Management*, 4: 3–6.

Comley, A.L. & DeMeyer, E. 2001, 'Assessing patient satisfaction with pain management through a continuous quality improvement effort', *Journal of Pain and Symptom Management*, 21(1): 278–40.

Cryer, B. & Feldman, M. 1998, 'Cyclooxygenase-1 and cyclooxygenase-2 selectivity of widely used nonsteroidal anti-inflammatory drugs', *American Journal of Medicine*, 104: 413–21.

Elliott, T.E. 1997, 'Pain Control at the End of Life', *Minnesota Medicine*, 80, 27–32.

Eisenberg, E., Carr, D.B. & Chalmers, T.C. 1995, 'Neurolytic celiac plexus block for treatment of cancer pain: A meta-analysis', *Anesthesia Analogue*, 80: 290–5.

Federation of State Medical Boards of the United States (FSMBUS), Inc. 1998, *Model Guidelines for the Use of Controlled Substances for the Treatment of Pain*, Author, Euless, USA.

Ferrell, B.R., Novy, D., Sullivan, M.D., Banja, J., Dubois, M.Y., Gitlin, M.C., Hamaty, D., Lebovits, A., Lipman, A.G., Lippe, P.M. & Livovich, J. 2001, 'Ethical dilemmas in pain management', *Journal of Pain*, 2(3): 171–80.

Ferris, D.J. 1999, 'Controlling myoclonus after high-dosage morphine infusions', *Home Care Exchange*, 56: 1009–10.

FSMBUS, *see* Federation of State Medical Boards of the United States, Inc. (FSMBUS).

Fulfaro, F., Casuccio, A., Ticozzi, C. & Ripamonit, C. 1998, 'The role of bisphosphonates in the treatment of painful metastatic bone disease: a review of phase III trials', *Pain* 78, 157–69.

Hanks, G.W., de Conno, F., Cherny, N., et al. 'Morphine and alternative opioids in cancer pain: the EAPC recommendations', *British Journal of Cancer*, 84(5): 587–593.

Holdsworth, M.T., Adams, V.R., Chavez, C.M., Vaughan, L.J. & Duncan, M.H. 1995, 'Continuous midazolam infusion for the management of morphine-induced myoclonus', *Annals of Pharmacotherapy*, 29: 25–9.

IASP, *see* International Association for the Study of Pain.

International Association for the Study of Pain Subcommittee on Taxonomy Pain Terms 1979, 'A list with definitions and notes on usage', *Pain* 6: 249–52.

Lichter, I. 1993, 'Results of anti-emetic management in terminal illness', *Journal of Palliative Care*, 9: 19–25.

Lillemoe, K.D., Cameron, J.L., Kaufman, H.S., Yeo, C.J., Pitt, H.A. & Sauter, P.K. 1993, 'Chemical splanchnicectomy in patients with unresectable pancreatic cancer: A prospective randomized trial', *Annals of Surgery*, 217(5): 447–55.

Maddocks, I., Somogyi, A., Abbott, F., Hayball, P. & Parker, D. 1996, 'Attenuation of morphine-induced delirium in palliative care by substitution with infusion of oxycodone', *Journal of Pain and Symptom Management*, 12(3): 182–9.

McCaffery, M. 1968, *Nursing Practice Theories Related to Cognition, Bodily Pain, and Man-environment Interactions*, p. 95, UCLA Student's Store, Los Angeles..

McCaffery, M, & Pasero, C. 1999, *Pain: Clinical Manual*, p. 60, Mosby, St Louis.

Portenoy, R.K. & Hagen, N.A. 1989, 'Breakthrough pain: Definition and management', *Oncology*, 3(Suppl 8): 25–9.

Porter, J. & Jick, H. 1980, 'Addiction rare in patients treated with narcotics', *New England Journal of Medicine*, 302(2): 123.

Rozan, J.P., Kahn, C.H. & Warfield, C.A. 1995, 'Epidural and intravenous opioid-induced neuroexcitation', *Anesthesiology*, 83: 860–3.

Seale, C. & Cartwright, A. 1994, *The Year Before Death*, Ashgate Publishing, Brookfield, USA.

Shiodt, F.V., Rochling, F.A., Casey, D.L. & Lee, W.M. 1997, 'Acetaminophen toxicity in an urban county hospital', *New England Journal of Medicine*, 337: 1112–17.

Spross, J. & Wolff, B.M. 1995, 'Nonpharmacological management of cancer pain', in McGuire, D.B., Yarbro, C.H. & Ferrell, B.R. (eds), *Cancer Pain Management*, pp 159–205, Jones & Bartlett, Boston.

Von Roenn, J.H., Cleeland, C.S., Gonin, R., Hatfield, A.K., Pandya, K.A. 1993, 'Physician attitudes and practice in cancer pain management. A survey from the Eastern Cooperative Oncology Group, *Annals of Internal Medicine*, 119(2): 121–6.

Warren, D. 1996, 'Practical use of rectal medications in palliative care', *Journal of Pain and Symptom Management*, 11(6): 378–87.

WHO, *see* World Health Organization.

World Health Organization (WHO) 1990, *Cancer Pain Relief and Palliative Care. Report of a WHO Expert Committee*, WHO, Geneva.

Yamamuro, M., Kusaka, K., Kato, M. & Takahashi, M. 2000, 'Celiac plexus block in cancer pain management', *Tohoku Journal of Experimental Medicine*, 192: 1–18.

Chapter 9 Breathlessness

Ahmedzai, S. 1993, 'Palliation of Respiratory Symptoms', in Doyle, D., Hanks, G.W. & Macdonald, N. (eds), *The Oxford Textbook of Palliative Medicine*, 9th edn, pp 349–78, Oxford University Press, Oxford.

Ahmedzai, S. & Davis, C. 1997, 'Nebulised drugs in palliative care', *Thorax*, 52: 2: pp 75–7.

Bailey, C.D. 1995, 'Nursing as therapy in the management of breathlessness in lung cancer', *European Journal of Cancer Care*, 4: pp 184–90.

Bass, C. 1994, 'Management of Patients with Hyperventilation-related Disorders', in Timmons, B.H. & Ley, R. (eds), *Behavioural and Psychological Approaches to Breathing Disorders*, pp 149–55, Plenum Press, New York.

Benner, P. & Wrubel, J. 1989, *The primacy of caring: stress and coping in health and illness*, Addison-Wesley Publishing Company, California.

Bion, W. 1962, *Seven Servants*, Jason Aronson, New York.

Bredin, M. 2001, CD-ROM, *A breath of fresh air: an interactive guide to managing breathlessness in patients with lung cancer*, Institute of Cancer Research, London (copies obtainable from Interactive Education Unit, <ieu@icr.ac.uk>).

Bredin, M., Corner, J., Krishnasamy, M., Plant, H., Bailey, C. & A'Hern, R. 1999, 'Multicentre randomised controlled trial of nursing intervention for breathlessness in patients with lung cancer', *British Medical Journal*, 318: pp 901–4.

Brown, M., Carrieri, V., Janson-Bjerklie, S. & Dodd, M.J. 1986, 'Lung cancer and dyspnoea: the patient's perception', *Oncology Nursing Forum*, 13: 5: pp 19–23.

Bruera E., Macmillan, K., Pither, J. & Macdonald, R.N. 1990, 'Effects of morphine on the dyspnoea of terminal cancer patients', *Journal of Pain and Symptom Management*, 5: 6: pp 341–4.

Carrieri, V.K., Janson-Bjerklie, S. & Jacobs, S. 1984, 'The sensation of dyspnoea: a review', *Heart and Lung*, 13 4: pp 436–46.

Corner, J. & O'Driscoll, M. 1999, 'Development of a breathlessness assessment guide for use in palliative care', *Palliative Medicine*, 13: pp 375–84.

Corner, J., Plant, H. & Warner, L. 1995, 'Developing a nursing approach to managing dyspnoea in lung cancer', *International Journal of Palliative Nursing*, 1: 1: pp 5–11.

Corner, J., Plant, H., A'Hern, R. & Bailey, C. 1996, 'Non-pharmacological intervention for breathlessness in lung cancer, *Palliative Medicine*, 10: pp 299–305.

Corner, J., Booth, S., Wilcock, A., Connolly, M., MacLeod, R. & Ahmedzai, S. 1997, 'The palliation of breathlessness in patients with cancer', conclusions from a consensus workshop at the European Congress for Palliative Care, London (unpublished document).

Cowcher, K. & Hanks, G.W. 1990, 'Long-term management of respiratory symptoms in advanced cancer', *Journal of Pain and Symptom Management*, 5: 5: pp 320–30.

Cohen, M.H., Johnston Anderson, A., Krasnow, S.H., Spagnolo, S.V., Citron, M.L., Payne, M., Fossieck, B.E. 1991, 'Continuous intravenous infusion of morphine for severe dyspnoea', *Southern Medical Journal*, 84: 2: pp 229–34.

Davis, C., Penn, K., A'Hern, R., Daniels, J. & Slevin, M. 1996, 'Single dose randomised controlled trial of nebulised morphine in patients with cancer-related breathlessness', *Palliative Medicine*, 10: 1, pp 64–5.

Davis, C. 1997, 'ABC of palliative care: breathlessness, cough, and other respiratory problems', *British Medical Journal*, 315: pp 931–4.

Dunlop, R. 1998, 'Management of Respiratory Symptoms', in *Cancer: Palliative Care*, pp 33–45, Springer-Verlag Ltd, London.

Gallo-Silver, L, & Pollack, B. 2000, 'Behavioural interventions for lung cancer related breathlessness', *Cancer Practice*, 8: 6: pp 268–73.

Gift, A. 1990, 'Dyspnoea', *Nursing Clinics of North America*, 25: 4: pp 955–65.

Gift, A., Moore, T. & Seoken, K. 1992, 'Relaxation to reduce dyspnoea and anxiety in COPD patients', *Nursing Research*, 41: 4: pp 242–6.

Heyes-Moore, L., Ross, V. & Mullee, M.A. 1991, 'How much of a problem is dyspnoea in advanced cancer?', *Palliative Medicine*, 5: pp 20–6.

Heyse-Moore, L. 1993, 'Respiratory Symptoms', in Saunders, C. & Sykes, N. (eds), *Management of Terminal Malignant Disease*, 3rd edn, pp 76–94, Hodder & Stoughton, Kent.

Higginson, I. & McCarthy, M. 1989, 'Measuring symptoms in terminal cancer: are pain and dyspnoea controlled?', *Journal of the Royal Society of Medicine*, 82: pp 264–7.

Janson-Bjerklie, S. & Clarke, E. 1982, 'The effects of biofeedback training on broncho diameter in asthma', *Heart and Lung*, 11 3: pp 200–7.

Krishnasamy, M., Corner, J., Bredin, M., Plant, H. & Bailey, C. 2001, 'Cancer nursing practice development: Understanding breathlessness', *Journal of Clinical Nursing*, 10: pp 103–8.

Lanceley, A. 2001, 'Therapeutic strategies in cancer care', in *Cancer Nursing Care in Context*, Corner, J. & Bailey, C. (eds), pp 120–38, Blackwell Science, Oxford.

Lewis, D. 1997, *The Tao of Natural Breathing*, pp 27–43, Mountain Wind Publishing, San Francisco..

O'Driscoll, M., Corner, J. & Bailey, C. 1999, 'The experience of breathlessness in lung cancer', *European Journal of Cancer Care*, 8: pp 37–43.

Renfroe, K. 1988, 'Effect of progressive relaxation on dyspnoea and state anxiety in patients with chronic obstructive pulmonary disease', *Heart and Lung*, 17: pp 408–13.

Reuben, D.B. & Mor, V. 1986, 'Dyspnoea in terminally ill cancer patients', *Chest*, 89: 2: pp 234–6.

Ripamonti, C. & Bruera, E. 1997, 'Dyspnoea: pathophysiology and assessment', *Journal of Pain and Symptom Management*, 13: 4: pp 220–32.

Roberts, D., Thorne, S.E. & Pearson, C. 1993, 'The experience of dyspnoea in late-stage cancer: patients' and nurses' perspectives', *Cancer Nursing*, 16: 4: pp 310–20.

Steele, B. & Shaver, J. 1992, 'The dyspnoea experience: nociceptive properties and a model for research and practice', *Advances in Nursing Science*, 15: 1: pp 64–76.

Twycross, R.G. & Lack, S.A. 1990, 'Respiratory Symptoms', in *Therapeutics in Terminal Cancer*, 2nd edn, pp 123–36, Churchill Livingston, Edinburgh.

Vainio, A. & Auvinen, A. 1996, 'Prevalence of symptoms among patients with advanced cancer: an international collaborative study', *Journal of Pain and Symptom Management*, 12: 1: pp 3–10.

Chapter 10 Fatigue

Aistars, J. 1987, 'Fatigue in the cancer patient: a conceptual approach to a clinical problem', *Oncology Nursing Forum*, 14(6): 25–9.

Berger, A. 1998, 'Patterns of fatigue and activity and rest during adjuvant breast cancer chemotherapy', *Oncology Nursing Forum*, 25(1): 51–62.

Berger, B.G. & Owen, D.R. 1992, 'Mood alteration with yoga and swimming: aerobic exercise may not be necessary', *Perceptual Motor and Skills*, 75(3 part 2): 1331–43.

Bower, J.E., Ganz, P.A., Desmond, K.A., Rowland, J.H., Meyerowitz, B.E. & Belin, T.R. 2000, 'Fatigue in Breast cancer survivors: Occurrence, correlates, and impact on quality of life', *Journal of Clinical Oncology*, 18(4): 743–53.

Brophy, L. & Sharp, E. 1991, 'Physical symptoms of biotherapy: a quality-of-life issue', *Oncology Nursing Forum*, 18 Suppl.: 25–30.

Bruera, E. & Schmitz, B., Pither, J., Neumann, C.M. & Hanson, J. 2000, 'The frequency and correlates of dyspnea in patients with advanced cancer, *Journal of Pain and Symptom Management*, 19(5): 357–62.

Byrne, A. & Byrne, D.G. 1993, 'The effect of exercise on depression, anxiety and other mood states: a review', *Journal of Psychosomatic Research*, 37(6), 565–74.

Carpenito, L.J. 1995, 'Fatigue', in Carpenito, L.J. (ed.), *Nursing Diagnosis: Application to Clinical Practice*, 6th edn, p. 379, Lippincott Company, Philadelphia.

Cramer, S.D., Neiman, D.C. & Lee, J.W. 1991, 'The effects of moderate exercise training on psychological well-being and mood state in women', *Journal of Psychosomatic Research*, 35: 437–49.

Doyne, E.J., Osip-Klein, D.J., Bowman, E.D., Osbron, K.M., McDougall-Wilson, I.B. & Neimeyer, R.A. 1987, 'Running versus weight-lifting in the treatment of depression', *Journal of Consultancy Clinical Psychology*, 55: 748–54.

Ferrell, B.R., Grant, M., Dean, G.E., Funk, B. & Ly, J. 1996, '"Bone tired": the experience of fatigue and its impact on quality of life', *Oncology Nursing Forum*, 23: 1539–47.

Funk, S.G., Tornquist, E.M. & Champagne, M.T. (eds) 1989, *Key Aspects of Comfort: Management of Pain, Fatigue and Nausea*, Springer Publishing, New York.

Glaus, A. 1993, 'Assessment of fatigue in cancer and non-cancer patients and in healthy individuals', *Journal of Supportive Care in Cancer*, 1: 305–15.

Glaus, A., Crow, R. & Hammond, S. 1996, 'A qualitative study to explore the concept of fatigue/tiredness in cancer patients and in healthy individuals', *European Journal of Cancer Care*, 5 Suppl. 2: 8–23.

Henriksson, M.M., Isometsa, E.T. & Hietanen, P.S. 1995, 'Mental disorders in cancer suicides', *Journal of Affective Disorders*, 36(1–2), 11–20.

Hopwood, P. & Stephens, R.J. 2000, 'Depression in Patients with Lung Cancer: Prevalence and Risk Factors Derived from Quality-of-Life Data, *Journal of Clinical Oncology*, 18(4): 893–903.

Irvine, D., Vincent, L., Thompson, L., Bubela, N. & Graydon, J.E. 1991, 'A critical appraisal of the research literature investigating fatigue in the individual with cancer', *Cancer Nursing*, 14: 188–199.

Irvine, D., Vincent, L., Graydon, J.E., Bubela, N. & Thompson, L. 1994, 'The prevalence and correlates of fatigue in patients receiving treatment with chemotherapy and radiotherapy', *Cancer Nursing*, 17: 367–78.

Juenger, J. 2002, 'The Fatigue of Biotherapy: A Qualitative Analysis', unpublished master's thesis, University of Missouri-Columbia, USA.

Johnson, J., Nail, L., Lauver, D., King, K. & Keys, H. 1988, 'Reducing the negative impact of radiation therapy on functional status', *Cancer*, 61: 46–51.

Kaempfer, S. & Lindsey, A. 1986, 'Energy expenditure in cancer: a review', *Cancer Nursing*, 9: 194–9.

Krishnasamy, M. 2000, 'Fatigue in advanced cancer—meaning before measurement?', *International Journal of Nursing Studies*, 37(5): 401–14.

Langendijk, J.A., Aaronson, N.K., de Jong, J.M.A., ten Velde, G.P.M., Muller, M.J., Lamers, R.J., Slotman, B.J. & Wouters, E.F.M. 2001, 'Prospective Study on Quality of Life Before and After Radical Radiotherapy in Non-Small-Cell Lung Cancer', *Journal of Clinical Oncology*, 19(8): 2123–33.

Lindsey, A. 1986, 'Cancer cachexia: effects of the disease and its treatment', *Seminars in Oncology Nursing*, 2: 19–29.

Love, R.R., Leventhal, H., Easterling, D.V. & Nerenz, D.R. 1989, 'Side effects and emotional distress during cancer chemotherapy', *Cancer*, 63, 604–12.

Luce, J.M. & Luce, J.A. 2001, 'Management of Dyspnea in Patients with Far-Advanced Lung Disease: "Once I Lose It, It's Kind of Hard to Catch It . . . "', *Journal of the American Medical Association*, 285(10), 1331–7.

Mays, M.Z. 1995, Impact of underconsumption on cognitive performance', in Marriott B.M. (ed.), *Not eating enough: Overcoming underconsumption of military operational rations*, National Academy Press, Washington D.C.

Miaskowski, C. & Portenoy, R.K. 1998, 'Update on the assessment and management of cancer-related fatigue', *Principles and Practice of Supportive Oncology Updates*, 1(2), 1–10.

Mooney, K.H., Ferrell, B.R., Nail, L.M., Benedict, S.C. & Haberman, M.R. 1991, 'Oncology Nursing Society Research Priorities Survey', *Oncology Nursing Forum*, 18(8): 1381–8.

Morrow, G. 2001, 'Reducing Depression Does Not Reduce Fatigue', American Society of Clinical Oncology Annual Meeting, May, San Francisco.

Muers, M.F. & Round, C.E. 1993, 'Palliation of symptoms in non-small cell lung cancer: A study by the Yorkshire Regional Cancer Organisation thoracic group', *Thorax*, 48(58): 339–43.

Nail, L.M., Jones, L.S. 1995, 'Fatigue side effects and treatment and quality of life', *Quality of Life Research*, 4 1: 8–16.

Nail, L. & Winningham, M. 1993, 'Fatigue', in Groenwald, S.L., Frogge, M., Goodman, M. & Yarbro, C. (eds), *Cancer Nursing: Principles and Practice*, 3rd edn, pp 608–19, Jones Bartlett, Boston.

Nail, L.M., Jones, L.S., Geene, D., Schipper, D. & Jensen, R. 1991, 'Use and perceived efficacy of self-care activities in patients receiving chemotherapy', *Oncology Nursing Forum*, 18: 883–7.

Oberle, K., Allen, M. & Lynkowski, P. 1994, 'Follow-up of same day surgery patients: a study of patient concerns', *AORN Journal*, 59(5): 1016–8, 1021–5.

Peck, A. & Boland, J. 1977, 'Emotional reactions to radiation treatment'. *Cancer*, 40: 180–4.

Piper, B. 1993, 'Fatigue', in Carrieri, V., Lindsey, A. & West, C. (eds), *Pathophysiological Phenomena in Nursing: Human Responses to Illness*, 2nd edn, pp 279–302, Saunders, Philadelphia.

Piper, B., Lindsey, A., Dodd, M., Ferketich, S, Paul, S. & Weller, S. 1989, 'Development of an Instrument to Measure the Subjective Dimension of Fatigue', in Funk, S., Tournquist, E., Champagne, M., Copp, L. & Wiese, R. (eds), *Key Aspects of Comfort: Management of Pain Fatigue and Nausea*, pp 199–208, Springer, New York.

Piper, B.F., Lindsey, A. & Dodd, M. 1987, 'Fatigue mechanisms in cancer patients: developing nursing theory', *Oncology Nursing Forum*, 14 6: 17–23.

Portenoy, R.K. & Itri, L.M. 1999, 'Cancer-related fatigue: guidelines for evaluation and management', *Oncologist*, 4(1): 1–10.

Porock, D. 1995, 'The effects of preparatory patient education on the anxiety and satisfaction of cancer patients receiving radiation therapy', *Cancer Nursing*, 18: 206–14.

Porock, D., Kristjanson, L., Tinnelly, K. & Blight, J. 2000, 'The effect of exercise on fatigue in patients with advanced cancer: A pilot study', *Journal of Palliative Care*, 16(3): 30–6.

Rhoten, D. 1982, 'Fatigue and the Postsurgical Patient', in Norris, C. (ed.), *Concepts Clarification in Nursing*, pp 277–300, Aspen, Rockville, USA.

Richardson, A. 1995, 'Fatigue in cancer patients: a review of the literature', *European Journal of Cancer Care*, 4: 20–32.

Richardson, A. & Ream, E. 1996, 'The experience of fatigue and other symptoms in patients receiving chemotherapy', *European Journal of Cancer Care*, 5 Suppl. 2: 24–30.

Ropka, M.E., Guterbock, T.M., Krebs, L.U., Murphy-Eade, K., Stetz, K.M., Summers, B.L., Bissonette, E., Given, B. & Mallory, G. 2002, 'Year 2000 Oncology Nursing Society Research Priorities Survey', *Oncology Nursing Forum*, 29(3): 481–91.

Selye, H. 1974, *Stress Without Distress*, Lippincott, Philadelphia.

Shippee, R., Friedl, K. & Kramer, T. 1994, 'Nutritional and immunological assessment of ranger students with increased caloric intake', US Army Research Institute of Environmental Medicine Technical Report T95-5, Natick, USA.

Simonson, E. 1971, *Physiology of Work Capacity and Fatigue*, Thomas, Springfield, USA.

Skalla, K. & Lacasse, C. 1992, 'Patient education for fatigue', *Oncology Nursing Forum*, 19: 1537–41.

Smets, E.M.A., Garssen, B., Cull, A. & de Haes, J.C.J.M. 1996, 'Application of the multidimensional fatigue inventory (MFI-20) in cancer patients receiving radiotherapy', *British Journal of Cancer*, 73: 241–5.

Stetz, K.M., Haberman, M.R., Holcombe, J. & Jones, L.S. 1994, 'Oncology Nursing Society Research Priorities Survey', *Oncology Nursing Forum*, 22(5): 785–9.

Stone, P., Hardy, J., Broadley, K., Tookman, A.J., Kurowaska, A. & A'Hern, R. 1999, 'Fatigue in advanced cancer: a prospective controlled cross-sectional study', *British Journal of Cancer*, 79(9–10), pp 1479–86.

Stoudemire, A., Bronheim, H. & Wise, T.N. 1998, 'Why guidelines for consultation-liaison psychiatry patients?', *Psychosomatics*, 39: S3–S7.

Stromgren, A.S., Goldschmidt, D., Groenvold, M., Petersen, M.A., Jensen, P.T., Pedersen, L., Hoermann, L., Helleberg, C. & Sjogren, P. 2002, 'Self-assessment in cancer patients referred to palliative care: a study of feasibility and symptom epidemiology', *Cancer*, 94(2): 512–20.

Watanabe, S. & Bruera, E. 1996, 'Anorexia and cachexia, asthenia, and lethargy', *Hematology Oncology Clinics of North America*, 10(1): 189–206.

Wheeler, V.S. 1997, 'Biotherapy', in Groenwald, S.L., Hansen Frogge, M., Goodman, M. & Yabro, C.H., *Cancer Nursing Principles and Practice,*, 4th edn, pp 426–58, Jones and Bartlett Publishers, Boston.

Winningham, M.L. 1991, 'Walking program for people with cancer', *Cancer Nursing*, 14: 270–6.

Winningham, M.L. 1999, 'Fatigue', in Yarbro, C.H., Frogge, M.H. & Goodman, M. (eds), *Cancer Symptom Management*, 2nd edn, p. 63, Jones & Bartlett Publishers, Sudbury.

Winningham, M.L., Nail, L.M., Burke, M.B., Brophy, L., Cimprich, B., Jones, L.S., Pickard-Holley, S., Rhodes, V., St Pierre, B., Beck, S., Glass, E.C., Mock, V.L., Mooney, D.H. & Piper, B. 1994, 'Fatigue and the cancer experience: the state of the knowledge', *Oncology Nursing Forum*, 21: 23–36.

Chapter 11 Constipation

Back, B.N. 2001, *Palliative Medicine Handbook* (3e). BPM Books, Cardiff.

Breitbart, W., Bruera, E., Chochinov, H. & Lynch, M. 1995, 'Psychiatric symptom management in terminal care', *Clinics in Geriatric Medicine*, 12: 329–47.

Bruera, E., Suarez-Almazor, M., Velasco, A., Bertolino, M., MacDonald, S. & Hanson, J. 1994, 'The assessment of constipation in terminal cancer patients admitted to a palliative care unit: a retrospective review', *Journal of Pain and Symptom Management*, 9 (8): 515–19.

Bruera, E. 2001, 'Confirming and Treating Constipation', *Oncology*, 15(1), 77–8.

Burke, A. 1994, 'The management of constipation in end-stage disease', *Australian Family Physician*, 23 (7): 1248–53.

Fallon, M. & Walsh, J. 1998, The management of gastrointestinal symptoms. In Faull Constipation, Cater Y., Woof R., eds. *Handbook of Palliative Care*, Blackwell Science, Oxford: 134–156.

Fallon, M. & O'Neill, B. (eds) 2000, 'Constipation and diarrhoea', *ABC of Palliative Care*, BMJ Books, London, 7: 23–6.

Goodman, M.L., Fellows, D. & Wilkinson, S.M. 2003a internal report 'A Study of the Management of Constipation Across the Marie Curie Cancer Care Centres'.

Goodman, M.L., Fellows, D. & Wilkinson, S.M. 2003b 'Laxatives for the management of constipation in palliative care patients': A Cochrane PAPAS Systematic Review.

McMillan, S.C. & Williams, F.A. 1989, 'Validity and reliability of the constipation assessment scale', *Cancer Nursing*, 12 (3): 183–8.

Maiskowski Constipation, 1995, Putting the cancer pain guideline into practice. *Capsules and Comments in Oncology Nursing* 3(1) 9–15.

O'Brien, T., Kelly, M. & Saunders, C.M. 1992, 'Motor neurone disease: a hospice perspective', *British Medical Journal*, 304: 471–3.

O'Mahoney, S., Coyle, N. & Payne, R. 2001, 'Current Management of Opioid-Related Side Effects', *Oncology*, 15(1): 61–73, 77; discussion 77–8, 80–2.

Robinson, C., Fritch, M. et al 2000, Development of a protocol to prevent opioid-induced constipation in patients with cancer—A research utilisation project. *Clinical Journal of Oncology Nursing* 4(2) 79–84.

Sykes, N.P., 1993, Constipation and diarrhoea. In Doyle D., Hanks G.W., MacDonald N. eds. *Oxford Textbook of Palliative Medicine* Chapter 4.

Thacker, E. 2001, Movicol in the Management of Constipation in Patients with Neurological Disease: an open study in nursing home residents. Presentation at the 21st Conference of the Association for Continence Advice.

Woodruff, R. 1999, 'Constipation', in *Palliative Medicine*, 3rd edn, Oxford University Press, Melbourne, pp 171–5.

Chapter 12 Nausea and Vomiting

Ashby, M.A. 1991, 'Percutaneous gastrostomy as a venting procedure in palliative care', *Palliative Medicine*, 5: 147–50.

Baines, M.J. 1997, 'Nausea, vomiting and intestinal obstruction', *British Medical Journal*, Vol. 315 1, Nov., 1148–50.

Brown, S., North, D., Marvel, M. & Fons, R. 1992, 'Acupressure wrist bands to relieve nausea and vomiting in hospice patients—Do they work?', *American Journal of Hospice and Palliative Care*, July/Aug. 25–9.

Chan, V. & McConigley, R. 2001, 'Nausea and Vomiting', in Chan, V., *Outline of Palliative Medicine*, 3rd edn, pp 61–9, Cabramatta, NSW.

Dibble, S.L., Chapman, J., Mack, K.A. & Shih, A. 2000, 'Acupressure for nausea: A pilot study', *Oncology Nursing Forum*, 27(1) 41–7.

Fessele, K. 1996, 'Managing the multiple causes of nausea and vomiting in the patient with cancer', *Oncology Nursing Forum*, Vol. 23 (9), 1409–14.

Fulder, S. 1988, 'The basic concepts of laternative medicine and their impact on our views of health', *Journal of Alternative and Complementary Medicine*, Summer, 4(2): 147–58.

Hudson, S. 1998, 'Natural therapies aid oncology nursing', *Australian Nursing Journal*, (5) April, 25.

Jenns. K. 1994, 'Importance of nausea', *Cancer Nursing*, 17 (6), pp 448–93.

Maxwell, J. 1997, 'The gentle power of acupressure', *RN Journal*, April, 53–6.

McMillan, C.M. & Dundee, J.W. 1991, 'The role of transcutaneous electrical stimulation of Neiguan antiemetic acupuncture point in controlling sickness after cancer chemotherapy', *Physiotherapy*, 77 (7), 499–502.

Rhodes, V. & McDaniel, R. 1999, 'The index of nausea, vomiting and retching: A new format of the index of nausea and vomiting,' *Oncology Nursing Forum*, Vol. 26, (5), pp 889–93.

Twycross, R. 1995, *Symptom management in advanced* cancer, pp 168–73, Radcliffe Medical Press, Oxford.

Walsh, D., Doona, M., Molnar, M. & Lipnickey, V. 2000, 'Symptom Control in Advanced Cancer: important drugs and routes of administration', *Seminars in Oncology*, 27 (1), 69–83.

Wilkinson, S. 1995, 'Aromatherapy and massage in palliative care', *International Journal of Palliative Care Nursing*, (1): 21–30.

Chapter 13 Nutrition and Hydration

American Dietetic Association 1992, 'Position of the American Dietetic Association: issues in feeding the terminally ill', *Journal of the American Dietetic Association*, 92: 996–1002.

American Medical Association 1986, 'Statement of the Council on Ethical and Judicial affairs: withholding or withdrawing life prolonging medical treatment', Chicago.

American Nurses Association 1992, 'Task force on the nurses role in end of life decisions: position statement: foregoing nutrition and hydration', Washington DC.

Andrews, M. & Levine, A. 1989, 'Dehydration in the terminal patient: perception of hospice nurses', *The American Journal of Hospice Care*, Jan/Feb, 31–4.

Arbolino, L. & Sacchet, D. 2000, 'Nutrition and cancer across the continuum—advanced cancer patient', *Topics in Clinical Nursing*, 15(2), pp 12–19.

Bozzetti, F, Amadori, D., Bruera, E. & Cozzeglio, L. 1996, 'Guidelines on artificial nutrition versus hydration in terminal cancer patients', *Nutrition*, 12: 163–7.

Bruera, E. & MacDonald, R.N. 1988, 'Nutrition in cancer patients: an update and review of our experience', *Journal of Pain and Symptom Management*, 3/30, 133–40.

Byrock, I. 1995, 'Patient refusal of nutrition and hydration: walking the ever-fine line', *The American Journal of Hospice & Palliative Care*, March/April, pp 8–13.

Craig, G.M. 1994, 'On withholding nutrition and hydration in the terminally ill: has palliative medicine gone too far?', *Journal of Medical Ethics*, 20: 139–43.

Dunlop, R.J., Ellershaw, J.E., Baines, M.J., Sykes, N. & Saunders, C.M. 1995, 'On withholding nutrition and hydration in the terminally ill: has palliative medicine gone too far? A reply', *Journal of Medical Ethics*, 21: 141–3.

Hastings Center 1987, *Guidelines on the termination of life-sustaining treatment and the care of the dying*, Briarcliff Manor, New York.

Jackson, K. C. II 2000, 'Nutrition & hydration problems in palliative care patients', *Journal of Pharmaceutical Care in Pain & Symptom Control*, Vol. 8, No. 1, pp 183–96.

Malone, N. 1994, 'Hydration in the terminally ill patient', *Nursing Standard*, 8: 29–32.

Meares, C.J. 2000, 'Nutritional issues in palliative care', *Seminars in Oncology Nursing*, Vol. 16, No. 2, pp 135–45.

National Council for Hospice & Specialist Palliative Care Services 1997, 'Articicial hydration (AH) for people who are terminally ill', *European Journal of Palliative Care*, 4: 124.

NCHSPCS, *see* National Council for Hospice & Specialist Palliative Care Services.

Noble-Adams, R. 1995, 'Dehydration: subcutaneous fluid administration', *British Journal of Nursing*, 4: 488–94.

Steiner, N. & Bruera, E. 1998, 'Methods of hydration in palliative care patients', *Journal of Palliative Care*, 14: 6–13.

Twycross, R.G. & Lack, S.A. 1990, *Therapeutics in Terminal Cancer*, Churchill Livingstone, UK.

Viola, R.A., Wells, G.A. & Peterson, J. 1997, 'The effects of fluid status and fluid therapy in the dying: a systematic review', *Journal of Palliative Care*, 13: 41–52.

Wade, R. 1998, 'Artificial hydration in terminally ill patients: is there a moral obligation?', *Caroline Chisholm Centre for Health Ethics*, Winter, Vol. 3, No.4.

Wilkes, E. 1994, 'On withholding nutrition and hydration in the terminally ill: has palliative medicine gone too far? A commentary', *Journal of Medical Ethics*, 20: 144–5.

Worrobee, F. & Brown, M.K. 1997, 'Hypodermoclysis therapy in a chronic care hospital setting', *Journal of Gerontological Nursing*, 23: 23–8.

Zerwekh, J. 1983, 'The dehydration question', *Nursing '83*, January, pp 47–51.

Chapter 14 Malignant Wounds

Ashford, R.F., Plant, G.T., Maher, J. & Teare, L. 1984, 'Double-blind trial of metronidazole in malodorous ulcerating tumours', *Lancet*, 1: 1232–3.

Back, I.N. & Finlay I 1995, 'Analgesic effect of topical opioids on painful skin ulcers' (letter), *Journal of Pain and Symptom Management*, 10(7): 493.

Bale, S. & Jones, V. 1997, *Wound Care Nursing A Patient-Centred Approach*, Ballière Tindall, London.

Benbow, M. 1995, 'Parameters of wound assessment', *British Journal of Nursing*, 4 (11): 647–51.

Boardman, M., Mellor, K. & Neville, B. 1993, 'Treating a patient with a heavily exuding malodorous fungating ulcer', *Journal of Wound Care*, 2(2): 74–6.

Boon, H., Brophy, J. & Lee, J. 2000, 'The community care of a patient with a fungating wound', *British Journal of Nursing*, 9(6): Tissue Viability Supplement S35–S38.

Bower, M., Stein, R., Evans, T.R.J., Hedley, A., Pert, P. & Coombes, R.C. 1992, 'A double-blind study of the efficacy of metronidazole gel in the treatment of malodorous fungating tumours', *European Journal of Cancer*, 28A (4/5): 888–9.

Bryan, G.T. 1994, 'Natural Histories of Cancers', in Love, R.R. (ed), *Manual of Clinical Oncology*, 6th edn, pp 18–34, Springer-Verlag, Berlin.

Bycroft, L. 1994, 'Care of a handicapped women with metastatic breast cancer', *British Journal of Nursing*, 3 (3): 126–33.

Carville, K. 1995, 'Caring for cancerous wounds in the community', *Journal of Wound Care*, 4(2): 66–8.

Collier, M. 1994, 'Assessing a wound', *Nursing Standard*, 8(49), RCN Nursing Update, 3–8.

Collier, M. 1997a, 'The assessment of patients with malignant fungating wounds—a holistic approach, part 1, *Nursing Times*, 93(44), Supplement 1–4.

Collier, M. 1997b, 'The assessment of patients with malignant fungating wounds—a holistic approach: part 2', *Nursing Times*, 93(46), Suppl. 1–4.

Collier, M. 2000, 'Management of patients with fungating wounds', *Nursing Standard*, 15 (11): 46–52.

Cooper, R. & Molan, P. 1999, 'The role of honey as an antiseptic in managing pseudomonas infection', *Journal of Wound Care*, 8(4): 161–4.

Cutting, K.F. 1998, *Educational Leaflet 5(2) Wounds and Infection*, The Wound Care Society, Huntingdon, UK.

Davis, V. 1995, 'Goal-setting aids care', *Nursing Times*, 91(39): 72–5.

Downing, J. 1999, *Pain in the Patient with Cancer, Nursing Times Clinical Monographs No 5*, NT Books, London.

Dunford, C. 2000, 'The use of honey in wound management', *Nursing Standard*, 15(11): 63–8.

Edwards, J. 2000, 'Wound management (2): managing malodorous wounds', *Journal of Community Nursing*, 14(4): <www.jcn.co.uk>.

Emflorgo, C.A. 1999, 'The assessment and treatment of wound pain', *Journal of Wound Care*, 8(8): 384–5.

Emflorgo, C. 1998, 'Controlling bleeding in fungating wounds' (letter), *Journal of Wound Care*, 7(5): 235.

Englund, F. 1993, 'Wound management in palliative care', *RCN Contact*, Winter: 2–3.

Esther, R.J., Lamps, L. & Schwartz, H.S. 1999, 'Marjolin ulcers: secondary carcinomas in chromic wounds', *Journal of the Southern Orthopaedic Association*, 8(3): 181–7.

Fairbairn, K. 1994, 'A challenge that requires further research: management of fungating breast lesions', *Professional Nurse*, 9(4): 272–7.

Fletcher, J. 1997, 'Update: wound cleansing', *Professional Nurse*, 12(11): 793–6.

Flock, P., Gibbs, L. & Sykes, N. 2000, 'Diamorphine-metronidazole gel effective for treatment of painful infected leg ulcers' (letter), *Journal of Pain and Symptom Management*, 20(6): 396–7.

Gallagher, J. 1995), 'Management of cutaneous symptoms', *Seminars in Oncology Nursing*, 11(4): 239–47.

Gilchrist, B. 1999, 'Wound infection', in Miller, M. & Glover, D. (eds), *Wound Management Theory and Practice*, pp 96–106, Nursing Times Books, London.

Goodman, M., Hilderley, L.J. & Purl, S. 1997, 'Integumentary and mucous membrane alterations', in Groenwald, S.L., Hansen Frogge, M., Goodman, M. & Henk Yarbro, C. (eds), *Cancer Nursing Principles and Practice*, 4th edn, pp 768–822, Jones & Bartlett Publishers, Sudbury, USA.

Gould, D. 1999, 'Wound management and pain control', *Nursing Standard*, 14(6): 47–54.

Grassi, L., Indelli, M., Maltoni, M., Falcini, F., Fabbri, L. & Indelli, R. 1996, 'Quality of life of homebound patients with advanced cancer: assessments by patients, family members, and oncologists', *Journal of Psychosocial Oncology*, 14(3): 31–45.

Grocott, P. 1993, 'Practical Changes', *Nursing Times*, 89(7): 64–70.

Grocott, P. 1995a, 'The palliative management of fungating malignant wounds', *Journal of Wound Care*, 4(5): 240–2.

Grocott, P. 1995b, 'Assessment of fungating malignant wounds', *Journal of Wound Care*, 4(7): 333–6.

Grocott, P. 1998, 'Controlling bleeding in fragile fungating tumours' (letter), *Journal of Wound Care*, 7(7): 342.

Grocott, P. 1999, 'The management of fungating wounds', *Journal of Wound Care*, 8(5): 232–4.

Grocott, P. 2000, 'Palliative management of fungating malignant wounds', *Journal of Community Nursing*, 14(3), <www.jcn.co.uk>.

Grocott, P. 2001, *Educational Booklet 8(2) The Palliative Management of Fungating Malignant Wounds*, Wound Care Society, Huntingdon, UK.

Haisfield-Wolfe, M.E. & Rund, C. 1997, 'Malignant cutaneous wounds: a management protocol', *Ostomy/Wound Management*, 43(1): 56–66.

Hallett, A. 1995, 'Fungating wounds', *Nursing Times*, 91(39): 81–5.

Hampton, J.P. 1996, 'The use of metronidazole in the treatment of malodorous wounds', *Journal of Wound Care*, 5(9): 421–6.

Hampton, S. & Collins, F. 2001, 'SuperSkin: the management of skin susceptible to breakdown', *British Journal of Nursing*, 10(11): 742–6.

Haughton, W. & Young, T. 1995, 'Common problems in wound care: malodorous wounds', *British Journal of Nursing*, 4(16): 959–63.

Hill, B.B., Sloan, D.A., Lee, E.Y., McGrath, P.C. & Kenady, D.E. 1996, 'Marjolin's ulcer of the foot caused by non-burn trauma', *Southern Medical Journal*, 89(7), <www.sma.org/smj/96jul11.htm>.

Hollinworth, H. 2000, *Educational Leaflet 7(2) Pain and wound care*, Wound Care Society, Huntingdon, UK.

Hollinworth, H. 1997, 'Less pain, more gain', *Nursing Times*, 93(46): 89–91.

Ingham, J. & Portenoy, R.K. 1998, 'The measurement of pain and other symptoms', in Doyle, D., Hanks, G.W.C. & MacDonald N (eds), *Oxford Textbook of Palliative Medicine*, 2nd edn, pp 203–19, Oxford University Press, Oxford.

Ivetić, O. & Lyne, P.A. 1990, 'Fungating and ulcerating malignant lesions: a review of the literature', *Journal of Advanced Nursing*, 15: 83–8.

Jones, M., Davey, J. & Champion, A. 1998, 'Dressing wounds', *Nursing Standard*, 12(39): 47–52.

Krajnik, M. & Zylicz, Z. 1997, 'Topical morphine for cutaneous cancer pain' (letter), *Palliative Medicine*, 11(4): 326.

Laverty, D., Cooper, J. & Soady, S. 2000, 'Wound Management', in Mallett, J. & Dougherty, L. (eds), *The Royal Marsden Hospital Manual of Clinical Nursing Procedures*, 5th edn, pp 681–710, Blackwell Science Publications, Oxford.

Leaper, D. 1996, 'Antiseptics in wound healing', *Nursing Times*, 92(39): 63–8.

Malheiro, E., Pinto, A., Choupina, M., Barroso, L., Reis, J. & Amarabte, J. 2001, 'Marjolin's ulcer of the scalp: case report and literature review', *Annals of Burns and Fire Disasters*, 14(1): <www.medbc.com/annals/review>.

Manning, M.P. 1998, 'Metastasis to skin', *Seminars in Oncology Nursing*, 14(3): 240–3.

Miller, C. 1998, 'Management of skin problems: nursing aspects', in Doyle, D., Hanks, G.W.C. & MacDonald, N. (eds), *Oxford Textbook of Palliative Medicine*, 2nd edn, pp 642–56, Oxford University Press, Oxford.

Molan, P.C. 1999, 'The role of honey in the management of wounds', *Journal of Wound Care*, 8(8): 415–18.

Moody, M. 1998, 'Metrotop: a topical antimicrobial agent for malodorous wounds', *British Journal of Nursing*, 7(5): 286–9.

Morgan, D.A. 2000, *Formulary of Wound Management Products: A Guide for Healthcare Staff*, 8th edn, Euromed Communications Ltd, Surrey, UK.

Mortimer, P.S. 1998, 'Management of skin problems: medical aspects', in Doyle, D., Hanks, G.W.C. & MacDonald, N. (eds), *Oxford Textbook of Palliative Medicine*, 2nd edn, pp 617–27, Oxford University Press, Oxford.

Naylor, W., Laverty, D. & Mallett, J. 2001, *The Royal Marsden Hospital Handbook of Wound Management in Cancer Care*, Blackwell Science Ltd, Oxford.

Naylor, W. 2001, 'Assessment and management of pain in fungating wounds', *British Journal of Nursing*, 10(22): Tissue Viability Supplement, S33–S56.

Neal, K. 1991, 'Treating fungating lesions', *Nursing Times*, 87(23): 84–6.

Newman, V., Allwood, M. & Oakes, R.A. 1989, 'The use of metronidazole gel to control the smell of malodorous lesions', *Palliative Medicine*, 34: 303–5.

Offer, G., Perks, G. & Wilcock, A. 2000, 'Palliative plastic surgery', *European Journal of Palliative Care*, 7(3): 85–7.

Oliver, L. 1997, 'Wound cleansing', *Nursing Standard*, 11(20): 47–51.

Price, E. 1996, 'The stigma of smell', *Nursing Times*, 92(20): 70–2.

Pudner, R. 1998), 'The management of patients with a fungating or malignant wound', *Journal of Community Nursing*, 12(9): <www.jcn.co.uk/septfung.htm>.

Ryman, L. & Rankin-Box, D. 2001, 'Relaxation and visualization', in Rankin-Box, D. (ed.), *The Nurse's Handbook of Complementary Therapies*, 2nd edn, pp 251–8, Baillière Tindall, London.

Sneeuw, K.C.A., Aaronson, N.K., Sprangers, M.A.G., Detmar, S.B., Wever, L.D.V. & Schornagel, J.H. 1999, 'Evaluating the quality of life of cancer patients: assessments by patients, significant others, physicians and nurses', *British Journal of Cancer*, 81(1): 87–94.

Stein, C. 1995, 'The control of pain in peripheral tissue by opioids', *The New England Journal of Medicine*, 332(25): 1685–90.

Sterling, C. 1996, 'Methods of wound assessment documentation: a study', *Nursing Standard*, 11(10): 38–41.

Thomas, S. 1989, 'Pain and wound management', *Community Outlook*, July: 11–15.

Thomas, S. 1992, *Current Practices in the Management of Fungating Lesions and Radiation Damaged Skin*, The Surgical Materials Testing Laboratory, Bridgend, Mid Glamorgan.

Thomas, S., Fischer, B., Fram, P.J. & Waring, M.J. 1998a, 'Odour-absorbing dressings', *Journal of Wound Care*, 7(5): 246–50.

Thomas, S., Vowden, K. & Newton, H. 1998b, 'Controlling bleeding in fragile fungating wounds', *Journal of Wound Care*, 7(3): 154.

Travis, S. 2000, 'Entonox administration', in Mallett, J. & Dougherty, L. (eds), *The Royal Marsden Hospital Manual of Clinical Nursing Procedures*, 5th edn, pp 261–5, Blackwell Science, Oxford.

Trevelyn, J. 1996, 'Wound cleansing: principles and practice', *Nursing Times*, 92(16): 46–8.

Twillman, R.K., Long, T.D., Cathers, T.A. & Mueller, D.W. 1999, 'Treatment of painful skin ulcers with topical opioids', *Journal of Pain and Symptom Management*, 17(4): 288–92.

Van Toller, S. 1994, 'Invisible wounds: the effects of skin ulcer malodours', *Journal of Wound Care*, 3(2): 103–5.

WHO, *see* World Health Organization.

Williams, C. 1998, '3M cavilon no sting barrier film in the protection of vulnerable skin', *British Journal of Nursing*, 7(10): 613–15.

Williams, C. 1999, 'Clinisorb activated charcoal dressing for odour control', *British Journal of Nursing*, 8(15): 1016–19.

World Health Organization 1996, *Cancer Pain Relief*, 2nd edn, WHO, Geneva.

Young, T. 1997, 'Wound care: the challenge of managing fungating wounds', *Community Nurse*, 3(9): Nurse Prescriber 41–4.

Chapter 15 Confusion and Terminal Restlessness

American Psychiatric Association (APA) 1994, *Diagnostic and Statistical Manual of Mental Disorders*, revised edn 4, APA, Washington.

APA, *see* American Psychiatric Association (APA).

Ashby, M., Martin, P. & Jackson, K. 1999, 'Opioid substitution to reduce adverse effects in cancer pain management', *Medical Journal of Australia*, 170: 68–71.

Back, I. 1992, 'Terminal restlessness in patients with advanced malignant disease', *Palliative Medicine*, 6: 293–8.

Barraclough, J. 1997, 'ABC of palliative care: depression, anxiety and confusion', *British Medical Journal*, 315 (7119): 1365–8.

Breitbart, W. & Cohen, K. 2000, *Handbook of psychiatry in palliative care*, H.M. Chochinov & W. Breitbart (eds), Oxford University Press, New York.

Burke, A. 1997, 'Palliative care: an update on "terminal restlessness"', *MJA*, 166: 39–42.

Caraceni, A., Nanni, O., Maltoni, M., Piva, L., Indelli, M., Arnoldi, E., Monti, M., Montanari, L., Amadori, D. & De Conno, F. 2000, 'Impact of delirium on the short-term prognosis of advanced cancer patients, *Cancer*, 89: 1145–9.

Casarett, D.J. & Inouye, S.K. 2001, 'Diagnosis and Management of Delirium near the End of Life', *Annals of Internal Medicine*, 135 : 32–40.

Davis, M., Walsh, D., Lawlor, P. & Gagnon, B. 2001, 'Clinical and ethical questions concerning delirium study on patients with advanced cancer/in reply', *Archives of Internal Medicine*, 161 (2): 161–7.

Folstein, M., Folstein, S. & McHugh, P. 1975, 'The Folstein Mini-Mental State Examination: a practical method for grading the cognitive state of patients for the clinician', *Journal of Psychiatric Research*, 12: 189–98.

Gagnon, P., Allard, P., Benoit, M. & DeSerres, M. 2000, 'Delirium in terminal cancer: a prospective study using daily screening, early diagnosis, and continuous monitoring', *Journal of Pain and Symptom Management*, 19 (6): 412–26.

Hardy, J. 2000, 'Sedation in terminally ill patients', *Lancet*, 356 (9245): 1866–7.

Inouye, S.K. 1990, 'Clarifying confusion: the Confusion Assessment Method', *Annals of Internal Medicine*, 113 (12): 941–8.

Lawlor, P., Fainsinger, R. & Bruera, E. 2000, 'Delirium at the end of life: critical issues in clinical practice and research', *JAMA* 284 (19): 2427–32.

Lindesay, J. 1999, 'The concept of delirium', *Dementia and geriatric cognitive disorders*, 10: 310–14.

Lindesay, J., MacDonald, A. & Starke, I. 1990, *Delirium in the Elderly*, Oxford University Press, Oxford.

McCaffery Boyle, D., Abernathy, G., Baker, L. & Conover Wall, A. 1998, 'End of life confusion in patients with cancer', *Oncology Nursing Forum*, 25(8): 1335–43.

Meagher, D. 2001, 'Delirium: optimising management', *British Medical Journal*, 322: 144–9.

Passik, D. & Cooper, M. 1999, 'Complicated delirium in a cancer patient successfully treated with olanzapine', *Journal of Pain and Symptom Management*, 17 (3): 219–23.

Randall, F. & Downie, R. 1999, *Palliative Care Ethics, A companion for all specialties*, 2nd edn, Oxford University Press, Oxford.

Ross, D. & Alexander, C. 2001, 'Management of common symptoms in terminally ill patients, Part 11: Constipation, delirium and dyspnea', *American Family Physician*, 64(6): 1019–26.

Williams, M. 1991, 'Delirium/acute confusional states: evaluation devices in nursing', *International Psychogeriatrics*, 3(2): 301–7.

Chapter 16 Psychological and Existential Distress

American Psychiatric Association (APA) 1994, *Diagnostic and Statistical Manual of Mental Disorders IV*, APA Press, Washington, D.C.

APA, *see* American Psychiatric Association (APA).

Beck, A.T., Kovacs, M. & Weisman, A.D. 1975, 'Hopelessness and suicidal behaviour', *Medical Journal of Australia*, 234: 1146–9.

Blazeby, J.M., Williams, M.H., Alderson, D. & Farndon, J.R. 1995, 'Observer variation in assessment of quality of life in patients with oesophageal cancer', *British Journal of Surgery*, 82: 1200–3.

Breitbart, W., Rosenfeld, B.D. & Passik, S.D. 1996, 'Interest in physician-assisted suicide among ambulatory HIV-infected patients', *American Journal of Psychiatry*, 153: 238–42.

Breitbart, W., Rosenfeld, B. & Pessin, H. 2000, 'Depression, hopelessness and the desire for hastened death in terminally ill patients with cancer', *Journal of the American Medical Association*, 284: 2907–11.

Butow, P.N., Kazemi, J.N. & Beeney, L.J. 1996, 'When the diagnosis is cancer. Patient communication experiences and preferences', *Cancer*, 77: 2630–7.

Cassell, E.J. 1982, 'The nature of suffering', *New England Journal of Medicine*, 306: 639–45.

Chochinov, H.M., Wilson, K.G., Enns, M. 1998, 'Depression, hopelessness and suicidal ideation in the terminally ill', *Psychosomatics*, 39: 366–70.

Chochinov, H.M., Wilson, K.G., Enns, M., Mowchun, N., Lander, S. & Levitt, M. 1995, 'Desire for death in the terminally ill', *American Journal of Psychiatry*, 152: 1185–91.

Chochinov, H.M., Tataryn, D., Clinch, J.J. & Dudgeon, D. 1999, 'Will to live in the terminally ill', *Lancet*, 354: 816–19.

Christakis, N.A. 1999, *Death Foretold. Prophecy and Prognosis in Medical Care*, The University of Chicago Press, Chicago.

Curtis, A.E. & Furnisher, J.I. 1989, 'Quality of life of oncology hospice patients: a comparison of patient and primary caregiver reports', *Oncology Nursing Forum*, 16: 49–53.

Ersek, M. 2001, 'The meaning of hope in the dying', in Ferrell, B. & Coyle, N. (eds), *Textbook of Palliative Nursing*, Oxford University Press, Oxford.

Grealish, L. 2000, 'Mini-Mental State Questionnaire: problems with its use in palliative care', *International Journal of Palliative Nursing*, 6(6): 298–302.

Herth, K. 1995, 'Engendering hope in the chronically and terminally ill: nursing intervention', *American Journal of Hospice and Palliative Care*, 12(5): 31–9.

Kissane, D.W., Clarke, D.M. & Street, A.F. 2001, 'Demoralisation syndrome: a relevant psychiatric diagnosis for palliative care', *Journal of Palliative Care*, 17: 12–21.

Kissane, D.W. 2001, 'Demoralisation: its impact on informed consent and medical care', *Medical Journal of Australia*, 175 (10): 537–9.

Kissane, D.W. & Bloch, S. 2002, *Family Focused Grief Therapy. A Model of Family-centred Care during Palliative Care and Bereavement*, Open University Press, Buckingham, UK.

Lloyd-Williams, M. 2001, 'Screening for depression in palliative care patients: a review', *European Journal of Cancer Care*, 10: 31–5.

Morita, T., Tsunoda, J., Inoue, S. & Chihara, S. 2000, 'An exploratory factor analysis of existential suffering in Japanese terminally ill patients', *Psycho-Oncology*, 9: 164–8.

National Breast Cancer Centre 2001, personal communication regarding referral of patients with breast cancer for specialist psychological assessment and treatment.

NBCC, *see* National Breast Cancer Centre.

Owen, C., Tennant, C., Levi, J. & Jones, M. 1994, 'Cancer patients' attitudes to final events in life: wish for death, attitudes to cessation of treatment, suicide and euthanasia', *Psycho-Oncology*, 3: 1–19.

Penson, J. 2000, 'A hope is not a promise: fostering hope within palliative care', *International Journal of Palliative Nursing*, 6(2): 94–8.

Seale, C. 1995, 'Heroic death', *Sociology*, 29: 597–613.

Sneeuw, K.C., Aaronson, N.K., Sprangers, M.S., Detmar, S.B., Wever, L.D. & Schornagel, J.H. 1997, 'Value of caregiver ratings in evaluation of quality of life of patients with cancer', *Journal of Clinical Oncology*, 15: 1206–17.

Stromgren, A., Groenvold, M., Sorensen, A. & Andersen, L. 2001, 'Symptom recognition in advanced cancer. A comparison of nursing records against patient self rating', *Acta Anaethesiologica Scandinavia*, 45: 1080–5.

Yalom, I.D. 1980, 'Death and Psychotherapy', in Yalom, I.D., *Existential Psychotherapy*, Basic Books, New York.

Chapter 17 Sexuality and Body Image

Annon, J.S. 1976, *The Behavioural Treatment of Sexual Problems, Vol. 1. Brief Therapy*, Harper & Row, New York.

Bruner, D.W. & Boyd, C.P. 1999, 'Assessing women's sexuality after cancer therapy: Checking assumptions with focus group techniques', *Cancer Nursing*, 21(6): 438–47.

Chamberlain Wilmoth, M.C. 1994, 'Strategies for becoming comfortable with sexual assessment', *Oncology Nursing News*, Spring: 6–7.

Clifford, D. 1998, 'Psychosexual awareness in everyday nursing', *Nursing Standard*, 12(3): 42–5.

Dennison, S. 2001, 'Sexuality and Cancer', in Corner, J. & Bailey, C. (eds), *Cancer Nursing: Care in Context*, Blackwell Science, London.

Fallowfield, L. 1992, 'The quality of life: sexual function and body image following cancer therapy', *Cancer Topics*, 9: 20–1.

Jenkins, B. 1988, 'Patients' reports of sexual changes after treatment for gynaecological cancer', *Oncology Nursing Forum*, 15(3): 349–54.

Kissane, D, White, K. & Cooper, K. 2002, 'Psychosocial support in the areas of sexuality and body image for women with breast cancer', National Breast Cancer Centre, Sydney.

Kutner, J.S., Kasner, C.T. & Nowels, D.E. 2001, 'Symptom Burden at the End of Life: Hospice Providers' Perceptions', *Journal of Pain and Symptom Management*, 21(6): 473–80.

Lawler, J. 1991, *Behind the screens. Nursing somology and the problem of body*, Churchill Livingstone, London.

Masters, W.H. & Johnson, V.E. 1980, *Human Sexual Response*, Little Brown & Co., Boston.

Massie, M.J. & Popkin, M.K. 1998, 'Depressive Disorders', in Holland, J.C. & Breitbart, W. (eds), *Psycho-oncology*, pp 518–40, Oxford University Press, New York.

Neuenschwander, H. & Bruera, E. 1998, 'Asthenia', in Doyle, D., Hanks, G.E. & Macdonald, N. (eds), *Oxford Textbook of Palliative Medicine*, 2nd edn, Oxford Medical Publications, London.

Rice, A. 2000, 'Sexuality in cancer and palliative care 2: exploring the issues',*International Journal of Palliative Nursing*, 6(9): 448–53.

Schover, L.R. 1991, 'The impact of breast cancer on sexuality, body image, and intimate relationships', *Ca: A Cancer Journal for Clinicians*, 41: 112–20.

Schover, L.R. 1997, *Sexuality and Fertility after Cancer*, John Wiley & Sons, New York.

Schover, L.R. 1999, 'Counselling cancer patients about changes in sexual function', *Oncology*, 13(11): 1585–92, 1595–6.

Schwartz, S. & Plawecki, H.M. 2002, 'Consequences of chemotherapy on the sexuality of patients with lung cancer', *Clinical Journal of Oncology Nursing*, 6(4): 212–16.

Shell, J.A. & Smith, C.K. 1994, 'Sexuality and the older person with cancer', *Oncology Nurses Forum*, 21: 553–58.

Waterhouse, J. & Metcalfe, M. 1991, 'Attitudes toward nurses discussing sexual concerns with patients', *Journal of Advanced Nursing*, 16(9): 1048–54.

Wilkinson, S. 1999, 'Communication: it makes a difference', Schering Plough clinical lecture, *Cancer Nursing*, 22(1): 17–20.

Woods, N.F. 1984, *Human Sexuality in Health and Illness*, 3rd edn, Mosby, St Louis.

Wright, P. 1996, 'Psychosocial dysfunction in women with gynaecological cancer receiving radiotherapy, and their management by health care professionals', unpublished MSc dissertation, University of Southampton, Southhampton.

Chapter 18 Complementary Therapies

Abrahm, J. 1998, 'Promoting symptom control in palliative care', *Seminars in Oncology Nursing*, 14(2), 95–109.

Australian Nursing Federation 1998, *Complementary therapies in nursing practice*, ANF Policy Statement.

Biley, F. 2000, 'The effects on patient well-being of music listening as a nursing intervention: a review of the literature', *Journal of Clinical Nursing*, 9(5), 668–77.

Brady, L., Henry, K., Luth, J. & Casper-Bruett, K. 2001, 'The effects of shiatsu on lower back pain, *Journal of Holistic Nursing*, 19(1), 57–70.

Brown, S., North, D., Marvel, M. & Fons, R. 1992, 'Acupressure wrist bands to relieve nausea and vomiting in hospice patients: Do they work?', *American Journal of Hospice and Palliative Care*, 9(4), 26–9.

Cheesman, S., Christian, R. & Cresswell, J. 2001, 'Exploring the value of shiatsu in palliative care day services', *International Journal of Palliative Nursing*, 7(5), 234–9.

Deane, K., Carman, M. & Fitch, M. 2000, 'The cancer journey: bridging art therapy and museum education', *Canadian Oncology Nursing Journal*, 10(4), 140–2.

Dibble, S., Chapman, J., Mack, K. & Shih, A. 2000, 'Acupressure for nausea: results of a pilot study, *Oncology Nursing Forum*, 27(1), 41–7.

Dossey, B., Keegan, L., Guzetta, K. & Kolkmeier, L. 1995, *Holistic nursing: a handbook for practice*, 2nd edn, Aspen Publishers, Gaithersburg, USA.

Fessele, K. 1996, 'Managing the multiple causes of nausea and vomiting in the patient with cancer', *Oncology Nursing Forum*, 23(9), 1409–17.

Freshwater, D. 1996, 'Complementary therapies and research in nursing practice', *Nursing Standard*, 10(38), 43–5.

Gadsby, J., Franks, A., Jarvis, P. & Dewhurst, F. 1997, 'Acupuncture-like transcutaneous electrical nerve stimulation within palliative care: a pilot study', *Complementary Therapies in Medicine*, 5, 13–18.

Gecsedi, R. & Decker, G. 2001, 'Incorporating alternative therapies into pain management: more patients are considering complementary approaches', *Oncology Nursing Update 2001 Supplement, American Journal of Nursing*, 101(4), S35.

Hadfield, N. 2001, 'The role of aromatherapy massage in reducing anxiety in patients with malignant brain tumours', *International Journal of Palliative Nursing*, 7(6), 279–85.

Harris, P. 1997, 'Acupressure: a review of the literature', *Complementary Therapies in Medicine*, 5(3), 156–61.

Hidderley, M. & Weinel, E. 1997, 'Effects of TENS applied to acupuncture points distal to a pain site', *International Journal of Palliative Nursing*, 3(4), 185–8.

Hirsch, S. & Meckes, D. 2000, 'Treatment of the whole person: incorporating emergent perspectives in collaborative medicine, empowerment, and music therapy', *Journal of Psychosocial Oncology*, 18(2), 65–77.

Hodgson, H. 2000, 'Does reflexology impact on cancer patients' quality of life?', *Nursing Standard*, 14(31), 33–8.

Hudson, S 1998, 'Natural therapies aid oncology nursing', *Australian Nursing Journal*, 5, 25.

Kanji, N. 2000, 'Management of pain through autogenic training', *Complementary Therapies in Nursing & Midwifery*, 6(3), 143–8.

Keller, V. 1995, 'Management of nausea and vomiting in children', *Journal of Pediatric Nursing*, 10(5), 280–6.

Kristjanson, L., Sloan, J., Dudgeon, D. & Adaskin, E. 1996, 'Family members' perceptions of palliative cancer care: predictors of family functioning and family members' health', *Journal of Palliative Care*, 12(4), 10–20.

Kwekkeboom, K. 2001, 'Pain management strategies used by patients with breast and gynecological cancer with postoperative pain', *Cancer Nursing*, 24(5), 378–86.

Lancaster, J. 2001. 'Legal and ethical aspects of CTs and complementary care', in P. McCabe (ed.), *Complementary therapies in nursing and midwifery: from vision to practice*, Ausmed Publications, Melbourne.

MacDonald, G. 1998, 'Massage as a respite intervention for primary caregivers', *The American Journal of Hospice & Palliative Care*, 15(1), 43–7.

Mackey, S. 1998, 'Massage as a nursing intervention: using reflection to achieve change in practice', *Contemporary Nurse*, 7(1), 18–22.

Maxwell, T., Givant, E. & Kowalski, M. 2001, 'Exploring the management of bone metastasis according to the Roy adaptation model', *Oncology Nursing Forum*, 28(7), 1173–9.

McCabe, P. 2001, 'Nursing and CTs: a natural partnership', in P. McCabe (ed.), *Complementary therapies in nursing and midwifery: from vision to practice*, Ausmed Publications, Melbourne.

NBV, *see* Nurses Board of Victoria

Nurses Board of Victoria (NBV) 1999, *Guidelines for use of CTs in nursing practice*, NBV, Melbourne.

O'Callaghan, C. 1996, 'Pain, music creativity and music therapy in palliative care', *Complementary Medicine International*, 3(2), 43–8.

Price, H., Lewith, G. & Williams, C. 1991, 'Acupressure as an antiemetic in cancer chemotherapy', *Complementary Medical Research*, 5, 93–4.

Rankin-Box, D. 1997, 'Therapies in practice: a survey assessing nurses' use of CTs', *Complementary Therapies in Nursing & Midwifery*, 3, 92–9.

RCNA, *see* Royal College of Nursing Australia.

Royal College of Nursing Australia (RCNA) 2000, *Position Statement: Complementary Therapies in Australian Nursing Practice*, RCNA, Canberra.

Scherer Australia 1998, *Vitamins, minerals, herbals and health supplements: usage data*, RP Scherer, Melbourne.

Shaw, R. & Wilkinson, S. 1996, 'Building the pyramids: palliative care patients' perceptions of making art', *International Journal of Palliative Nursing*, 2(4), 217–21.

Shenton, D. 1996, 'Does aromatherapy provide an holistic approach to palliative care?' *International Journal of Palliative Nursing*, 2(4), 187–91.

Sloman, R., Brown, P., Aldana, E. & Chee, E. 1994, 'The use of relaxation for the promotion of comfort and pain relief in persons with advanced cancer', *Contemporary Nursing*. 3(1), 6–12.

Sparber, A. & Lin, E. 2000, 'Issues in clinical trials management. Clinical trials and subject use of complementary and alternative therapies: implications for nurses working in research settings', *Research Practitioner*, 1(6).

Stephenson, N., Weinrich, S. & Tavakoli, A. 2000, 'The effects of foot reflexology on anxiety and pain in patients with breast and lung cancer', *Oncology Nursing Forum*, 27(1), 67–72.

Stevensen, C. 1995, 'The role of shiatsu in palliative care', *Complementary Therapies in Nursing & Midwifery*, 1, 51–8.

Taylor, B. 2001, 'Research issues in CTs and holistic care', in P. McCabe (ed.), *Complementary therapies in nursing and midwifery: from vision to practice*, Ausmed Publications, Melbourne.

Turton, P. & Cooke, H. 2000, 'Meeting the needs of people with cancer for support and self management', *Complementary Therapies in Nursing & Midwifery*, 6(3), 130–7.

Vickers, A. 1996a, 'Can acupuncture have specific effects on health? A systematic literature review of acupuncture antiemesis trials', *Journal of the the Royal Society of Medicine*, 89, 303–11.

Vickers, A. 1996b, 'Complementary therapies in palliative care', *European Journal of Palliative Care*, 3(4), 150–3.

Vickers, A. 2000, 'Researching complementary medicine', *British Journal of Therapy and Rehabilitation.*, 7(1), 26–9.

Weitzner, M., Moody, L. & McMillan, S. 1997, 'Symptom management issues in hospice care, *The American Journal of Hospice & Palliative Care*, 14(4), 190–5.

Wilkinson, S. 1995, 'Aromatherapy and massage in palliative care', *International Journal of Palliative Care Nursing*, 1(1), 21–30.

Chapter 19 Working with Families

Bergen, A. 1991, 'Nurses caring for the terminally ill in the community: A review of the literature', *International Journal of Nursing Studies*, 28: 89–101.

Blanchard, C.G., Albrecht, R.L. & Ruckdeschel, J.C. 1997, 'The crisis of cancer: psychological impact of family caregivers', *Oncology*, 11, 189–94.

Bucher, J.A., Trostle, G.B. & Moore, M. 1999, 'Family reports of cancer pain, pain relief, and prescription access', *Cancer Practitioner*, 7(2), 71–7.

Buehler, J.A. & Lee, H.J. 1992, 'Exploration of home care resources for rural families with cancer', *Cancer Nursing*, 15, 299–308.

Cobbs, E.L. 1998, 'Health of older women', *Medical Clinical of North America*, 82(1), 127–44.

Ferrell, B.R. 1998, 'The family', in Doyle, C., Hanks, G.W.C. & McDonald, N., *Oxford Textbook of Palliative Medicine*, 2nd edn, pp 909–17, Oxford University Press, Oxford.

Ferrell, B.R., Rhiner, M., Cohen, M. & Grant, M. 1991, 'Pain as a metaphor for illness. Part I: impact of pain on family caregivers', *Oncology Nursing Forum*, 18(8), 1303–9.

Ferrell, B., Grant, M., Chan, J., Ahn, C. & Ferrell, B. 1995, 'The impact of cancer pain education on family caregivers of elderly patients', *Oncology Nursing Forum*, 22(8), 1211–18.

Gaugler, J., Kane, R. & Langlois, J. 2000, 'Assessment of family caregivers of older adults', in Kane, R. & Kane, R. (eds), *Assessing older persons: Measures, meaning and practical applications*, pp 320–59, Oxford University Press, New York.

Given, B.A. & Given, C.W. 1998, 'Health promotion for family caregivers of chronically ill elders', *Annual Review of Nursing Resources*, 16, 197–217.

Glajchen, M., Fitzmartin, R.D., Blum, D. & Swanton, R. 1995, 'Psychosocial barriers to cancer pain relief', *Cancer Practitioner*, 3(2), 76–82.

Grbich, C., Parker, D. & Maddocks, I. 2000, 'Communication and information needs of care-givers of adult family members at diagnosis and during treatment of terminal cancer', *Progress in Palliative Care*, 8(6), 345–50.

Hilton, B.A. 1996, 'Getting back to normal: The family experience during early stage breast cancer', *Oncology Nursing Forum*, 23(4), 605–14.

Higginson, I.J., Wade, A.M. & McCarthy, M. 1992, 'Effectiveness of two palliative support teams', *Journal of Public Health Medicine*, 14(1), 50–6.

Hudson, P. nd, *Support for family caregivers of dying cancer patients: A randomised controlled trial*, unpublished PhD thesis, University of Melbourne.

Hudson, P., Aranda, S. & McMurray, N. 2002, 'Intervention development for enhanced lay palliative caregiver support—the use of focus groups, *European Journal of Cancer Care*, vol. 11, issue 4, pp 262–70.

Hull, M.M. 1992, 'Coping strategies of family caregivers in hospice home care', *Oncology Nursing Forum*, 19(8), 1179–87.

Jensen, S. & Given, B.A. 1991, 'Fatigue affecting family caregivers of cancer patients', *Cancer Nursing*, 14(4), 181–7.

Kelleher, A. 1999, *Health Promoting Palliative Care*, Oxford University Press, Melbourne.

Kissane, D.W., Bloch, S., Burns, W.I., Patrick, J.D., Wallace, C.S. & McKenzie, D.P. 1994, 'Perceptions of family functioning and cancer', *Psycho-Oncology*, 3, 259–69.

Kristjanson, L.J. 1986, 'Indicators of quality of palliative care from a family perspective', *Journal of Palliative Care*, 2, 1, 7–19.

Kristjanson, L.J. 1989, 'Quality of terminal care: Salient indicators identified by families', *Journal of Palliative Care*, 5, 21–8.

Kristjanson, L.J. & Avery, L. 1994, 'Vicarious pain: The family's perspective', *Pain Management Newsletter*, 7(3), 1–2.

Kristjanson, L.J. & Sloan, J.A. 1991, 'Determinants of the grief reactions among survivors', *Journal of Palliative Care*, 7(4), 51–6.

Kristjanson, L.J. & White, K. 2002, 'Clinical Support for Families in the Palliative Care Phase of Hematological or Oncological Illness', *Hematology/Oncology Clinics of North America*, 16(3), 745–62.

Kristjanson, L.J., Sloan, J.A., Dudgeon, D.J. & Adaskin, E. 1996, 'Family members' perceptions of palliative cancer care: Predictors of family functioning and family members' health, *Journal of Palliative Care*, 12(4), 10–20.

Leis, A., Kristjanson, L.J., Koop, P. & Laizner, A. 1997, 'Family health and the palliative care trajectory: A research agenda', *Canadian Journal of Clinical Oncology*, I(5), 352–60.

Nolan, M. 2001, 'Positive aspects of caring', in Payne, S. & Ellis-Hill, C. (eds), *Chronic and terminal illness: New perspectives on caring and carers*, Oxford University Press, Oxford.

Palliative Care Australia (PCA) 2000, *Australia's future in palliative care research: A collaborative approach*, PCA, Canberra.

PCA, *see* Palliative Care Australia.

Ramirez, A., Addington Hall, J. & Richards, M. 1998, 'ABC of palliative care. The carers', *British Medical Journal*, 316(7126): 208–11.

Scott, G. 2001, 'A study of family carers of people with a life-threatening illness 2: the implications of the needs assessment', *International Journal of Palliative Nursing*, 7(7), 323–30.

Scott, G., Whyler, N. & Grant, G. 2001, 'A study of family carers of people with a life-threatening illness 1: the carers' needs analysis', *International Journal of Palliative Nursing*, 7(6), 290–330.

Smeenk, F., van Haastregt, J., de Witte, L. & Crebolder, H. 1998, 'Effectiveness of home care programmes for patients with incurable cancer on their quality of life and time spent in hospital: systematic review', *British Medical Journal*, 316, 1939–44.

Stetz, K.M. & Hanson, W.K. 1992, 'Alterations in perceptions of caregiving demands in advanced cancer during and after the experience', *Hospice Journal*, 8, 21–34.

Thorne, S.E. & Robinson, C.A. 1988, 'Reciprocal trust in health care relationships', *Journal of Advanced Nursing*, 13, 782–9.

Vachon, M. 1998, 'Psychosocial needs of patients and families', *Journal of Palliative Care*, 14(3), 49–56.

Wilkes, L., White, K., & O'Riordan, L. 2000, 'Empowerment through information: Supporting rural families of oncology patients in palliative care', *Australian Journal of Rural Health*, 8, 41–6.

Weitzner, M.A., McMillan, S.C. & Jacobsen, P.B. 1999, 'Family caregiver quality of life: Differences between curative and palliative care treatment settings', *Journal of Pain Symptom Management*, 17(6).

World Health Organization 1990, *Cancer pain relief and palliative care*, Report of a WHO Expert Committee, WHO, Geneva.

Yang, C. & Kirschling, J.M. 1992, 'Exploration of factors related to direct care and outcomes of caregiving: caregivers of terminally ill older person', *Cancer Nursing*, 15, 173–81.

Yeager, K.A., Miaskowski, C., Dibble, S.L. & Wallhagen, M. 1995, 'Differences in pain knowledge and perception of the pain experience between outpatients with cancer and their family caregivers', *Oncology Nursing Forum*, 22(8), 1235–41.

Chapter 20 Bereavement

Aranda, S. & Milne, D. 2000, *Guidelines for the Asssessment of Complicated Bereavement Risk in Family Members of People Receiving Palliative Care*, Centre for Palliative Care, Melbourne.

Bourke, M.P. 1984, 'The continuum of pre- and post-bereavement grieving', *British Journal of Medical Psychology*, 57: 121–5.

Cleiren, M. 1993, *Bereavement and adaptation. A comparative study of the aftermath of death*, Hemisphere Publishing, Washington.

Gamino, L.A., Sewell, K.W. & Easterling, L.W. 1998, 'Scott & White Greif Study: an empirical test of predicators of intensified mourning', *Death Studies*, 22: 333–55.

Kavanaugh, R. 1974, *Facing Death*, Penguin Books, Baltimore.

Kissane, D.W. & Bloch, S. 1994, 'Family Grief', *British Journal of Psychiatry*, 164: 728–40.

Kissane, D.W., Bloch, S., McKenzie, M., McDowall, A.C. & Nitzan, R. 1998, 'Family Grief Therapy: A Preliminary Account of a New Model to Promote Healthy Family Functioning During Palliative Care and Bereavement', *Psycho-Oncology*, 7: 14–25.

Lewis, C.S. 1976, *A Grief Observed*, Bantam, New York; first published under the psudonym N.W. Clerk 1961, Faber & Faber, England.

McKissock, M. & McKissock, D. 1998, *Bereavement Counselling Guidelines for Practitioners*, Bereavement CARE Centre, NSW.

Moos, H.H. & Moos, B.S. 1981, *Family Environment Scale Manual*, Psychologists Press, California.

Parkes, C.M. 1975, 'Determinants of outcome following bereavement', *Omega*, 6(4): 303–23.

Parkes, C.M. 1980, 'Bereavement counselling: Does it work?', *British Medical Journal*, 281: 3–10.

Parkes, C.M. 1993, 'Bereavement', in Doyle, D., Hanks, G.W.C. & MacDonald, N. (eds), *Oxford Textbook of Palliative Medicine*, pp 665–78, Oxford University Press, Oxford.

Parkes, C.M., Laungani, P. & Young, B. 1997, *Death and Bereavement Across Cultures*, Routledge, London.

Prior, D. 1999, 'Palliative care in marginalised communities', *Progress in Palliative Care*, 7(3): 109–15.

Ramsden, I. 1998, 'After Kia-Ora—What Next?', paper presented at Hospice New Zealand Conference, Wellington, New Zealand, 24–28 June.

Rando, T. 1984, *Grief Dying and Death*, Research Press Company, Illinois.

Rando, T.A. 1993, 'Clinical assessment of grief and mourning. Treatment of complicated mourning', pp 243–66, Research Press, Illinois.

Raphael, B. 1982, *The Anatomy of Bereavement*, Basic Books, New York.

Rosenblatt, P.C. 1993, 'Grief: The social context of private feelings', in Stroebe, M.S., Stroebe, W. & Hansson, R.O., *Handbook of Bereavement: Theory, Research, and Intervention*, pp 102–11, Cambridge University Press, Cambridge.

Walshe, C. 1997, 'Whom to help? An exploration of the assessment of grief', *International Journal of Palliative Nursing*, 3 (3): 132–7.

Zisook, S. & Lyons, L. 1989, 'Bereavement and Unresolved Grief in Psychiatric Outpatients', *Omega*, 20 (4): 307–22.

Zisook, S., Shuchter, S.R. & Lyons, L.E. 1987, 'Predictors of psychological reactions during the early stages of widowhood', *Psychiatric Clinics of North America*, 10 (3): 355–68.

Chapter 21 Palliative Care in Chronic Illness

Addington-Hall, J.M., Lay, M., Altmann, D. & McCarthy, M. 1997, 'Community care for stroke patients in the last year of life: results of a national retrospective survey of surviving family, friends and carers', *Health and Social Care in the Community*, 6: 112–19.

Addington-Hall, J.M. 1998, *Reaching out: Specialist Palliative Care for Adults with Non-malignant Disease*, National Council for Hospices and Specialist Palliative Care Services, London.

Addington-Hall, J.M., Fakhoury, W. & McCarthy, M. 1998, 'Specialist palliative care in non-malignant disease', *Palliative Medicine*, 12: 417–27.

Ahmedzai, S. 1998, 'Palliation of respiratory symptoms', in Doyle, D., Hanks, G.W.C., MacDonald, N. (eds), *Oxford Textbook of Palliative Medicine*, 2nd edn, Oxford University Press, Oxford.

Anderson, H., Ward, C., Earley, A., Gomm, S.A., Connolly, M., Coppinger, T., Corgie, D., Williams, J.L. & Makin, W.P. 2001, 'The concerns of patients under palliative care and a heart failure clinic are not being met', *Palliative Medicine*, 15: 279–86.

Barby, T. & Leigh, P.N. 1995, 'Palliative care in motor neurone disease', *International Journal of Palliative Nursing*, 1: 183–8.

Bosanquet, N. & Salisbury, C. 1999, *Providing a Palliative Care Service: towards an evidence base*', Oxford University Press, Oxford.

Cassel, C.K. & Vladek, B.C. 1996, 'Sounding board. ICD-9 code for palliative or terminal care', *New England Journal of Medicine*, 335: 1232.

Cohen, L.M., McCue, J.D., Germain, M. & Kjellstrand, C.M. 1995, 'Dialysis discontinuation. A good death?' *Archives of International Medicine*, 155: 42–7.

Costain Schou, K. & Hewison, J. 1997, *Experiencing Cancer: Quality of Life in Treatment*, Open University Press, Buckingham.

Edmonds, P., Karlsen, S., Khan, S. & Addington-Hall, J. 2001, 'A comparison of the palliative care needs of patients dying from respiratory diseases and lung cancer', *Palliative Medicine*, 15; 287–95.

Eve, A., Smith, A.M. & Tebbit, P. 1997, 'Hospice and palliative care in the UK 1994–1995, including a summary of trends 1990–1995, *Palliative Medicine*, 11: 31–43.

Froggatt, K.A. 2001, 'Palliative care and nursing homes: where next?', *Palliative Medicine*, 15: 42–8.

Hanrahan, P., Luchins, D.J. & Murphy, K. 2001, 'Palliative care for patients with dementia', in Addington-Hall, J.M. & Higginson, I.J. (eds), *Palliative care for non-cancer patients*, Oxford University Press, Oxford.

Haste, F.H. & MacDonald, L.D. 1992, 'The role of the specialist in community nursing: perceptions of specialist and district nurses', *International Journal of Nursing Studies*, 29: 37–47.

Heneghan, M.A. & O'Grady, J.G. 2001, 'Palliative care in liver disease', in Addington-Hall, J.M. & Higginson, I.J. (eds), *Palliative care for non-cancer patients*, Oxford University Press, Oxford.

Holmes, S., Pope, S. & Lamond, D. 1997, 'General nurses' perceptions of palliative care', *International Journal of Palliative Nursing*, 3: 92–9.

Hoyert, D.L. 1996, 'Mortality trends for Alzheimer's disease: 1979–1991', *Vital Health Statistics*, 28: 1–23.

Hunt, R.W. & Maddocks, I. 1997, 'Terminal care in South Australia: historical aspects and equity issues', in Clark, D., Hockley, J. & Ahmedzai, S. eds, *New Themes in Palliative Care*, Open University Press, Buckingham.

Lloyd-Williams, M. 1996, 'An audit of palliative care in dementia', *European Journal of Cancer Care*, 5: 53–5.

Maddocks, I. 1998, 'Chronic heart failure: a malignant condition', *Medical Journal of Australia*, 168: 200.

Maddocks, I. & Parker, D. 2001, 'Palliative care in nursing homes', in Addington-Hall, J.M. & Higginson, I.J. (eds), *Palliative care for non-cancer patients*, Oxford University Press, Oxford.

McCarthy, M., Lay, M. & Addington-Hall, J.M. 1996, 'Dying from heart disease', *Journal of the Royal College of Physicians*, 30: 325–8.

McCarthy, M., Lay, M. & Addington-Hall, J.M. 1997, 'Communication and choice in dying from heart disease', *Journal of the Royal Society of Medicine*, 90: 128–31.

Morgan, M. & Singh, S. 1997, *Practical pulmonary rehabilitation*, Chapman and Hall Medical, London.

Murray, C.J. & Lopez, A.D. 1997, 'Alternative projections of mortality and disability by cause 1990–2020: Global Burden of Disease Study', *Lancet*, 349: 1498–504.

National Council for Hospice and Specialist Palliative Care Services (NCHSPCS) (2001), *What do we mean by palliative care?* NCHSPCS, London.

NCHSPCS, *see* National Council for Hospice and Specialist Palliative Care Services.

Nolan, M., Grant, G. & Keady, J. 1996, *Understanding family care: a multidimensional model of caring and coping*,Open University Press, Buckingham.

ONS, *see* Office for National Statistics.

Office for National Statistics (ONS) (1997), *Series DH1 (28) mortality statistics: General 1993, 1994 and 1995*, Stationary Office, London.

Porock, D. 1999, 'Fatigue', in Aranda, S. & O'Connor, M. (eds), *Palliative Care Nursing: a guide to nursing practice*, Ausmed Publications, Melbourne.

Simon, J. & Gibbs, R. 2001, 'Heart Disease', in Addington-Hall, J.M. & Higginson, I.J. (eds), *Palliative care for non-cancer patients*, Oxford University Press, Oxford.

Skilbeck, J., Mott, L., Smith, D., Page, H. & Clark, D. 1997, 'Nursing care for people dying from chronic obstructive airways disease', *International Journal of Palliative Nursing*, 3: 100–6.

Skilbeck, J., Mott, L., Smith, D., Page, H. & Clark, D. 1998, 'Palliative care in chronic obstructive airways disease: a needs assessment', *Palliative Medicine*, 12: 245–54.

Chapter 22 Ageing, Dementia, and Palliative Care

Abbey, J. 1995, 'Death and late-stage dementia in institutions: a cultural analysis', PhD thesis, Deakin University, Geelong.

Abbey, J., De Bellis, A., Piller, N., Easterman, A., Parker, D. & Lowcay, B. 2001, 'When "Tell me if it's hurting doesn't work"—a pain scale for people with dementia who cannot verbalize', report of a research study funded by the Gunn Foundation, South Australia, Geriaction Inc. National Conference, 'Sustaining the changes: Directions in Aged Care', 11–13 October, Brisbane.

Ashby, M. & Stoffell, B. 1991, 'Therapeutic ratio and defined phases: proposal of ethical framework for palliative care', *British Medical Journal*, Vol. 302, 1 June, p. 1323.

Billings, J. 1985, 'Comfort Measures for the Terminally Ill. Is Dehydration Painful?', editorial, *Journal of the American Geriatrics Society*, November, Vol. 33, No. 11, pp 808–10.

Madson, S. 1993, 'Patient Self-Determination Act, Implications for Long-Term Care', *Journal of Gerontological Nursing*, February, pp 15–24.

McCue, J. 1995, 'The naturalness of dying', *Journal of the American Medical Association*, 5 April, 273(13), pp 1039–43.

McCullough, L. & Wilson, N. (eds) 1995, *Long-Term Care Decisions, Ethical and Conceptual Dimensions*, The Johns Hopkins University Press, Baltimore.

Starck, P.L. 1992, 'The management of suffering in a nursing home: an ethnographic study', in Starck, P.C. & Mc Govern, J.P. (eds), *The Hidden Dimension of Illness: Human Suffering*, p. 149, National League for Nursing Press, New York.

Watson, R. 1994, 'Measuring feeding difficulty in patients with dementia: developing a scale', *Journal of Advanced Nursing*, 19, pp 257–63.

Chapter 23 Caring for Dying People in Critical Care

Audit Commission 1999, *Critical to success: the place of efficient and effective critical care services within the acute hospital*, Audit Commission, London.

Block, S.D. 2001, 'Helping the clinician cope with death in the ICU', in Randall-Curtis & Rubenfeld 2001, op. cit..

de Raeve, L. 1996, 'Dignity and integrity at the end of life', *International Journal of Palliative Nursing*, 2: 71–6.

Hall, K. 2002, 'Medical decision-making; an argument for narrative and metaphor', *Theoretical Medicine and Bioethics*, 23(1): 55–73.

Johnson, N, Cook, D., Giacomini, M. & Willms, D. 2000, 'Towards a "good" death: end of life narratives constructed in an intensive care unit', *Culture, Medicine and Psychiatry*, 24: 275–95.

McNamara, B. 2001, *Fragile Lives. Death, Dying and Care*, Open University Press, Buckingham.

Miles, S.H. 2001, 'The role of the physician in sacred end of life rituals in the ICU', in Randall-Curtis & Rubenfeld 2001, op. cit..

Prendergast, T.J. & Luce, J.M. 1997, 'Increasing incidence of withholding and withdrawal of life support from the critically ill', *American Journal of Respiratory Care Medicine*, 155: 15–20.

Puntillo, K.A. 2001, 'The role of critical care nurses in providing and managing end of life care', in Randall-Curtis & Rubenfeld 2001, op. cit..

Randall-Curtis, J. & Rubenfeld, G.D. 2001 (eds), *Managing Death in the Intensive Care Unit. The Transition from Cure to Comfort*, Oxford University Press, Oxford.

Saunders, J.M. & Valente, S.M. 1994, 'Nurses' grief', *Cancer Nursing*, 17: 318–25.

Seymour, J.E. 2000, 'Negotiating natural death in intensive care', *Social Science and Medicine*, 51: 1241-1252.

Seymour, J.E. 2001, *Critical Moments: Death and Dying in Intensive Care*, Open University Press, Buckingham.

Chapter 24 Paediatric Palliative Care

Black, D. 1998, 'Bereavement', in Goldman, A. (ed.), *Care of the Dying Child*, Oxford University Press, New York.

Colleau, D. 2001, 'Easing the pain of seriously ill children: a progress report', *Cancer Pain*, 14: 2–8.

Dominica, F. 1998, 'The development of paediatric palliative care: Development in the United Kingdom', in Doyle, D., Hanks, G.W.C. & MacDonald, N. (eds), *Oxford Textbook of Palliative Medicine*, Oxford University Press, Oxford.

Faulkner, K.W. 1997, 'Talking about death with a dying child', *American Journal of Nursing*, 97: 64–9.

Frager, G. 1996, 'Pediatric palliative care: building the model, bridging the gaps', *Journal of Palliative Care*, 12: 9–12.

Goldman, A. 1996, 'Home care of the dying child', *Journal of Palliative Care*, 12: 16–19.

Goldman, A. 1998, 'Life threatening illnesses and symptom control in children', in Doyle, D., Hanks, G.W.C. & MacDonald, N. (eds), *Oxford Textbook of Palliative Medicine*, Oxford University Press, Oxford.

Hunt, A.M. 1990, 'A survey of signs, symptoms and symptom control in 30 ill children', *Developmental Medicine and Child Neurology*, 32: 341–6.

Kane, J.R. & Primomo, M. 2001, 'Alleviating the suffering of seriously ill children', *American Journal of Hospice & Palliative Care*, 18: 161–9.

Levetown, M. 1996, 'Ethical aspects of pediatric palliative care', *Journal of Palliative Care*, 12: 35–9.

Liben, S. 1996, 'Pediatric palliative medicine: obstacles to overcome', *Journal of Palliative Care*, 12: 24–8.

Liben, S. & Goldman, A. 1998, 'Home care for children with life threatening illness', *Journal of Palliative Care*, 14: 33–8.

McGrath, P.A. 1996, 'Development of the World Health Organisation guidelines on cancer pain relief and palliative care in children', *Journal of Pain and Symptom Management*, 12: 87–92.

McQuillan, R. & Finlay, I. 1996, 'Facilitating the care of terminally ill children', *Journal of Pain and Symptom Management*, 12: 320–4.

Rando, T.A. 1983, 'An investigation of grief and adaptation in parents whose children have died from cancer', *Journal of Pediatric Psychology*, 18: 3–20.

Sahler, O.J.Z., Frager, G., Levetown, M., Cohn, F.G. & Lipson, M.A. 2000, 'Medical education about end-of-life care in the pediatric setting: Principles, challenges, and opportunities', *Pediatrics*, 105: 575–84.

Schonfeld, D.J. 1993, 'Talking with children about death', *Journal of Pediatric Health Care*, 7: 269–74.

Stevens, M.M., Jones, P. & O'Riordan, E. 1996, 'Family responses when a child with cancer is in palliative care', *Journal of Palliative Care*, 12: 51–5.

TG, *see* Therapeutic Guidelines Limited.

Therapeutic Guidelines Limited 2001, *Therapeutic Guidelines: Palliative Care, Version 1*, Therapeutic Guidelines Limited, North Melbourne.

Vickers, J. & Carlisle, C. 2000, 'Choices and control: parental experiences in pediatric terminal home care', *Journal of Pediatric Oncology Nursing*, 17: 12–21.

Whaley, L.F. & Wong, D.L. 1997, *Whaley and Wong's Essentials of Pediatric Nursing*, 5th edn, Mosby-Year Book Inc., St Louis.

Wolfe, J., Holcombe, E.G., Klar, N., Levin, S.B., Ellenbogen, J.M. & Salem-Scatz, S. 2000, 'Symptoms and suffering at the end of life in children with cancer', *New England Journal of Medicine*, 342: 326–33.

Index